Colon Cancer

Editor

MARK W. ARNOLD

SURGICAL ONCOLOGY CLINICS OF NORTH AMERICA

www.surgonc.theclinics.com

Consulting Editor
TIMOTHY M. PAWLIK

April 2018 • Volume 27 • Number 2

ELSEVIER

1600 John F. Kennedy Boulevard • Suite 1800 • Philadelphia, Pennsylvania, 19103-2899

http://www.theclinics.com

SURGICAL ONCOLOGY CLINICS OF NORTH AMERICA Volume 27, Number 2
April 2018 ISSN 1055-3207, ISBN-13: 978-0-323-58330-5

Editor: John Vassallo (j.vassallo@elsevier.com)
Developmental Editor: Sara Watkins

Surgical Oncology Clinics of North America (ISSN 1055-3207) is published quarterly by Elsevier Inc., 360 Park Avenue South, New York, NY 10010-1710. Months of publication are January, April, July, and October. Business and Editorial Offices: 1600 John F. Kennedy Blvd., Ste. 1800, Philadelphia, PA 19103-2899. Customer Service Office: 3251 Riverport Lane, Maryland Heights, MO 63043. Periodicals postage paid at New York, NY and additional mailing offices. Subscription prices are $296.00 per year (US individuals), $505.00 (US institutions) $100.00 (US student/resident), $337.00 (Canadian individuals), $638.00 (Canadian institutions), $205.00 (Canadian student/resident), $418.00 (foreign individuals), $638.00 (foreign institutions), and $205.00 (foreign student/resident). Foreign air speed delivery is included in all *Clinics* subscription prices. All prices are subject to change without notice. **POSTMASTER:** Send address changes to *Surgical Oncology Clinics of North America,* Elsevier Health Science Division, Subscription Customer Service, 3251 Riverport Lane, Maryland Heights, MO 63043. **Customer Service: 1-800-654-2452 (US and Canada). 314-447-8871 (outside US and Canada). Fax: 314-447-8029. E-mail: journalscustomerservice-usa@elsevier.com (for print support); journalsonline support-usa@elsevier.com (for online support).**

Reprints. For copies of 100 or more, of articles in this publication, please contact the Commercial Reprints Department, Elsevier Inc., 360 Park Avenue South, New York, New York 10010-1710. Tel. 212-633-3874; Fax: 212-633-3820; E-mail: reprints@elsevier.com.

Surgical Oncology Clinics of North America is covered in *MEDLINE/PubMed (Index Medicus)* and *EMBASE/ Excerpta Medica, Current Contents/Clinical Medicine, and ISI/BIOMED.*

Contributors

CONSULTING EDITOR

TIMOTHY M. PAWLIK, MD, MPH, PhD, FACS, FRACS (Hon)
Professor and Chair, Department of Surgery, The Urban Meyer III and Shelley Meyer Chair for Cancer Research, Professor of Surgery, Oncology, and Health Services Management and Policy, The Ohio State University Wexner Medical Center, Columbus, Ohio

EDITOR

MARK W. ARNOLD, MD
Professor of Clinical Surgery, The Ohio State University Wexner Medical Center, Columbus, Ohio

AUTHORS

JEAN ASHBURN, MD
Associate Staff, Assistant Professor of Surgery, Department of Colorectal Surgery, Cleveland Clinic, Cleveland, Ohio

TANIOS BEKAII-SAAB, MD
Professor of Medicine, Co-Leader, Gastrointestinal Cancer Program, Mayo Clinic Cancer Center, Mayo Clinic, Phoenix, Arizona

JEFFERY CHAKEDIS, MD
Fellow, Complex General Surgical Oncology, Division of Surgical Oncology, Department of Surgery, The Ohio State University Wexner Medical Center, The James Cancer Hospital and Solove Research Institute, Columbus, Ohio

JOHN A. DUMOT, DO
Director, UH Digestive Health Institute, University Hospitals Cleveland Medical Center, Professor of Medicine, Case Western Reserve University, Cleveland, Ohio

WENDY L. FRANKEL, MD
Kurtz Chair and Distinguished Professor, Department of Pathology, The Ohio State University Wexner Medical Center, Columbus, Ohio

SRIHARSHA GUMMADI, MD
Division of Colorectal Surgery, Lankenau Medical Center, Wynnewood, Pennsylvania

NATHAN C. HALL, MD, PhD
Associate Professor, Department of Radiology, Hospital of the University of Pennsylvania, Service Chief, Diagnostic Imaging, Acting Section Chief, Nuclear Medicine, Corporal Michael J. Crescenz VAMC, Philadelphia, Pennsylvania; Adjunct Professor, Department of Surgery, Division of Surgical Oncology, The Ohio State University Wexner Medical Center, Columbus, Ohio

HEATHER HAMPEL, MS, LGC
Associate Director, Division of Human Genetics, Professor, Department of Internal Medicine, The Ohio State University Comprehensive Cancer Center, Columbus, Ohio

EMINA HUANG, MD
Staff, Professor of Surgery, Departments of Colorectal Surgery and Stem Cell Biology and Regenerative Medicine, Cleveland Clinic, Cleveland, Ohio

MING JIN, MD, PhD
Assistant Professor, Department of Pathology, The Ohio State University Wexner Medical Center, Columbus, Ohio

JOHN H. MARKS, MD
Chief, Division of Colorectal Surgery, Director of Minimally Invasive Colorectal Surgery Rectal Cancer Management Fellowship, Lankenau Medical Center, Wynnewood, Pennsylvania

KABIR MODY, MD
Assistant Professor of Medicine, Associate Member, Gastrointestinal Cancer Program, Mayo Clinic Cancer Center, Mayo Clinic, Jacksonville, Florida

GUY R. ORANGIO, MD, FACS, FASCRS
Professor of Clinical Surgery, Chief of Section of Colon and Rectal Surgery, LSU Department of Surgery, LSU School of Medicine, New Orleans, Louisiana

PAN PAN, PhD
Postdoctoral Fellow, Department of Medicine, Division of Hematology and Oncology, Medical College of Wisconsin, Milwaukee, Wisconsin

ALEXANDER T. RUUTIAINEN, MD
Section Chief, Diagnostic Radiology, Corporal Michael J. Crescenz VAMC, Philadelphia, Pennsylvania

JEAN F. SALEM, MD
Division of Colorectal Surgery, Lankenau Medical Center, Wynnewood, Pennsylvania

CARL R. SCHMIDT, MD
Associate Professor, Department of Surgery, Division of Surgical Oncology, The Ohio State University Wexner Medical Center, The James Cancer Hospital and Solove Research Institute, Columbus, Ohio

SHERIEF SHAWKI, MD
Assistant Staff, Assistant Professor of Surgery, Department of Colorectal Surgery, Cleveland Clinic, Cleveland, Ohio

STEVEN A. SIGNS, PhD
Research Associate, Assistant Staff, Assistant Professor, Department of Stem Cell Biology and Regenerative Medicine, Cleveland Clinic, Cleveland Clinic Lerner Research Institute, Cleveland, Ohio

JOHN F. SULLIVAN, MD
Fellow, Department of Gastroenterology and Liver Disease, University Hospitals Cleveland Medical Center, Cleveland, Ohio

LI-SHU WANG, PhD
Associate Professor, Department of Medicine, Division of Hematology and Oncology, Medical College of Wisconsin, Milwaukee, Wisconsin

CHRISTINA WU, MD
Associate Professor of Hematology/Oncology, Winship Cancer Institute of Emory University, Atlanta, Georgia

JIANHUA YU, PhD
Associate Professor, Department of Internal Medicine, Division of Hematology, College of Medicine, Comprehensive Cancer Center, The James Cancer Hospital and Solove Research Institute, The Ohio State University, Columbus, Ohio

Contents

Foreword: Colon Cancer   xiii

Timothy M. Pawlik

Preface: Colon Cancer: The Road Traveled   xv

Mark W. Arnold

Systemic Therapy for Colon Cancer   235

Christina Wu

> Systemic treatments for patients with colon cancer has expanded broadly beyond 5-fluorouracil-based chemotherapy. For patients with early-stage colon cancer who are considering adjuvant chemotherapy, multiple factors such as the risk of disease recurrence, absolute survival benefit of chemotherapy, treatment toxicity, and patient comorbid medical conditions must be taken into account. In the metastatic setting, biomarkers such as KRAS/NRAS/BRAF mutation, microsatellite instability status, and left- versus right-sided colon cancer have helped oncologists to tailor systemic treatment regimens, which include chemotherapy, targeted therapy, and immunotherapy.

Colon Cancer: What We Eat   243

Pan Pan, Jianhua Yu, and Li-Shu Wang

> A higher incidence of colorectal cancer (CRC) is observed in Oceania and Europe, whereas Africa and Asia have a lower incidence. CRC is largely preventable by adapting a healthy lifestyle, such as healthy diet, adequate physical activity, and avoiding obesity. This article summarizes the latest work available, mainly epidemiologic studies, to examine the relationship between diet and CRC. Higher intake of red/processed meat could increase the CRC risk, whereas fibers, especially from whole grains and cereals, as well as fruit and vegetables may decrease the CRC risk. Heterogeneity and inconsistency among studies or individuals, however, need to be taken into consideration.

Colon Cancer: Inflammation-Associated Cancer   269

Sherief Shawki, Jean Ashburn, Steven A. Signs, and Emina Huang

> Colitis-associated cancer is a relatively rare form of cancer with an unclear pathogenesis. Colitis-associated cancer serves as a prototype of inflammation-associated cancers. Advanced colonoscopic techniques are considered standard of care for surveillance in patients with long-standing colitis, especially those with other risk factors, including sclerosing cholangitis and a family history of colorectal cancer. When colitis-associated cancer is diagnosed, the standard operation involves total proctocolectomy. Restorative procedures and surveillance after colectomy require special considerations. In these contexts, new 3-dimensional human models may be used to usher in personalized medicine.

Colorectal Cancer: Imaging Conundrums   289

Nathan C. Hall and Alexander T. Ruutiainen

> Progressive technologic advancements in imaging have significantly improved the preoperative sensitivity for the detection of very small foci of regionally or hematogenously metastatic colorectal cancer. Unfortunately, this information has not translated to continued linear gains in patient survival and might even result in the false-positive upstaging of some cases: these are two conundrums in the imaging of colorectal cancer. Both conundrums might be resolved by the widespread use of real-time imaging guidance during operative procedures, and this might open the way for the widespread use of fluorodeoxyglucose PET/CT for the initial staging of patients with colorectal cancer.

Minimally Invasive Surgical Approaches to Colon Cancer   303

Jean F. Salem, Sriharsha Gummadi, and John H. Marks

> Colon cancer remains the most common abdominal visceral malignancy affecting both men and women in America. Open colectomy has been the standard of care for patients with colon cancer in the past 100 years; although this method is highly effective, the major trauma associated with it has a significant morbidity rate and represents a large operation for patients to recover from. Minimally invasive colon surgery was developed as a new and alternative option, and surgeons aim to continue to make it simpler, more reproducible, and easier to teach and learn. We describe herein the current state of minimally invasive colorectal surgery for colon cancer and compare it with open surgery to offer insights to future directions.

Population Screening for Hereditary Colorectal Cancer   319

Heather Hampel

> Colorectal cancer can be caused by hereditary cancer syndromes such as Lynch syndrome and the polyposis syndromes. Tumor screening for Lynch syndrome has been recommended by several professional organizations. In addition, it has been shown that patients with microsatellite unstable colorectal cancer can benefit from immunotherapy. Unfortunately, universal tumor screening for Lynch syndrome has not been implemented at all hospitals yet. More recent studies have found that the prevalence of all hereditary cancer syndromes is around 10%, and for those diagnosed under age 50 years, it is closer to 16%. It may be time to consider offering genetic counseling and testing to all patients with colorectal cancer.

The Economics of Colon Cancer   327

Guy R. Orangio

> The economic burden of cancer on the national health expenditure is billions of dollars. The economic cost is measured on direct and indirect medical costs, which vary depending on the stage at diagnosis, patient age, type of medical services, and site of service. Costs vary by region, physician behavior, and patient preferences. When analyzing the economic burden of survivors of colon cancer, one cannot forget the societal burden. Post-acute care and readmissions are major economic burdens. People with colon cancer have to be followed up for their lifetime. Economic models are being studied to give cost-effective solutions to this problem.

Clinical Trials and Progress in Metastatic Colon Cancer   349

Kabir Mody and Tanios Bekaii-Saab

Colorectal cancer (CRC) is a leading cause of cancer-related deaths worldwide, but associated mortality has declined in recent decades. Genomic profiling of the disease has resulted in the definition of subsets of patients, for example, KRAS, NRAS, or BRAF mutated; Her2 amplified; and mismatch repair deficient, which has enabled personalization of therapeutic decision making. These subsets are guiding drug development and combination therapy approaches using both targeted therapies and immunotherapies. Further refinement based on molecular discoveries and the emergence of newer technologies to enable new discoveries allow for great optimism for the future on behalf of patients with colon cancer.

Maximizing the Effectiveness of Colonoscopy in the Prevention of Colorectal Cancer   367

John F. Sullivan and John A. Dumot

Colonoscopy is a proven screening test for colorectal cancer; maximizing its effectiveness is the best way to decrease interval colorectal cancer. The adenoma detection rate can be improved by monitoring physician detection rates. Assistive devices and innovative endoscopic equipment may also decrease adenoma miss rates. Complete polypectomy of adenomatous lesions and recommending the proper date for the next examination are important considerations. Advanced polypectomy techniques, including endoscopic mucosal resection and endoscopic submucosal dissection, have a clear role in the nonsurgical management of large laterally spreading adenomatous polyps that previously would have required surgical resection.

Surgical Treatment of Metastatic Colorectal Cancer   377

Jeffery Chakedis and Carl R. Schmidt

Surgical treatment of metastatic colorectal cancer offers a chance for cure or prolonged survival, particularly for those with more favorable prognostic factors and limited tumor burden. The treatment plan requires multidisciplinary evaluation because multiple therapy options exist. Advanced surgical techniques, adjuncts to resection, and modern chemotherapy all contribute to best outcomes for patients with hepatic metastases. Although cure is less common for patients with metastasis to lung or peritoneum, surgical resection for the former and cytoreduction and intraperitoneal chemotherapy for the latter may help to achieve cancer control in selected patients.

Lymph Node Metastasis in Colorectal Cancer   401

Ming Jin and Wendy L. Frankel

Pathologic examination of lymph nodes in patients with cancer remains crucial for postoperative treatment and prognosis prediction. In this article, the authors aim to review several important and challenging issues regarding lymph node metastasis in colorectal cancer using the AJCC staging manual, College of American Pathologists cancer protocol, as well as the literature. These topics include lymph node staging, the definition and controversies in tumor deposits, isolated tumor cells in lymph node and micrometastasis, lymph node ratio as a prognostic stratification factor, and neoadjuvant treatment effect in rectal cancer. Updates from the most recent AJCC 8th edition are included.

SURGICAL ONCOLOGY
CLINICS OF NORTH AMERICA

FORTHCOMING ISSUES

July 2018
Peritoneal Malignancies
Edward A. Levine, *Editor*

October 2018
Measuring Quality in a Shifting Payment
Landscape: Implications for Surgical
Oncology
Caprice C. Greenberg and
Daniel E. Abbott, *Editors*

January 2019
Minimally Invasive Oncologic Surgery, Part I
James Fleshman and Claudius Conrad,
Editors

RECENT ISSUES

January 2018
Changing Paradigms in Breast Cancer
Diagnosis and Treatment
Kelly K. Hunt, *Editor*

October 2017
Clinics Trials in Surgical Oncology
Elin Sigurdson, *Editor*

July 2017
Emerging Updates of Radiation Oncology
for Surgeons
Adam Raben, *Editor*

RELATED INTEREST

Surgical Clinics, June 2017 (Vol. 97, No. 3)
Advances in Colorectal Neoplasia
Sean J. Langenfeld, *Editor*
Available at: www.surgical.theclinics.com

THE CLINICS ARE AVAILABLE ONLINE!
Access your subscription at:
www.theclinics.com

Foreword
Colon Cancer

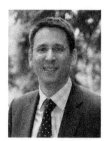

Timothy M. Pawlik, MD, MPH, PhD, FACS, FRACS (Hon)
Consulting Editor

This issue of the *Surgical Oncology Clinics of North America* is devoted to colon cancer. Over the last decade, there has been a dramatic increase in our knowledge and treatment of this disease. In addition, there have been signficant surgical innovations, including the increased utilization of laparoscopy and robotic approaches. The guest editor is Mark W. Arnold, MD, FACS. Dr Arnold is Professor and Chief of the Division of Colorectal Surgery at The Ohio State University. Dr Arnold has over three decades' worth of experience treating patients with colorectal cancer and is widely considered an expert in the management of this disease. Having treated hundreds of patients with colorectal cancer, as well as having trained multitudes of residents and fellows in colorectal surgical techniques, Dr Arnold is ideally suited to be the guest editor of this important issue of the *Surgical Oncology Clinics of North America*.

This issue covers a number of important topics, including such interesting matters as systemic therapy and imaging, as well as minimally invasive surgical approaches to colon cancer. This issue covers other subjects, such as population-based screening for hereditary colorectal cancer, and updates the readership on clinical trials and progress in metastatic colon cancer. In addition, less often discussed, yet equally important, topics such as the impact of diet on colon cancer, and the economics of colon cancer are covered. In sum, this is a fantastic, comprehensive, and thorough state-of-the-art review on a wide range of topics relevant to colon cancer. To accomplish this goal, Dr Arnold relied on an incredible group of authors who are the respective leaders in

Surg Oncol Clin N Am 27 (2018) xiii–xiv
https://doi.org/10.1016/j.soc.2017.11.013
1055-3207/18/© 2017 Published by Elsevier Inc.

surgonc.theclinics.com

their field. I would like to thank Dr Arnold and his colleagues for an excellent issue of the *Surgical Oncology Clinics of North America* and for taking on such an important topic.

Timothy M. Pawlik, MD, MPH, PhD, FACS, FRACS (Hon)
Professor and Chair
Department of Surgery
The Urban Meyer III and Shelley Meyer Chair for Cancer Research
The Ohio State University
Wexner Medical Center
395 West 12th Avenue, Suite 670
Columbus, OH 43210, USA

E-mail address:
Tim.Pawlik@osumc.edu

Preface

Colon Cancer: The Road Traveled

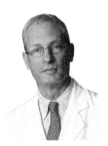

Mark W. Arnold, MD
Editor

Each Wednesday at 5 PM, a group of 15 to 20 physicians, nurse practitioners, residents, and medical students, representing medical oncology, radiation oncology, interventional radiology, pathology, surgical oncology, and colorectal surgery, meets on the second floor conference room of the Arthur G. James Cancer Hospital for the Colon and Rectal Cancer Tumor Board. Patient care plans are made and revised so that each patient with cancer has the best opportunity for cure, palliation, and long-term survival. In addition, complicated patients, interesting cases, clinical trials, and new studies are presented. This multidisciplinary approach to colon cancer has made a huge difference in the lives of these patients and in the effectiveness of the therapies offered. It was not always this way.

When I first started as a young colorectal surgeon 30 years ago, a patient diagnosed with colon cancer was typically referred to a surgeon, regardless of the presence of metastatic disease, and was almost always offered resection of the primary tumor first. Then, after recovery, if the patient was unfortunate enough to have lymph nodal or distant metastatic disease, there was a referral to a medical oncologist. Chemotherapeutic treatments were primarily fluorouracil based with limited effectiveness. Even so, overall survival was good, because early-stage colon cancers were often cured by surgery alone. Successful outcomes, however, had not significantly changed since Dukes and Bussey[1] published their landmark article, "The Spread of Rectal Cancer and Its Effect on Prognosis" 60 years ago.

That study was validation of the A, B, and C staging system, first described by the same authors in 1932 and designed at the St Marks Hospital. It was an extensive single-hospital retrospective study, spanning 25 years and 3596 patients with rectal cancer, of which 2447 were treated by extirpation of the primary tumor. The crude overall five-year survival was 48.3%. Survival stage by stage was A, 81.2%; B, 64%; and C, 27.4%. These were excellent results for the state of medical care development at that time. It was also the first advanced staging system for colon and rectal cancer

https://doi.org/10.1016/j.soc.2017.11.012
1055-3207/18/© 2017 Published by Elsevier Inc.
surgonc.theclinics.com

and made it possible to accurately judge the effectiveness, success and failure, of changes in therapy by stage. This work was the beginning of the modern era for colon cancer treatment.

There have been other important milestones that have advanced our understanding of colon cancer, a few of which are especially noteworthy in that they have changed the treatment of the disease and are routinely incorporated into our practices today. Carcinoembryonic antigen (CEA) is an excellent example.

In 1965, Gold and Freedman[2] published their landmark article, "Demonstration of Tumor-Specific Antigens in Human Colonic Carcinomata by Immunological Tolerance and Absorption Techniques." Using specimens of human colon cancer, with normal colonic mucosa as controls, they were able to identify the presence of the tumor marker, CEA, using sera with tumor-specific antibodies obtained from animals immunized with human colon cancer cells.

CEA is expressed primarily on human colon and rectal adenocarcinomas; therefore, measurement of its level became a practical way to longitudinally follow patients with colon cancer and identify those developing metastatic disease. A rise in CEA is often apparent prior to a recurrence being detectable with imaging. This led Martin and colleagues[3] to begin a program of CEA-directed second-look surgery in patients being monitored for recurrence. In 139 of their initial 146 patients, reoperation for a rising CEA resulted in finding metastatic disease. Eighty-one of those patients were re-resected for potential cure. This change in the surgical treatment of colon cancer made it possible for patients with locally recurrent cancer or isolated metastatic disease to have a second chance at cure.

CEA is still routinely used to follow patients with colon cancer, to check for recurrence, and to gauge the effectiveness of therapeutic chemotherapy. It is often more sensitive than the imaging studies and can detect a response earlier to that seen on PET or CT. Other advances in technology have also played an important role in diagnosis and treatment. The introduction of the flexible colonoscope and its widespread use proved that that adenomatous colon polyps were the precursor to colon cancer.[4] Today, surveillance protocols by colonoscopy are standard and are both diagnostic and preventive. Through education and outreach, it is now a basic part of the public's understanding of health care that everyone should have a colonoscopy at age 50.

Improvements in surgical technique over the last 25 years have changed the surgical practice of colon cancer for the better. In 1991, Jacobs and colleagues[5] published a series of 20 patients who successfully underwent laparoscopic colectomy. Laparoscopy surgery was controversial at the time, having only recently been introduced as an option for cholecystectomy. Many surgeons were reluctant to adapt it and considered the technique inappropriate for cancer surgery. In their series, 12 of the 20 patients had either a large villous adenoma or colon cancer. This article, demonstrating the feasibility of minimally invasive surgery for colectomy, was rapidly followed by others. Two subsequent large trials, the Clinical Outcomes of Surgical Therapy Study Group and the Colon Cancer Laparoscopic or Open Resection trial, with 872 and 1248, respectively, randomized patients, showed that laparoscopy was as safe and as effective as open surgery with shorter recovery and hospital stays, leading to decreased cost.[6,7] There were no significant changes in either long-term survival or complications. Minimally invasive surgery, laparoscopy and robotics, combined with specific Colon-Enhanced Recovery after Surgery Protocols, has become the default choice for most colon and rectal cancer surgeons, resulting in less complications, better results, and quicker recoveries.[8]

Advances in chemotherapy are also making a significant impact on survival. Publication of the MOSAIC trial, Oxaliplatin, Fluororuracil, and Leucovorin as Adjuvant

Treatment for Colon Cancer in 2004, demonstrated that the addition of Oxaliplatin to previous protocols of 5-FU-based therapy for adjuvant and therapeutic purposes significantly improves survival.[9] This approach has been validated by multiple other prospective randomized studies.[10] Earlier diagnosis, more advanced surgical techniques, and highly effective chemotherapy are resulting in more patients surviving longer and leading higher-quality lives. For patients whose initial diagnosis is stage IV metastatic disease, the standard now is to initiate chemotherapy first and to choose surgery only for significant symptoms or signs of obstruction.

It is challenging to create an issue of *Surgical Oncology Clinics of North America* that is primarily about colon cancer without covering rectal cancer too, as there are more similarities than differences and large areas of overlap, but the main focus of this effort is on the colon cancer side. There has already been a lot written in the literature focusing on rectal cancer. In this issue, I have also tried to expand the discussion beyond the usual focus of diagnosis, surgery, and chemotherapy to include articles on environmental factors, pathology, associated inflammation, imaging, and the economic toll this disease takes. Colon cancer is best treated by a broad and multidisciplinary approach.

Mark W. Arnold, MD
The Ohio State University
Wexner Medical Center
410 West 10th Avenue
Columbus, OH 43210, USA

E-mail address:
mark.arnold@osumc.edu

REFERENCES

1. Dukes CE, Bussey HJR. The spread of rectal cancer and its effect on prognosis. Br J Cancer 1958;12:309–20.
2. Gold P, Freedman SO. Demonstration of tumor-specific antigens in human colonic carcinomata by immunological tolerance and absorption techniques. J Exp Med 1965;121:439–62.
3. Martin EW Jr, Minton JP, Carey LC. CEA-directed second-look surgery in the asymptomatic patient after primary resection of colorectal carcinoma. Ann Surg 1985;202(3):310–7.
4. Stryker SJ, Wolff BG, Culp CE, et al. Natural history of untreated colon polyps. Gastroenterology 1987;93:1009–13.
5. Jacobs M, Verdega JC, Goldstein HS. Minimally invasive colon resection (laparoscopic colectomy). Surg Laparosc Endosc 1991;1(3):144–50.
6. The Clinical Outcomes of Surgical Therapy Study Group. A comparison of laparoscopically assisted and open colectomy for colon cancer. N Engl J Med 2004; 350:2050–9.
7. Velkamp R, Kuhry E, Hop WC, et al. COlon cancer Laparoscopic or Open Resection Study Group (COLOR) laparoscopic surgery versus open surgery for colon cancer: short term outcome of a randomized trial. Lancet Oncol 2005;6:477–84.
8. Carmichael JC, Keller DS, Baldini G, et al. Clinical practice guidelines for enhanced recovery after colon and rectal surgery from the American Society of Colon and Rectal Surgeons and Society of American Gastrointestinal and Endoscopic Surgeons. Dis Colon Rectum 2017;60:761–84.

9. André T, Boni C, Navarro M, et al. Improved overall survival with oxaliplatin, fluo-rouracil, and leucovorin as adjuvant treatment in stage II or III colon cancer in the MOSAIC trial. J Clin Oncol 2009;27(19):3109–16.

10. Schmoll HJ, Twelves C, Sun W, et al. Effect of adjuvant capecitabine or fluoro-uracil, with or without oxaliplatin, on survival outcomes in stage III colon cancer and the effect of oxaliplatin on post-relapse survival: a pooled analysis of individ-ual patient data from four randomized controlled trials. Lancet Oncol 2014;15(13): 1481–92.

Systemic Therapy for Colon Cancer

Christina Wu, MD

KEYWORDS

- Irinotecan • Oxaliplatin • 5-fluorouracil
- Antiepidermal growth factor receptor antibody
- Vascular endothelial growth factor antibody • Immunotherapy • Regorafenib
- Trifluridine/tipiracil

KEY POINTS

- Determining the suitable adjuvant chemotherapy for colon cancer patients depends on the tumor stage, presence of high-risk pathologic features, microsatellite instability status, patient age, and performance status.
- Systemic treatment for colon cancer patients with metastatic disease includes chemotherapy, targeted therapy, and immunotherapy.
- Prognostic and predictive biomarkers have been developed to help better tailor treatment regimens for patients.

INTRODUCTION

Colorectal cancer is the fourth most common cancer in the United States, with an estimated 135,430 new cases in 2017. Colon cancer is the second leading cause of cancer deaths in Western countries.[1] Most colon cancer patients will be diagnosed with regional or distant metastasis, and thus will need adjuvant chemotherapy after their surgery or palliative chemotherapy for their metastatic disease. In the adjuvant setting, we have improved our ability to identify patients who will benefit the most from chemotherapy by examining patient and tumor characteristics. In the metastatic setting, there are chemotherapy drugs, biologic agents targeting the vascular endothelial growth factor (VEGF) pathway and epidermal growth factor receptor (EGFR) pathway, and immunotherapy to offer patients. Oncologists are better able to tailor systemic therapy for their patients based on predictive and prognostic biomarkers, which include: right- versus left-sided cancer and tumor biomarkers such as microsatellite instability-high (MSI-high), KRAS, NRAS, and BRAF mutations.

Disclosure Statement: No financial disclosures.
Emory University, Department of Hematology/Oncology, Winship Cancer Institute, 1365-C Clifton Road, Northeast, Atlanta, GA 30322, USA
E-mail address: Christina.Wu@emoryhealthcare.org

Surg Oncol Clin N Am 27 (2018) 235–242
https://doi.org/10.1016/j.soc.2017.11.001
1055-3207/18/© 2017 Elsevier Inc. All rights reserved.

surgonc.theclinics.com

LOCALLY ADVANCED COLON CANCER AND ADJUVANT CHEMOTHERAPY

The 3 chemotherapy agents utilized to treat patients with early stage colon cancer are 5-fluorouracil (5FU), capecitabine (Xeloda), and oxaliplatin (Eloxatin).

5FU is a nucleotide analogue that can inhibit thymidylate synthase (TS), an enzyme crucial for pyrimidine nucleotide synthesis. The 5FU metabolite, fluorodeoxyuridine triphosphosphate (FdUTP), also disrupts RNA synthesis. 5FU may be administered as an intravenous infusion or bolus schedule, with prolonged infusion inhibiting TS and bolus infusion leading to incorporation of FdUTP into RNA.[2] Leucovorin is administered with 5FU to enhance clinical activity.[3]

Capecitabine is the oral pro-drug for 5FU, and thus both have been shown to have equal efficacy in the adjuvant and metastatic setting.

Oxaliplatin is a platinum drug, and is an alkylating agent that inhibits DNA synthesis. It may be administered intravenously in combination with either 5FU or capecitabine.

Adjuvant therapy is given over the course of 6 months, either single-agent 5FU or capecitabine, or doublet combination of 5FU/oxaliplatin or capecitabine/oxaliplatin.

Adjuvant Therapy for Stage II Colon Cancer

When patients are diagnosed with early stage colon cancer, oncologists determine whether they should recommend adjuvant chemotherapy largely based on the risk of cancer recurrence and the amount of benefit the patients will receive with treatment. Patients with stage II colon cancer generally have good prognosis and survival (5-year overall survival is estimated to be 80%), and the added benefit in survival with adjuvant chemotherapy may not be more than 5%.[4] The QUASAR study randomized patients with stage II colon cancer to observation versus 5FU therapy, and reported a small absolute improvement in survival of 3.6% (95% confidence interval [CI] 1.0–6.0) for patients who received chemotherapy.[5] Two phase III clinical trials for patients with stage II and III colon cancer, the Multi-center International Study of Oxaliplatin/ 5-Fluorouracil/Leucovorin in the Adjuvant Treatment of Colon Cancer (MOSAIC) and the National Surgical Adjuvant Breast and Bowel Project (NSABP) C07, randomized patients to receive 5FU versus 5FU and oxaliplatin. Patients with stage II colon cancer in the MOSAIC trial had 6-year overall survival of 87% in both treatment arms, thus did not benefit from the addition of oxaliplatin to 5FU.[6] The NSABP C07 study also did not show a difference in survival in both treatment arms for patients with stage II colon cancer.[7] Based on the results from these phase III trials, patients with stage II colon cancer do not receive great benefit from either single-agent 5FU or doublet chemotherapy with 5FU/oxaliplatin over observation alone.

Microsatellite Instability High and Stage II Colon Cancer

If patients with stage II colon cancer are identified to have MSI-high tumors, they have been shown in a large retrospective study to have improved survival outcome over patients with microsatellite stable (MSS) tumors. In addition, patients with MSI-high colon cancer do not benefit from adjuvant 5FU chemotherapy.[8] Mismatch repair (MMR) proteins are responsible for correcting mistakes made by DNA polymerase during DNA synthesis. MMR protein deficiency leads to MSI, which is an accumulation of errors within short repetitive sequences of DNA, called microsatellites. MSI status is checked by either immunohistochemistry (IHC) staining for the mismatch repair proteins or by polymerase chain reaction to detect instable and shortened microsatellites. MSI-high tumors would have missing MMR protein(s) by IHC and shortened/instable microsatellites. MMR protein deficiency is caused by either germline mutation of the MMR genes (hereditary Lynch syndrome) or sporadic silencing of the MMR genes.

High-Risk Features in Stage II Colon Cancer

5FU or 5FU/oxaliplatin chemotherapy may be offered if the following high-risk tumor features are identified in the pathology report: T4 stage, bowel perforation, bowel obstruction, poorly differentiated histology (and MSS), lymphovascular invasion, perineural invasion, less than 12 lymph nodes examined, close or positive surgical margins.[4] These features would indicate a higher-risk of cancer recurrence; however there are no data to prove that these patient subsets benefit any more than others from adjuvant therapy. Ultimately, the clinician will have to factor in all the good and poor risk features of the patient's tumor, and then engage the patient in a thorough discussion about the risks and benefits of undergoing adjuvant therapy.

Adjuvant Therapy for Stage III Colon Cancer

For stage III colon cancer, the risk of recurrence after surgery is 50% to 60%, and adjuvant 5FU/oxaliplatin chemotherapy can reduce the risk of death by 20%. In the phase III MOSAIC trial, in which patients were randomized to either 5FU or 5FU/oxaliplatin treatment, patients with stage III colon cancer had an improved 6-year overall survival with 5FU/oxaliplatin over 5FU alone, 73% versus 69%, respectively.[6] NSABP C07 showed improved survival outcome for stage III colon cancer patients with 5FU/oxaliplatin as well.[7] Although the phase III trials show a survival benefit from adjuvant 5FU/oxaliplatin therapy, retrospective subgroup analysis of elderly patients (defined as ages 70–75 years) in the MOSAIC trial showed that 5FU/oxaliplatin was not superior to 5FU.[9] Although the elderly population made up a small fraction of the total patients enrolled on the study, age and comorbid medical conditions should be taken into account when deciding on suitable adjuvant chemoregimen. Retrospective studies examining MSI-high stage III colon cancer patients show that patients have improved prognosis, but still benefit from adjuvant 5FU/oxaliplatin therapy.[10]

3 Versus 6 Months of FOLFOX for Stage III Colon Cancer

Adjuvant 5FU/oxaliplatin was studied in phase III trials to be administered for 6 months; however often in clinical practice the duration of treatment is limited due to oxaliplatin-induced neuropathy. Thus, a prospective pooled analysis of 6 phase III trials investigating 3 versus 6 months of 5FU/oxaliplatin therapy for patients with stage III colon cancer was recently reported as part of the International Duration Evaluation of Adjuvant Chemotherapy (IDEA) collaboration. The results showed noninferiority was not established with 3 months of 5FU/oxaliplatin therapy compared with 6 months, but subgroup analysis did show noninferiority with 3 months of therapy for low-risk stage III (T1-3 N1) colon cancers. Thus, stage III colon cancers are now subdivided into low-risk (T1-3 N1) and high-risk (T4 or N2), and patients will be offered different duration of therapy accordingly.[11]

METASTATIC COLORECTAL CANCER
First- and Second-Line Chemotherapy

Chemotherapy agents used in the first- and second-line metastatic settings are 5FU, capecitabine (Xeloda), oxaliplatin (Eloxatin), and irinotecan.

Irinotecan is a DNA topoisomerase I inhibitor that leads to DNA damage and cell death. It is administered intravenously, either as a single agent or in combination with infusional 5FU. Irinotecan is generally not combined with capecitabine because of the overlapping toxicity of diarrhea.

The chemotherapy backbone in the metastatic setting is generally the combination of infusional 5FU/irinotecan (FOLFIRI) or 5FU/oxaliplatin (FOLFOX) with the addition of a biologic targeted agent. Both chemoregimens have been shown to be equally effective, the GERCOR C97 - 3 trial randomized patients to either start with FOLFIRI followed by FOLFOX, or the opposite sequence. There was no difference in response rates (RR), time to progression (TTP), or overall survival (OS) between the 2 arms.[12] Oncologists often determine which chemoregimen to start with based on chemotherapy toxicities and patients' existing comorbid medical conditions and preferences. Oxaliplatin causes cold sensitivity and neuropathy, whereas irinotecan treatment leads to hair loss and diarrhea.

Single-agent 5FU or Xeloda may be given with a biologic agent if the patient's performance status is not good enough to tolerate doublet chemotherapy. The phase III CAIRO study randomized patients to either (sequential therapy) first-line capecitabine, second-line irinotecan, or third-line capecitabine/oxaliplatin versus (combination) first-line capecitabine/irinotecan and second-line capecitabine/oxaliplatin. Median overall survival was 16.3 months for sequential therapy and 17.4 months for combination therapy, $P=.3281$.[13] The trial showed that sequential therapy was as good as combination therapy, and that survival was the same if patients were exposed to all agents.

Triplet chemotherapy, with 5FU/oxaliplatin/irinotecan (FOLFOXIRI) may be considered in patients with high tumor burden and rapidly progressing disease, in order to improve RR and OS, although this intense therapy also leads to increased toxicities such as fatigue, nausea and vomiting, and cytopenias. The phase 3 TRIBE study compared FOLFOXIRI/bevacizumab versus FOLFIRI/bevacizumab, and reported improved median OS of 29.8 months 95% CI 26.0–34.3 in the FOLFOXIRI/bevacizumab arm versus 25.8 months (95% CI 22.5–29.1) in the FOLFIRI/bevacizumab treatment arm.[14]

Antibody Therapy Targeting Vascular Endothelial Growth Factor Pathway

VEGF is a growth factor that is secreted by tumor cells and their adjacent stromal cells to promote angiogenesis and cancer metastasis. Monoclonal antibodies have been developed to target either the VEGF ligand itself or the VEGF receptors (VEGFR).

Bevacizumab (Avastin) is a monoclonal antibody that binds the ligand VEGF-A, and the first biologic agent to be approved in the treatment of metastatic colorectal cancer (mCRC). The phase III trial compared bolus 5FU/irinotecan/bevacizumab and bolus 5FU/irinotecan in the first-line setting, and an increased OS was shown with the addition of bevacizumab, 20.3 versus 15.6 months, hazard ratio (HR) 0.66, $P<.004$.[15] Bevacizumab is approved by the US Food and Drug Administration (FDA) to be used in the first- and second-line setting in combination with 5FU-containing chemotherapy, and is also effective when given beyond progression (eg, FOLFOX/bevacizumab followed by FOLFIRI/bevacizumab).

Additional agents that target the VEGF pathway are ziv-aflibercept (Zaltrap) which is a recombinant fusion protein that has binding domains of VEGFR-1 and VEGFR-2, and targets VEGF-A, VEGF-B, and PIGF. The phase III VELOUR trial showed that in the second-line setting, FOLFIRI/ziv-aflibercept versus FOLFIRI had improved OS, 12.5 months (95% CI 10.8–15.5) versus 11.7 months (95% CI 9.8–13.8), respectively, for patients who had prior bevacizumab therapy.[16]

Ramucirumab (Cyramza) is a monoclonal antibody that targets VEGR-2, and in the phase III RAISE trial, it was shown to improve OS when patients were treated with FOLFIRI/ramucirumab versus FOLFIRI alone, 13.3 months (95% CI 12.4–14.5) versus 11.7 months (95% CI 10.8–12.7).

Both ziv-aflibercept and ramucirumab are FDA approved in the second-line setting in combination with chemotherapy.

Bevacizumab, ziv-aflibercept, and ramucirumab are administered in combination with chemotherapy, but not given as single agents. There is no biomarker to select for patients who benefit the most from anti-VEGF therapy.

Antibody Therapy Targeting Epidermal Growth Factor Receptor Pathway

The EGFR pathway plays an important role in colorectal carcinogenesis. EGFR is a member of the human epidermal growth factor family of receptor tyrosine kinases. EGFR is expressed on colorectal cancers, and it can lead to activation of signaling pathways such as the RAS-RAF mitogen-activated protein kinase (MAPK), phosphatidylinositol 3-kinase (PI3K), and phospholipase C pathways that lead to tumor proliferation, metastasis, and survival.

Cetuximab (Erbitux) and panitumumab (Vectibix) are monoclonal antibodies developed to bind and inhibit EGFR activation, both approved by the FDA for the treatment of mCRC. They are administered intravenously, and may be given in combination with chemotherapy and as a single agent.

KRAS, NRAS, and BRAF proteins are downstream of EGFR in the MAPK pathway. BRAF mutation is indicative of poor prognosis and aggressive tumors. Oncologists often choose to treat patients with triplet FOLFOXIRI chemotherapy due to the presence of BRAF mutation, indicating a poor prognosis. At present, there are ongoing clinical trials to target tumors with BRAF mutation, including BRAF and MEK inhibitors in combination with chemotherapy (**Table 1**).

KRAS and NRAS mutations are indicative of poor prognosis as well, but also negative predictive biomarkers of the efficacy of cetuximab and panitumumab. KRAS and NRAS mutations lead to constitutive activation of the MAPK signaling pathway downstream of EGFR; thus inhibition of EGFR by cetuximab and panitumumab upstream to KRAS and NRAS is not effective. In the Panitumumab Randomized trial In combination with chemotherapy for Metastatic colorectal cancer to determine Efficacy (PRIME) phase III study, patients were randomized to treatment with FOLFOX and panitumumab versus FOLFOX. Patients who had KRAS and NRAS wild-type tumors benefited from the addition of panitumumab; PFS was 10.1 months with FOLFOX/panitumumab versus 7.9 months with FOLFOX (HR 0.72, 95% CI 0.58–0.90 $P=.004$).[17] Patients who harbored KRAS or NRAS mutation had worse PFS with the addition of panitumumab, 7.3 months with FOLFOX/panitumumab versus 8.7 months with FOLFOX (HR 1.31, 95% CI 1.07–1.60, $P=.008$).

Recently, there have been findings that the location of the primary colon cancer, right versus left side, may be prognostic and predictive of the efficacy of anti-EGFR antibody. Biology of right- and left-sided colon cancers may be different because of differing embryonic origins of midgut versus hindgut. A retrospective study of 6

Table 1	
Biomarkers in colon cancer	
Biomarker	**Prognostic and/or Predictive Qualities**
MSI-high[8,21]	Improved prognosis for stage II colon cancer
	Positive predictive biomarker for pembrolizumab or nivolumab therapy
KRAS mutation[17] (exon 1,2,3,4)	Worse prognosis
	Negative predictive biomarker for cetuximab or panitumumab
NRAS mutation[17] (exon 1,2,3,4)	Worse prognosis
	Negative predictive biomarker for cetuximab or panitumumab
BRAF mutation[17] (exon 15)	Worse prognosis

randomized trials comparing chemotherapy with EGFR antibody therapy versus chemotherapy alone showed striking differences. In patients treated with chemotherapy, a worse prognosis is seen with patients with right-sided tumors when compared with left-sided tumors, OS HR 2.03, (95% CI, 1.69–2.42).[18] Patients with left-sided tumors had improved OS with chemotherapy and panitumumab versus chemotherapy alone OS HR 0.75 (0.67–0.84). Right-sided tumors had no significant benefit with the addition of panitumumab to chemotherapy OS HR 1.12 (0.87–1.45).

Anti-EGFR antibody therapy is most efficacious in patients with tumors that are KRAS/NRAS wild-type and left-sided.

Refractory Colon Cancer

Regorafenib and trifluridine/tipiracil are FDA-approved agents for patients who have progressed on prior 5FU, oxaliplatin, irinotecan, and anti-EGFR therapy (if eligible). The choice of a specific drug is largely based on the toxicity profile that patients' can best tolerate.

Regorafenib is a receptor tyrosine kinase inhibitor that targets multiple angiogenic tyrosine kinases, including VEGFR, fibroblast growth factor receptor (FGFR), and platelet derived-growth factor (PDGFR), as well as RET, KIT, and BRAF mutation. In the phase III CORRECT trial, patients with refractory mCRC were randomized to best supportive care and regorafenib versus best supportive care alone. An improved OS was seen with regorafenib, 6.6 versus 5 months, HR 0.773 (95% CI 0.635–0.941, $P=.0051$).[19] The drug is administered orally as a single agent. The main toxicities are hand-foot syndrome, hypertension, elevated liver function tests, and fatigue.

Although trifluridine is a thymidine-based nucleotide, similar to 5FU, it differs in mechanism of action, because it is incorporated into DNA and ultimately leads to DNA damage. Tipiracil inhibits thymidine phosphorylase, which in turn inhibits the breakdown of trifluridine. Trifluridine/tipiracil is an oral drug, administered as a single agent. The phase III RECOURSE study randomized patients to placebo versus trifluridine/tipiracil, and an improvement on OS was seen with 5.3 months versus 7.1 months, HR 0.68 (95% CI 0.58–0.81, $P<.001$).[20] Trifluridine/tipiracil is given orally as a single agent. The clinically significant toxicities seen were neutropenia and leukopenia.

Immunotherapy for Microsatellite Instability-High Cancers

One of the most exciting advancements in mCRC therapy has been the FDA approval of programmed death 1(PD-1) inhibitors pembrolizumab (Keytruda) and nivolumab (Opdivo) for MSI-high tumors and MSI-high mCRC, respectively (see **Table 1**). The PD-1 pathway negatively regulates the cytotoxic immune response to cancer cells. Thus, tumors that have upregulation of PD-1 and programmed-death ligand-1 (PD-L1) escape the host immune system. Because of DNA mismatch repair deficiencies, MSI-high tumors have increased amounts of mutations and neoantigens, and are also found to have increasing tumor infiltrating lymphocytes (TILs) which have higher expression of PD-1, PDL-1, and checkpoint ligands such as cytotoxic T lymphocyte-associated 4 (CTLA-4). Thus, it is hypothesized that when PD-1 inhibitors activate the host immune response toward cancer cells, they are especially effective in MSI-high cancers because of the high number of neoantigens, TILs, and associated immune infiltrate at the tumor-invasive fronts. In the landmark phase II study of pembrolizumab, patients with MSI-high mCRC, MSS mCRC, and MSI-high solid tumors were treated with pembrolizumab.[21] Only the patients with MSI-high CRC and MSI-high solid tumors had a durable response to therapy (objective radiographic responses in 53% of patients, complete responses in 21% of patients) with improved survival.[22] Pembrolizumab and nivolumab are administered intravenously, and tolerated better overall better than chemotherapy agents. Their toxicity profile is related to autoimmune side effects, such as thyroid hormone disturbance, adrenal insufficiency, autoimmune colitis, dermatitis, and arthralgias. The challenge has been that only 5% mCRCs are MSI-high. Thus, much work is needed to identify ways to stimulate the immune system in the many patients who have MSS mCRC so that they may be sensitive to PD-1 inhibitors also.

REFERENCES

1. Howlader N, Noone AM, Krapcho M, et al. SEER cancer statistics review, 1075–2014. Bethesda (MD): National Cancer Institute; Available at: https://seer.cancer.gov/csr/1975_2014. Accessed october 15, 2017.

2. Harstrick A, Gonzales A, Schleucher N, et al. Comparison between short or long exposure to 5-fluorouracil in human gastric and colon cancer cell lines: biochemical mechanism of resistance. Anticancer Drugs 1998;9:625–34.

3. Modulation of fluorouracil by leucovorin in patients with advanced colorectal cancer: evidence in terms of response rate. Advanced Colorectal Cancer Meta-Analysis Project. J Clin Oncol 1992;10:896–903.

4. Benson AB, Schrag D, Somerfield MR, et al. American Society of Clinical Oncology recommendations on adjuvant chemotherapy for stage II colon cancer. J Clin Oncol 2004;22:3408–19.

5. Quasar Collaborative Group, Gray R, Barnwell J, McConkey C, et al. Adjuvant chemotherapy versus observation in patients with colorectal cancer: a randomised study. Lancet 2007;370:2020–9.

6. Andre T, Boni C, Navarro M, et al. Improved overall survival with oxaliplatin, fluorouracil, and leucovorin as adjuvant treatment in stage II or III colon cancer in the MOSAIC trial. J Clin Oncol 2009;27:3109–16.

7. Yothers G, O'Connell MJ, Allegra CJ, et al. Oxaliplatin as adjuvant therapy for colon cancer: updated results of NSABP C-07 trial, including survival and subset analyses. J Clin Oncol 2011;29:3768–74.

8. Sargent DJ, Marsoni S, Monges G. Defective mismatch repair as a predictive marker for lack of efficacy of fluorouracil-based adjuvant therapy in colon cancer. J Clin Oncol 2010;38:3219–26.

9. Tournigand C, André T, Bonnetain F, et al. Adjuvant therapy with fluorouracil and oxaliplatin in stage II and elderly patients (between ages 70 and 75 years) with colon cancer: subgroup analyses of the multicenter international study of oxaliplatin, fluorouracil, and leucovorin in the adjuvant treatment of colon cancer trial. J Clin Oncol 2012;30:3353–60.

10. Sinicrope FA, Foster NR, Thibodeau SN, et al. DNA mismatch repair status and colon cancer recurrence and survival in clinical trials of 5-fluoruacil-based adjuvant therapy. J Natl Cancer Inst 2011;1-3:863–75.

11. Shi Q, Sobrero AF, Shields AF, et al. Prospective pooled analysis of six phase III trials of investigation duration of adjuvant oxaliplatin-based therapy (3 vs 6 months) for patients with stage III colon cancer: the IDEA (International Duration Evaluation of Adjuvant chemotherapy) collaboration. J Clin Oncol 2017;35 [abstract LBA1].

12. Tournigand C, Andre T, Achille E, et al. FOLFIRI followed by FOLFOX6 or the reverse sequence in advanced colorectal cancer: a randomized GERCOR study. J Clin Oncol 2004;22:229–37.

13. Koopman M, Antonini NF, Douma J, et al. Sequential versus combination chemo-therapy with capecitabine, irinotecan, and oxaliplatin in advanced colorectal can-cer (CAIRO): a phase III randomized controlled trial. Lancet 2007;370:135–42.
14. Cremolini C, Loupakis F, Antoniotti C, et al. FOLFIRIS plus bevacizumab versus FOLFIRI plus bevacizumab as first-line treatment of patients with metastatic colo-rectal cancer: updated overall survival and molecular subgroup analyses of the open-label, phase 3 TRIBE study. Lancet Oncol 2015;16:1306–15.
15. Hurwitz H, Fehrenbacher L, Novotny W, et al. Bevacizumab plus irinotecan, fluo-rouracil, and leucovorin for metastatic colorectal cancer. N Engl J Med 2004;350: 2335–42.
16. Tabernero J, Van Cutsem E, Lakomy R, et al. Aflibercept versus placebo in com-bination with fluorouracil, leucovorin, and irinotecan in the treatment of previously treated metastatic colorectal cancer: prespecified subgroup analysis from the VELOUR trial. Eur J Cancer 2014;50:320–31.
17. Douillard J-Y, Oliner KS, Siena S, et al. Panitumumab-FOLFOX4 Treatment in RAS Mutations in Colorectal Cancer. N Engl J Med 2013;369:1023–34.
18. Arnold D, Lueza B, Douillard J-Y, et al. Prognostic and predictive value of primary tumor side in patients with RAS wild-type metastatic colorectal cancere treated with chemotherapy and EGFR directed antibodies in six randomized trials. Ann Oncol 2017;28:1719–29.
19. Grothey A, Van Cutsem E, Sobrero A, et al. Regorafenib monotherapy for previ-ously treated metastatic colorectal cancer (CORRECT): an international, multi-center, randomized, placebo-controlled, phase 3 trial. Lancet 2013;381:303–12.
20. Mayer RJ, Van Cutsem E, Falcone A, et al. Randomized trial of TAS-102 for refrac-tory metastatic colorectal cancer. N Engl J Med 2015;372:1909–19.
21. Le DT, Uram JN, Wang H, et al. PD-1 blockade in tumors with mismatch-repair deficiency. N Engl J Med 2015;372:2509–20.
22. Le DT, Durham JN, Smith KN, et al. Mismatch repair deficiency predicts response of solid tumors to PD-1 blockade. Science 2017;367:409–13.

Colon Cancer: What We Eat

Pan Pan, PhD[a], Jianhua Yu, PhD[b], Li-Shu Wang, PhD[a,*]

KEYWORDS

- Colorectal cancer • Diet • Red/processed meat • Fish • Fiber • Fruit and vegetables
- Vitamins and minerals • Coffee and tea

KEY POINTS

- Colorectal cancer has a higher incidence in Oceania and Europe and a lower incidence in Africa and Asia.
- Colorectal cancer is largely preventable by adapting a healthy lifestyle including healthy diet, adequate physical activity, and avoiding obesity.
- What is eaten affects the risk of developing colorectal cancer: red/processed meat could increase the risk whereas fibers, fruit and vegetables may decrease the risk.
- Other foods, such as fish, vitamins and minerals, and coffee, might have potential effects on the risk of developing colorectal cancer.

INTRODUCTION

Cancer is the second leading cause of death worldwide, having caused 8.8 million deaths in 2015.[1] Among all cancers, colorectal cancer (CRC) is the third most common cancer in men (accounting for 10% of all male cancers) and the second in women (accounting for 9.2% of all female cancers).[2] The estimated age-standardized incidence rate of CRC is 20.6 per 100,000 for men and 14.3 per 100,000 for women, and the mortality rate is 10.0 for men and 6.9 for women.[2] A higher incidence of CRC is observed in Oceania and Europe, ranging from 30 or more per 100,000, whereas Africa and Asia have a lower incidence, at less than 5 per 100,000.[3,4] Countries with the highest economic development are likely to have higher incidences and mortality rates, and these are rising in countries becoming more developed.[2]

CRC is largely preventable. The higher incidence in more developed countries can be attributed, at least partially, to the Western lifestyle, with its high intake of red and processed meat, which has been reported to associate positively with higher risk of CRC.[5,6] The global cancer reports published by the World Cancer Research Fund

Disclosure Statement: This article was partially supported by an National Institute of Health grant (5 R01 CA148818) and an American Cancer Society grant (RSG-13-138-01–CNE to L.-S. Wang).
[a] Division of Hematology and Oncology, Department of Medicine, Medical College of Wisconsin, 8701 Watertown Plank Road, Milwaukee, WI 53226, USA; [b] Division of Hematology, Department of Internal Medicine, College of Medicine, Comprehensive Cancer Center, The James Cancer Hospital, The Ohio State University, 460 West 12th Avenue, Columbus, OH 43210, USA
* Corresponding author.
E-mail address: liswang@mcw.edu

Abbreviations	
AHS	Adventist Health Study
ALA	α-linolenic acid
AICR	American Institute for Cancer Research
ATBC	Alpha-Tocopherol, Beta-Carotene Cancer Prevention Study
CI	Confidence interval
CRC	Colorectal cancer
DCH	Danish Diet, Cancer and Health cohort study
DHA	Docosahexaenoic acid
EPA	Eicosapentaenoic acid
EPIC	European Prospective Investigation into Cancer and Nutrition
FFQ	Food frequency questionnaire
HPFS	Health Professionals Follow-up Study
HR	Hazard ratios
IRR	Incidence rate ratios
JACC	Japan Collaborative Cohort
JPHC	Japan Public Health Center-based Prospective Study
MCC	Melbourne Collaborative Cohort
NHS	Nurses' Health Study
NIH-AARP DHS	National Institutes of Health-American Association for Retired Persons Diet and Health Study
NLCS	Netherlands Cohort Study
NOWAC	Norwegian Women and Cancer
NSHDS	Northern Sweden Health and Disease Study
OR	odds ratios
PHS	Physicians' Health Study
PLCO	Prostate, Lung, Colorectal, and Ovarian Cancer Screening Trial
PUFAs	polyunsaturated fatty acids
RR	relative risk
SCFAs	short-chain fatty acids
SMC	Swedish Mammography Cohort
SWHS	Shanghai Women's Health Study
WCRF	World Cancer Research Fund
WHS	Women's Health Study

(WCRF) and the American Institute for Cancer Research (AICR) in 2007 and updated in 2011 listed red and processed meat as "convincing" factors that increase the risk of CRC.[4,7] Many other dietary factors, such as fiber, fruit, and vegetables, may associate inversely with CRC risk.[4,7]

This review aims to summarize the latest work available, mainly epidemiologic studies, to examine the relationship between diet and CRC. The largest studies of dietary consumption and CRC risk conducted worldwide include the National Institutes of Health–American Association of Retired Persons Diet and Health Study (NIH-AARP DHS); the Prostate, Lung, Colorectal, and Ovarian Cancer Screening Trial (PLCO); the Nurses' Health Study (NHS); the Health Professionals Follow-Up Study (HPFS); and the Physicians' Health Study (PHS) from the United States. From Europe, the European Prospective Investigation into Cancer and Nutrition (EPIC) was included and from Asia the Japan Public Health Center-based Prospective (JPHC) study and the Shanghai Women's Health Study (SWHS) were selected. Many other regional studies have also added to our understanding of the diet–CRC interaction.

MATERIALS AND METHODS

The authors conducted a PubMed search for human studies published up to 2017, using the key words—colorectal cancer, diet, nutrition, and epidemiology—giving preference to studies that reported risk estimates (hazard ratio [HR], odds ratio [OR], relative risk [RR], or incidence rate ratio [IRR]) of CRC as well as measures of variability (95% confidence interval (CI)). Articles and clinical trials that described and compared the impact of diets on CRC were first screened according to abstracts and titles; then the full-text articles were assessed for eligibility. Reference lists from the studies selected by the electronic search were manually searched to identify further relevant reports. Reference lists from all available review articles and primary studies were also considered. Analysis included only the most common foods across different cultures, including meat, fish, dietary fiber, fruit and vegetables, vitamins and minerals, and coffee and tea.

Red Meat and Processed Meat

During the past 3 decades, many large epidemiologic studies have investigated the association of red/processed meat with the risk of CRC. Although these studies varied in terms of analytical model, gender, sublocation of the tumor, and meat subtype, the majority observed a positive association of high intake of red/processed meat with the risk of developing CRC.[8–17] Therefore, the WCRF/AICR listed red/processed meat as "convincing" factors for increasing CRC risk.[4,7]

The NIH-AARP DHS analyzed approximately 500,000 participants aged 50 years to 71 years at baseline (1995–1996), and followed them until the end of 2003, using a 124-item food frequency questionnaire (FFQ). Individuals in the highest quintile, compared with those in the lowest quintile, of red meat (HR 1.24; 95% CI, 1.12–1.36; P trend <0.001) and processed meat (HR 1.20; 95% CI, 1.09–1.32; P trend <0.001) intake had an increased risk of CRC. The positive association for both types of meat was more robust for rectal cancer than for colon cancer.[18,19]

The PLCO study was a large population-based randomized trial of 154,952 participants aged 55 years to 74 years in 1993. The subjects were randomly assigned to an intervention arm with trial screening or a control arm with standard care, and they were followed for 6 years, using a 137-item FFQ. Some suggestive positive associations of red meat (OR 1.22; 95% CI, 0.98–1.52; P trend = 0.12) and processed meat (OR 1.23, 95% CI, 0.99–1.54; P trend = 0.12) were observed when the highest quartiles were compared with the lowest quartiles.[20]

The NHS included 121,700 US female registered nurses aged 30 years to 55 years in 1976, and the HFPS included 51,529 US male health care professionals (dentists, pharmacists, optometrists, osteopaths, podiatrists, and veterinarians) aged 40 years to 75 years in 1986. These 2 large studies used a 131-item FFQ every 4 years until they ended in 2010. Only higher intake of processed red meat was associated significantly with a higher risk of distal colon cancer in both age-adjusted and multivariable-adjusted models (HR 1.36; 95% CI, 1.09–1.69; P trend = 0.006). Unprocessed red meat intake was associated inversely with the risk of distal colon cancer (HR 0.75; 95% CI, 0.68–0.82; P trend <0.001) but only after adjustments for calcium, folate, and fiber intake. No significant gender difference was observed.[21]

The EPIC study was one of the largest cohort studies worldwide; 366,521 women and 153,457 men aged 35 years to 70 years at baseline (1992–1998) from 10 European countries were followed for almost 15 years. Red and processed meat were associated significantly with increased CRC risk (HR 1.35; 95% CI, 0.96–1.88; P trend = 0.03), but the associations were not significant in specific sublocations of tumors.[22] After correction for measurement errors, red and processed meat intake was significantly associated with higher CRC risk (HR 1.55; 95% CI, 1.19–2.02; P trend = 0.001).[22]

The JPHC study involved 2 cohorts with a total of 46,026 men and 52,485 women aged 45 years to 74 years in 1995 to 1998. The participants were surveyed with a 138-item FFQ until 2006. The analysis found statistically significant positive associations between higher intake of red meat (HR 1.48; 95% CI, 1.01–2.17; P trend = 0.03) and beef (HR 1.62; 95% CI, 1.12–2.34; P trend = 0.04) with colon cancer risk in women. In particular, higher intake of beef was associated positively with risk of proximal colon cancer in women (HR 2.52; 95% CI, 1.53–4.14; P trend = 0.01) and with distal colon cancer in men (HR 1.36; 95% CI, 0.90–2.06; P trend = 0.04). No significant association was observed between processed meat and risk of CRC.[23]

In the SWHS, approximately 75,000 women aged 40 years to 70 years in 1997 to 2000 were surveyed by an FFQ every 2 years until the end of 2005. Neither total meat intake nor red meat intake was associated with the risk of CRC cancer. This study also compared the various popular cooking methods in China, such as deep frying, stir frying, roasting, smoking, and salting. Only smoking was positively associated with risk of CRC (RR 1.4; 95% CI, 1.1–1.9; P trend = 0.01).[24]

Some regional studies produced inconsistent results, however. For example, the Danish Diet, Cancer and Health (DCH) cohort study, which was part of the overall EPIC study (although EPIC included only 18% of this Danish cohort), found no overall significant association between red/processed meats with risk of CRC. The only positive associations were between lamb and colon cancer (IRR 1.35; 95% CI, 1.07–1.71; P trend = 0.01) and pork and rectal cancer (IRR 1.63; 95% CI, 1.11–2.39; P trend = 0.03).There was a significant negative association between beef and rectal cancer (IRR 0.75; 95% CI, 0.52–1.09; P trend = 0.03).[25]

The Alpha-Tocopherol, Beta-Carotene Cancer Prevention (ATBC) study in Finland found no significant associations between meat, different types of meat, or fried meat and risk of CRC.[26] The Melbourne Collaborative Cohort Study (MCC) in Australia observed no significant associations between red/processed meat and the risk of CRC.[27] On the other hand, the Swedish Mammography Cohort (SMC) observed a significant positive association between red meat intake and risk of distal colon cancer (RR 2.22; 95% CI, 1.34–3.68; P trend = 0.001).[28] A Canadian case-control study reported increased risk of both colon cancer (OR 1.5; 95% CI, 1.2–1.8; P trend <0.0001) and rectal cancer (OR 1.5; 95% CI, 1.2–2.0; P trend = 0.001) with higher intake of processed meat.[29,30]

In summary, currently available epidemiologic evidence indicates positive associations between red/processed meat and CRC risk, although it does not rule out contributions from other confounding factors, such as higher fat intake and lack of physical activity. The associations tend to be stronger for rectal cancer than colon cancer and for processed meat than red meat as well as for men than women. Potential underlying mechanisms of the elevated CRC risk by red/processed meat include carcinogenic chemical byproducts made during cooking and processing, such as heterocyclic amines, polycyclic aromatic hydrocarbons, and N-nitroso compounds. Controlled studies, however, need to delineate the mechanisms of action of these carcinogenic chemicals. Characteristics of studies of red/processed meat intake and CRC risk are shown in **Table 1**.

Fish

Fish consumption may decrease the risk of CRC development, partially because fish contains high levels of polyunsaturated fatty acids (PUFAs). Although many epidemiologic studies have examined the possible association between fish consumption and risk of CRC, highly inconsistent results among studies were reported.[31,32] Therefore, in 2011, the WCRF/AICR changed fish consumption from "suggestive" to "no conclusion."[4,7]

The EPIC study observed significantly inverse associations between fish consumption and the risk of CRC (HR 0.69; 95% CI, 0.54–0.88; P trend <0.001). The trend for this inverse association was due mainly to the decreased risk for the left side of the colon (P trend = 0.02) and for the rectum (P trend <0.001).[22]

Table 1
Characteristics of studies of red/processed meat and colorectal cancer

Study	Number of Study Participants	Ages of Participants (Y)	Follow-up Years	Colorectal Cancer Incidence (No. of cases)	Analytical Category	Analytical Comparison, High vs Low Intake	Relative Risk (95% CI)	Reference
NIH-AARP DHS	294,724 men and 199,312 women	50–71	1995–2003	5107 (CRC)	Red meat	62.7 g/1000 kcal vs 9.8 g/1000 kcal	CRC: 1.24 (1.12–1.36), P<.001	Cross et al,[18] 2007
					Processed meat	22.6 g/1000 kcal vs 1.6 g/1000 kcal	CRC: 1.20 (1.09–1.32), P<.001	
HPFS and NHS	47,389 men and 87,108 women	40–75/30–55	1986–2010/ 1980–2010	1968 (colon), 589 (rectum)	Processed red meat	>5 servings/wk vs 0	Distal colon cancer: 1.36 (1.09–1.69), P =.006	Bernstein et al,[21] 2015
					Unprocessed red meat	>5 servings/wk vs 0	Distal colon cancer: 0.75 (0.68–0.82), P<.001	
EPIC	47,8040 men and women	35–70	1992–2002	855 (colon), 474 (rectum)	Red and processed meat	≥160 g/d vs <10 g/d	CRC: 1.35 (0.96–1.88), P =.03	Norat et al,[22] 2005
						Per 100-g increase	CRC: 1.55 (1.19–2.02), P =.001	
JPHC	80,658 men and women	45–74	1995–2006	788 (colon), 357 (rectum)	Red meat	≥93 g/d vs <14 g/d	Women—colon cancer: 1.48 (1.01–2.17), P =.03	Takachi et al,[23] 2011
					Beef	≥28 g/d vs <0.1 g/d	Women—colon cancer: 1.62 (1.12–2.34), P =.04 Women—proxima colon cancer: 2.52 (1.53–4.14), P =.01	
						≥34 g/d vs <0.2 g/d	Men—distal colon cancer: 1.36 (0.90–2.06), P =.04	

(continued on next page)

Table 1
(continued)

Study	Number of Study Participants	Ages of Participants (Y)	Follow-up Years	Colorectal Cancer Incidence (No. of cases)	Analytical Category	Analytical Comparison, High vs Low Intake	Relative Risk (95% CI)	Reference
SWHS	73,224 women	40–70	1997–2005	236 (colon), 158 (rectum)	Smoking method of cooking	Ever vs never	Colon cancer: 1.4 (1.1–1.9), P = .01	Lee et al,[24] 2009
DCH	25,832 men and 28,156 women	50–64	1993–2009	644 (colon), 345 (rectum)	Lamb Pork Beef	>8 g/d vs ≤5 g/d >54 g/d vs ≤27 g/d >45 g/d vs ≤22 g/d	Colon cancer: 1.35 (1.07–1.71), P = .01 Rectal cancer: 1.63 (1.11–2.39), P = .03 Rectal cancer: 0.75 (0.52–1.09), P = .03	Egeberg et al,[25] 2013
SMC	61,433 women	40–75	1987–2003	389 (colon), 230 (rectum)	Red meat	≥94 g/d vs <50 g/d	Distal colon cancer: 2.22 (1.34–3.68), P = .001	Larsson et al,[28] 2005
Case-control	—	20–76	—	1727 (colon), 1447 (rectum), 5039 (control)	Processed red meat	≥5.42 servings/wk vs ≤0.94 servings/wk	Colon cancer: 1.5 (1.2–1.8), P<.0001 Rectal cancer: 1.5 (1.2–2.0), P = .01	Hu et al,[29] 2011
ATBC	27,111 men (all smokers)	50–69	1985–1993	185 (CRC)	Total red meat Processed meat	≥203 g/d vs <79 g/d ≥122 g/d vs ≤26 g/d	Nonsignificant associations Nonsignificant associations Nonsignificant associations	Pietinen et al,[26] 1999
PLCO	17,072 men and women	55–74	1993–2001	1008 (distal colorectal adenoma)	Red meat Processed meat	60.1 g/1000 kcal vs 13.5 g/1000 kcal 15.5 g/1000 kcal vs 1.5 g/1000 kcal	Nonsignificant associations Nonsignificant associations Nonsignificant associations	Ferrucci et al,[20] 2012
MCC	37,112 men and women	40–69	1990–1994	283 (colon), 169 (rectum)	Fresh red meat Processed meat	>6.5 times/wk vs <3 times/wk >4 times/wk vs <1.5 times/wk	Nonsignificant associations Nonsignificant associations Nonsignificant associations	English et al,[27] 2004

The PHS also revealed significantly inverse associations between fish intake and the risk of CRC (RR 0.63; 95% CI, 0.42–0.95; P trend = 0.02). More importantly, this inverse association was not due solely to the substitution of fish for red meat,[33] suggesting that fish has a potentially protective effect.

However, 3 large US prospective studies found no significant overall associations. The NHS and HPFS found no overall association between fish, ω-3 PUFA, or ω-6 PUFA intake and CRC. Surprisingly, ω-3 PUFAs, such as α-linolenic acid (ALA), eicosapentaenoic acid (EPA), docosahexaenoic acid (DHA), and docosapentaenoic acid, which are generally considered to protect against cancer, were associated positively with risk of CRC in the NHS (HR 1.36; 95% CI, 1.03–1.80; P trend = 0.04).[34] The NIH-AARP DHS reported no significant association between fish intake and risk of CRC.[35]

Similarly, many regional studies showed mixed results. For example, no associations were observed in the ATBC study[26] in Finland, the Japan Collaborative Cohort Study (JACC)[36] and the Ohsaki Cohort Study[37] in Japan, the SMC study[28] in Sweden, the Oxford Vegetarian Study[38] in the United Kingdom, the Norwegian Women and Cancer (NOWAC) study[39] in Norway, or a Canadian population-based case-control study.[30] A significant lower risk of CRC was observed in Finnish professional fishermen and their wives, who consume large amounts of fish, but that might have been due to their high physical activity during fishing.[40] Although no association was observed between total fish intake and the risk of CRC in the SWHS in China, higher consumption of eel (P trend = 0.01) and shellfish (P trend = 0.04) were found to increase the risk of CRC.[24] High levels of arachidonic acid, a ω-6 PUFA, also were associated with a higher risk of CRC (RR 1.39; 95% CI, 0.97–1.99; P trend = 0.03).[41]

Encouragingly, 1 meta-analysis that pooled 27 prospective cohort studies observed a moderate but significant reduction in the risk of CRC (RR 0.93; 95% CI, 0.87–0.99; P trend <0.01),[31] and the association was stronger for rectal cancer (RR 0.85; 95% CI, 0.75–0.95) than for colon cancer (RR 0.95; 95% CI, 0.91–0.98). Another meta-analysis that pooled 22 prospective cohorts and 19 case-control studies observed a 12% decrease in the risk of CRC with the highest fish intake (OR 0.88; 95% CI, 0.80–0.95).[32] Both analyses, however, found significant ($P<0.001$) heterogeneity among the included studies, suggesting the contribution of other confounding factors and possible nonresponsiveness to fish consumption. Collectively, understanding the mechanisms of how PUFAs might benefit human health could explain the nonresponsiveness in some studies. Fish oil, which is rich in EPA and DHA, was reported to improve cancer patients' quality of life,[42] suggesting that it might be a useful dietary supplement for CRC patients on standard therapies. Characteristics of studies of fish intake and CRC risk are shown in **Table 2**.

Fibers from All Sources

In 1969, Burkitt[43] proposed that high fiber consumption might reduce the risk of CRC after observing that African blacks who consumed a high-fiber/low-fat diet had a lower incidence of colon cancer and mortality than their white counterparts who ate a low-fiber/high-fat diet. Fiber includes heterogeneous plant material composed of cellulose, hemicellulose, and pectin.[10] Its potential protective effects include reducing fecal transit time, diluting fecal carcinogens, affecting bile acid metabolism, maintaining colonic epithelial cell integrity, absorbing heterocyclic amines, and stimulating bacterial anaerobic fermentation to promote the production of short-chain fatty acids (SCFAs).[10,16] SCFAs, such as acetate, propionate, and butyrate, have been shown to decrease colonic pH[44,45] and inhibit colon carcinogenesis.[46–50]

Pooling multiple studies (1 meta-analysis of 13 case-control studies,[51] 1 analysis of 25 prospective studies,[52] and 1 analysis of 16 case-control and 4 cohort studies[53]) uncovered significant inverse associations between dietary fiber intake and risk of CRC, but

Table 2
Characteristics of studies of fish and colorectal cancer

Study	Number of Study Participants	Ages of Participants	Follow-up Years	Colorectal Cancer Incidence	Analytical category	Analytical Comparison, High vs Low Intake	Relative Risk (95% CI)	Reference
EPIC	47,8040 men and women	35–70	1992–2002	855 (colon), 474 (rectum)	Fish	≥80 g/d vs <10 g/d	CRC: 0.69 (0.54–0.88), P<.001	Norat et al,[22] 2005
PHS	21,406 men and women	40–84	1982–1995	500 (CRC)	Fish	≥5 times/wk vs <1 time/wk	CRC: 0.63 (0.42–0.95), P = .02	Hall et al,[33] 2008
Finnish fishermen cohort	6410 men and 4260 women	—	1980–2011	79 (colon), 68 (rectum)	Fish	—	Men—colon cancer: 0.72 (0.52–0.98)	Turunen et al,[40] 2014
SWHS	73,242 women	40–70	1997–2005	396 (CRC)	Arachidonic acid	≥0.09 g/d vs <0.02 g/d	CRC: 1.39 (0.97–1.99), P = .03	Murff et al,[41] 2009
SWHS	73,224 women	40–70	1997–2005	236 (colon), 158 (rectum)	Eel / Shellfish	≥0.35 g/d vs 0 / ≥0.6 g/d vs 0	CRC: 1.3 (0.9–1.7), P = .01 / CRC: 1.3 (1.0–1.6), P = .04	Lee etal,[24] 2009
22 prospective cohort and 19 case-control studies	—	—	—	—	Fish	—	CRC: 0.88 (0.80–0.95)	Wu et al,[32] 2012
27 prospective cohort studies	2,325,040 men and women	—	—	—	Fish	—	CRC: 0.93 (0.87–0.99) Colon cancer: 0.95 (0.91–0.98) Rectal cancer: 0.85 (0.75–0.95)	Yu et al,[31] 2014

Study	Population	Age	Years	Cases	Exposure	Comparison	Results	Reference
HPFS and NHS	47,143 men and 76,386 women	40–75/30–55	1986–2010/1980–2010	1,773B (colon), 525 (rectum), 158 (unspecific)	Fish	Men: ≥46 g/d vs <16 g/d; Women: ≥40 g/d vs <15 g/d	Nonsignificant associations	Song et al,[34] 2014
					Marine ω-3	≥0.3 g/d vs <0.15 g/d	Women—distal colon cancer: 1.36 (1.03–1.80), P = .04	
NIH-AARP DHS	293,466 men and 198,720 women	50–71	1995–2003	5095 (colon), 1884 (rectum)	Fish	≥21.4 g/100 kcal vs <3.6 g/1000 kcal	Nonsignificant associations	Daniel et al,[35] 2011
ATBC	27,111 men (all smokers)	50–69	1985–1993	185 (CRC)	Fish	≥68 g/d vs <13 g/d	Nonsignificant associations	Pietinen et al,[26] 1999
JACC	45,181 men and 62,643 women	40–79	1988–1997	284 (colon), 173 (rectum)	Fish	Everyday vs <2 d/wk	Nonsignificant associations	Kojima et al,[36] 2004
Ohsaki Cohort Study	18,858 men and 20,640 women	40–79	1995–2003	566 (CRC)	Fish	Men: ≥96.4 g/d vs <26.2 g/d; Women: ≥81.4 g/d vs <26.6 g/d	Nonsignificant associations	Sugawara et al,[37] 2009
SMC	61,433 women	40–75	1987–2003	389 (colon), 230 (rectum)	Fish	≥2 servings/wk vs <0.5 servings/wk	Nonsignificant associations	Larsson et al,[28] 2005
Oxford Vegetarian Study	4162 men and 6836 women	16–89	1980–1999	95 (CRC)	Fish	>1 time/wk vs never	Nonsignificant associations	Sanjoaquin et al,[38] 2004
NOWAC	63,914 women	40–70	1996–2004	254 (CRC)	Fish	>53.4 g/d vs <29.1 g/d	Nonsignificant associations	Engeset et al,[39] 2007
Case-control	—	20–76	—	1727 (colon), 1447 (rectum), 5039 (control)	Fish	—	Nonsignificant associations	Hu et al,[30] 2008

this association was not seen in the Pooling Project of Prospective Studies of Diet and Cancer.[54] In addition, some individual large prospective studies, including the EPIC study (RR 0.83; 95% CI, 0.72–0.96; P trend = 0.013)[55,56] and the PLCO study (for distal colon cancer: HR 0.62; 95% CI, 0.41–0.94; P trend = 0.03),[57] observed significant inverse associations, which were not seen in others, such as the NHS, the HPFS,[58] and the Women's Health Study (WHS).[59] Even in the same populations, different studies showed discrepant results. For example, a case-control study in China[60] observed a significant inverse association between total dietary fiber and the risk of CRC (OR 0.38; 95% CI, 0.27–0.55; P trend <0.01), whereas the prospective SWHS in China[61] showed no significant results. Similarly, the JACC in Japan[62] reported a significant decreasing trend of dietary fiber intake with the risk of colon cancer (RR 0.73; 95% CI, 0.51–1.03; P trend = 0.028), whereas the JPHC study in Japan[63] showed no association. Methodological differences might be one reason. For example, 1 case-control study within 7 UK cohort studies reported a significant inverse association when food diaries but not FFQs[64] were used. Food diaries may provide more details of dietary intake, whereas FFQs provide only a short list (100–200 items) that combines several sources into 1 category. Food diaries, however, may introduce greater bias and measurement error into a study. Therefore, confounding factors and limitations in study design need to be considered when interpreting results from either individual studies or pooled meta-analyses.

Fiber from Whole Grains and Cereals

Whole grains and cereals are major sources of dietary fiber, and accumulating evidence suggests that high fiber intake from whole grains and cereals associates with a lower risk of CRC. This association was seen in the EPIC study (cereals: RR 0.87; 95% CI, 0.77–0.99; P trend = 0.003),[55] the NIH-AARP DHS (grain: RR 0.51; 95% CI, 0.29–0.89; P trend = 0.01),[65] and the Scandinavian HELGA study (whole-grain wheat: IRR 0.65; 95% CI, 0.50–0.84).[66,67] The HELGA study included 3 prospective cohorts: the NOWAC study, the Northern Sweden Health and Disease Study (NSHDS), and the DCH study. In Scandinavia, whole-grain food consumption is high. No consistent associations were observed, however, within individual studies.[68,69] One analysis that used plasma alkylresorcinol concentration (a biomarker of whole-grain wheat and rye intake) alone or combined with FFQ showed inverse associations with distal colon cancer, but using only an FFQ was not powerful enough.[70] Accordingly, these studies suggest a decreasing trend between high intake of fiber from whole grains and cereals with the risk of CRC. Characteristics of studies of fiber intake and CRC risk are shown in **Table 3**.

Fruit and Vegetables

Fruit and vegetables, which are rich in polyphenol compounds, flavonoids, soluble fiber, vitamins, and minerals, have been highly recommended for CRC prevention, although the results of epidemiologic studies are weak, possibly because of the variability within the category "fruit and vegetables."[10,11,15,16,36] The WCRF/AICR listed fruit and vegetables as "suggestive" factors for decreasing CRC risk.[4]

The EPIC study observed a lower risk of CRC with higher consumption of fruit and vegetables combined (HR 0.86; 95% CI, 0.75–1.00; P trend = 0.04).[55,71] Further analysis found that this association was dependent on smoking status: the association was inverse in never and former smokers, whereas it became positive in current smokers.[71] When dietary consumption was converted into flavonoid intake, however, no association was observed.[72]

The NHS and HPFS also examined flavonoid intake and found no significant association with CRC.[73] In another US study, the NIH-AARP DHS, which used servings per 1000 kcal per day for analysis, observed a significantly reduced risk of CRC for the

Table 3
Characteristics of studies of fiber and colorectal cancer

Study	Number of Study Participants	Ages of Participants	Follow-up Years	Colorectal Cancer Incidence	Analytical Category	Analytical Comparison, High vs Low Intake	Relative Risk (95% CI)	Reference
13 case-control studies	—	—	—	5225 (CRC), 10,349 (control)	Total fiber	>31.2 g/d vs <10.1 g/d	CRC: 0.53 (0.47–0.61), P<.0001	Howe et al,[51] 1992
16 case-control and 4 cohort studies	10,948 men and women	—	—	—	Total fiber	Per 100-g increase	CRC: 0.72 (0.63–0.83)	Ben et al,[53] 2014
25 prospective studies	—	—	—	—	Total fiber	—	CRC: 0.90 (0.86–0.94)	Aune et al,[52] 2011
EPIC	142,250 men and 335,062 women	35–70	1992–2002	2869 (colon), 1266 (rectum)	Total fiber Cereal fiber	≥28.5 g/d vs <16.4 g/d ≥12.3 g/d vs <4.64 g/d	CRC: 0.83 (0.72–0.96), P = .013 CRC: 0.87 (0.77–0.99), P = .003	Murphy et al,[56] 2012
EPIC	131,985 men and 320,770 women	35–70	1992–2002	2,819 (CRC)	Total fiber	—	CRC: 0.86 (0.75–1.00), P = .04	Bradbury et al,[55] 2014
PLCO	57,774 men and women	55–74	1993–2001	733 (CRC)	Total fiber	≥12.8 g/1000 kcal vs <9.9 g/1000 kcal	Distal colon cancer: 0.62 (0.41, 0.94), P = .03	Kunzmann et al,[57] 2015
Case-control	—	30–75	—	341 (colon), 265 (rectum), 613 (control)	Total fiber	Men: >14.92 g/d vs <7.73 g/d Women: >12.65 g/d vs <6.52 g/d	CRC: 0.38 (0.27–0.55), P<.01	Zhong et al,[60] 2014
JACC	16,636 men and 26,479 women	40–79	1988–1997	291 (colon), 142 (rectum)	Total fiber	—	CRC: 0.73 (0.51–1.03), P = .028	Wakai et al,[62] 2007

(continued on next page)

Table 3
(continued)

Study	Number of Study Participants	Ages of Participants	Follow-up Years	Colorectal Cancer Incidence	Analytical Category	Analytical Comparison, High vs Low Intake	Relative Risk (95% CI)	Reference
NIH-AARP DHS	291,988 men and 197,623 women	50–71	1995–2000	2974 (CRC)	Fiber from grains	>5.7 g/1000 kcal vs <1.7 g/1000 kcal	CRC: 0.86 (0.76–0.98), $P = .01$	Schatzkin et al,[65] 2007
HELGA	38,841 men and 69,159 women	40–65	1991–2002	680 (colon), 399 (rectum)	Whole-grain wheat	Men: >9 g/d vs ≤1 g/d; Women: >36 g/d vs <3 g/d	CRC: 0.65 (0.50–0.84)	Kyro et al,[66] 2013
13 prospective cohort studies	725,628 men and women	—	6–20 y	—	Total fiber	>30 g/d vs <10 g/d	Nonsignificant associations	Park et al,[54] 2005
HPFS and NHS	47,279 men and 76,947 women	40–75/30–55	1986–2010/ 1980–2010	1202 (colon), 310 (rectum)	Total fiber	>14 g/1000 kcal vs <8 g/1000 kcal	Nonsignificant associations	Michels et al,[58] 2005
WHS	36,976 women	45+	1993–2003	223 (CRC)	Total fiber	≥23.1 g/d vs <12.5 g/d	Nonsignificant associations	Lin et al,[59] 2005
SWHS	73,314 women	40–70	1997–2005	283 (CRC)	Total fiber	>13.45 g/d vs <7.3 g/d	Nonsignificant associations	Shin et al,[61] 2006
JPHC	65,803 men and 67,520 women	45–74	1995–2006	742 (colon) and 375 (rectum)	Total fiber	Men: >18.7 g/d vs <6.4 g/d; Women: >20 g/d vs <8.3 g/d	Nonsignificant associations	Otani et al,[63] 2006
DCH	26,630 men and 29,189 women	50–64	1993–2009	461 (colon), 283 (rectum)	Total whole grain	>160 g/dat vs ≤75 g/d	Nonsignificant associations	Egeberg et al,[68] 2010
NOWAC	78,254 women	40–70	1996–2006	509 (colon), 218 (rectum)	Whole-grain bread	180–240 g/d vs 0	Nonsignificant associations	Bakken et al,[69] 2016

highest intake of vegetables among men (RR 0.82; 95% CI, 0.71–0.94; P trend = 0.03), mainly from distal colon cancer (RR 0.76; 95% CI, 0.59–0.98; P trend = 0.04).A significantly increased risk of rectal cancer for the highest intake of fruit among women was also observed (RR 1.59; 95% CI, 1.04–2.44; P trend = 0.01). When subtypes of vegetables were considered, green leafy vegetables were associated with a lower risk of CRC among men (RR 0.86; 95% CI, 0.74–0.99; P trend = 0.04).[74]

Although some regional studies have reported nonsignificant results, including the Netherlands Cohort Study–Meat Investigation Cohort (NLCS-MIC),[75,76] the Western Australian Bowel Health Study,[77] and a meta-analysis in a Japanese population,[78] pooled studies resulted in a weak decreasing trend between higher consumption of fruit and vegetables and the risk of CRC.[79,80] Promisingly, a meta-analysis that focused only on cruciferous vegetables and included 24 case-control and 11 prospective studies found a significantly inverse association (RR 0.82; 95% CI, 0.75–0.90) between cruciferous vegetables intake and the risk of CRC.[81]

Some studies have classified subjects as vegetarians (including vegan, lacto-ovo vegetarian, pescatarian, and semivegetarian) and nonvegetarians. The Adventist Health Study 2 observed an overall lower risk of CRC among vegetarians than in nonvegetarians (HR 0.78; 95% CI, 0.64–0.95; P trend = 0.01), in particular pesco-vegetarians (HR 0.57; 95% CI, 0.40–0.82; P trend = 0.002).[82] After combining 6 cohort studies, a meta-analysis found that the association between a vegetarian diet and the risk of CRC was not significant.[83] Semivegetarians and pesco-vegetarians, however, showed a lower risk of CRC.[83] This potential protection observed in pesco-vegetarians might be due to the beneficial effects of fish consumption. The EPIC-Oxford study reported an opposite trend: a higher incidence in vegetarians than in nonvegetarians (IR 1.49; 95% CI, 1.09–2.03) or meat eaters (IRR 1.39; 95% CI, 1.01–1.91).[84]

Accordingly, higher consumption of fruit and vegetables might have the potential to decrease the risk of CRC. More research is needed, however, to explain the heterogeneity among studies. Many factors easily influence the outcomes of analyses, such as the way food intake is measured, analytical method, and other confounding factors. It is also highly debatable whether an analysis should accept "fruit and vegetables" as a category or delineate it into subtypes. Characteristics of studies of intake of fruit and vegetables and CRC risk are shown in **Table 4**.

Vitamins and Minerals

Vitamins and minerals are important micronutrients that support bodies and benefit health. The relationship between their intake and disease, however, is far from clear. A Canadian study observed overall beneficial effects of multiple vitamins (OR 0.7; 95% CI, 0.4–1.3; P trend = 0.03), B-complex vitamins (OR 0.4; 95% CI, 0.2–0.7; P trend = 0.0005), vitamin E (OR 0.6; 95% CI, 0.4–0.9; P trend = 0.002), calcium (OR 0.4; 95% CI, 0.3–0.6; P trend <0.0001), iron (OR 0.6; 95% CI, 0.4–1.0; P trend = 0.03), and zinc (OR 0.4; 95% CI, 0.2–0.9; P trend = 0.03) against distal colon cancer among women taking these nutrients as supplements.[85]

It could be argued, however, that more is not always better[86] and that a balanced combination with the right doses would maximize the beneficial effects. For example, the MCC study obtained interesting results after analyzing the risk of CRC with dietary intake of B vitamins, finding a U-shaped association between vitamin B_6 and colon cancer and an inverse U-shaped association between vitamin B_{12} and rectal cancer.[87] Vitamin B_6 was also found to significantly increase the risk of rectal cancer among Dutch women (RR 3.57; 95% CI, 1.56–8.17; P trend = 0.01).[88] Folate, however, a form of vitamin B, was shown associated with a lower risk of CRC in the DCH study (IRR 0.83; 95% CI, 0.57–1.21; P trend = 0.04).[89] This association

Table 4
Characteristics of studies of fruit and vegetables and colorectal cancer

Study	Number of Study Participants	Ages of Participants	Follow-up Years	Colorectal Cancer Incidence	Analytical Category	Analytical Comparison, High vs Low Intake	Relative Risk (95% CI)	Reference
EPIC	131,985 men and 320,770 women	35–70	1992–2006	2, 819 (CRC)	Fruit and vegetables	>603.6 g/d vs <221.1 g/d	CRC: 0.86 (0.75–1.00), P = .04	Bradbury et al,[55] 2014; van Duijnhoven et al,[71] 2009
NIH-AARP DHS	291,094 men and 196,949 women	50–71	1995–2000	2972 (CRC)	Vegetables	Men: >2.8 servings/1000 kcal vs <0.6 servings/1000 kcal	Men—CRC: 0.82 (0.71–0.94), P = .03 Men—distal colon cancer: 0.76 (0.59–0.98), P = .04	Park et al,[74] 2007
			—		Fruit	Women: >3.5 servings/1000 kcal vs <0.6 servings/1000 kcal	Women—rectal cancer: 1.59 (1.04–2.44), P = .01	
			—		Green leafy vegetables	—	Men—CRC: 0.86 (0.74–0.99), P = .04	
19 prospective studies	—	—	—	—	Fruit and vegetables	—	CRC: 0.92 (0.86–0.99)	Aune et al,[79] 2011
24 case-control and 11 prospective studies	1,295,063 men and women	—	1978–2012	24,275 (CRC)	Cruciferous vegetable	—	CRC: 0.82 (0.75–0.90)	Wu et al,[81] 2013
EPIC	477,312 men and women	35–70	1992–2006	2869 (colon), 1648 (rectum)	Total flavonoids and flavonoid	—	Nonsignificant associations	Zamora-Ros et al,[72] 2017

Study	Population	Age	Years	Cases	Exposure	Comparison	Result	Reference
HPFS and NHS	42,478 men and 76,364 women	40–75/ 30–55	1986–2010/ 1980–2010	2519 (CRC)	Flavonoid	—	Nonsignificant associations	Nimptsch et al,[73] 2016
NLCS-MIC	58,279 men and 62,573 women	55–69	1986–2000	1678 (colon), 572 (rectum)	Total flavonol and flavone	—	Nonsignificant associations	Simons et al,[75] 2009
Case-control	—	40–79	—	834 (CRC), 939 (control)	Fruit and vegetables	>10.82 servings/day vs <5.77 servings/day	Nonsignificant associations	Annema et al,[77] 2011
6 cohorts and 11 case-control	—	—	—	—	Fruit and vegetables	—	Nonsignificant associations	Kashino et al,[78] 2015
14 cohort studies	756,217 men and women	—	6–20 y	5383 (colon)	Fruit and vegetables	—	Nonsignificant associations	Koushik et al,[80] 2007
6 cohorts	686,629 men and women	—	—	4062 (CRC)	Semi-vegetarian diet	Versus nonvegetarian diet	CRC: 0.86 (0.79–0.94)	Godos et al,[83] 2017
					Pesco-vegetarian diet	Versus nonvegetarian diet	CRC: 0.67 (0.53–0.83)	
AHS II	77,659 men and women	—	2002–2009	380 (colon), 110 (rectum)	Vegetarian diet	Versus non-vegetarian diet	CRC: 0.78 (0.64–0.95), P = .01	Orlich et al,[82] 2015
					Pesco-vegetarian diet	Versus nonvegetarian diet	CRC: 0.57 (0.40–0.82), P = .002	
EPIC-Oxford	12,230 men and 40,476 women	20–89	1993–2005	290 (CRC)	Vegetarian	Versus nonvegetarian	CRC: 1.49 (1.09–2.03)	Key et al,[84] 2009
					Vegetarian or vegan	Versus meat eater	CRC: 1.39 (1.01–1.91)	

Table 5
Characteristics of studies of vitamins and minerals and colorectal cancer

Study	Number of Study Participants	Ages of Participants	Follow-up Years	Colorectal Cancer Incidence	Analytical Category	Analytical Comparison, High vs Low Intake	Relative Risk (95% CI)	Reference
Case-control	—	—	—	1723 (colon), 3097 (control)	Multiple vitamins	>5 y vs nerver or <1 y	Women—colon cancer: 0.7 (0.4–1.3), P = .03	Hu et al,[85] 2007
					B-complex vitamins		Women—colon cancer: 0.4 (0.2–0.7), P = .0005	
					Vitamin E		Women—colon cancer: 0.6 (0.4–0.9), P = .002	
					Calcium		Women—colon cancer: 0.4 (0.3–0.6), P<.0001	
					Iron		Women—colon cancer: 0.6 (0.4–1.0), P = .03	
					Zinc		Women—colon cancer: 0.4 (0.2–0.9), P = .03	
Case-control	—	—	—	2349 (CRC), 4168 (control)	Vitamin B6	>5 mg/d vs <1 mg/d	Women—rectal cancer: 3.57 (1.56–8.17), P = .01	de Vogel et al,[88] 2008
DCH	56,332 men and women	50–64	1993–2009	465 (colon), 283 (rectum)	Dietary folate	—	CRC: 0.83 (0.57–1.21), P = .04	Roswall et al,[89] 2010
					Supplemental folate	—	CRC: 0.83 (0.58–1.20), P = .76	

was significant only when the vitamin was obtained from the diet but not from supplements.[89]

Several studies have suggested that magnesium seems to associate with a lower risk of CRC.[90–93] Calcium was shown to reduce the risk of CRC in some studies,[94,95] but it did not correlate with vitamin D.[94,96] Characteristics of studies of intake of vitamins and minerals and CRC risk are shown in **Table 5**.

Coffee and Tea

Although coffee and tea are popular worldwide, only a few studies have investigated their effects on the risk of CRC. One meta-analysis of 41 prospective studies[97] and another of 87 databases[98] found no significant associations between tea consumption and the risk of CRC. Several other regional studies also reported nonsignificant results.[99–102] The SWHS showed a dose-response relationship between green tea consumption and a lower risk of CRC,[103] whereas the Singapore Chinese Health Study observed an increased risk of CRC among male green tea drinkers.[104] The subjects in these 2 studies are generally considered the same (Chinese), which may suggest a gender difference in response to green tea. In addition, other confounding factors also affect the results. For example, the NIH-AARP DHS found an inverse association between the risk of proximal colon cancer with both caffeinated coffee and decaffeinated coffee, but the subjects who drank decaffeinated coffee happened to consume less alcohol, fewer calories, less red meat, and more fruit and vegetables. They also, however, exercised less and smoked more.[102]

SUMMARY/DISCUSSION

Does cancer occur because of genes, environmental factors, or merely bad luck?[105] A surprisingly high correlation ($r = 0.80$) was observed between normal stem cell divisions and cancer incidence in an analysis of 17 different cancer types in 69 countries, representing 4.8 billion people.[106] For colon cancer, 26.1% of the driver gene mutations were induced by the environment, only 2.5% were heredity, and the remaining 71.4% were attributable to random mistakes during normal DNA replication.[106] Although it could be argued that this was only a statistical analysis and that the model might be too ideal, this randomness might explain the heterogeneity and inconsistency among studies or even individuals.

This review focuses mainly on large prospective studies and meta-analyses. The literature research supports the WCRF/AICR's recommendations,[4,7] although some variants exist, especially regarding dietary fiber, a complex substance that is difficult to define. This review is also limited because the WCRF/AICR's cancer reports include many more studies. In addition, all studies are subject to design bias and measurement errors to a certain degree. Therefore, results from different studies should be carefully interpreted and compared.

REFERENCES

1. Cancer key facts. Available at: http://www.who.int/mediacentre/factsheets/fs297/en/. Accessed April 6, 2017.
2. Stewart BW, WC. World cancer report 2014. Available at: http://publications.iarc.fr/Non-Series-Publications/World-Cancer-Reports/World-Cancer-Report-2014. Accessed April 6, 2017.
3. World Cancer Research Fund International. Available at: http://www.wcrf.org/int/cancer-facts-figures/data-specific-cancers/colorectal-cancer-statistics. Accessed April 10, 2017.

4. World Cancer Research Fund/American Institute for Cancer Research. Continuous update project report. Food, nutrition, physical activity, and the prevention of colorectal cancer. Available at: http://www.aicr.org/continuous-update-project/reports/Colorectal-Cancer-2011-Report.pdf. Accessed April 10, 2017.

5. Bouvard V, Loomis D, Guyton KZ, et al. Carcinogenicity of consumption of red and processed meat. Lancet Oncol 2015;16(16):1599–600. Available at: http://www.sciencedirect.com/science/article/pii/S1470204515004441.

6. Aune D, Chan DS, Vieira AR, et al. Red and processed meat intake and risk of colorectal adenomas: a systematic review and meta-analysis of epidemiological studies. Cancer Causes Control 2013;24(4):611–27. Available at: https://link.springer.com/article/10.1007%2Fs10552-012-0139-z.

7. World Cancer Research Fund/American Institute for Cancer Research expert report. Food, nutrition, physical activity, and the prevention of cancer: a global perspective. Washington, DC: AICR; 2007. Available at: http://www.aicr.org/assets/docs/pdf/reports/Second_Expert_Report.pdf.

8. Alexander DD, Cushing CA. Red meat and colorectal cancer: a critical summary of prospective epidemiologic studies. Obes Rev 2011;12(5):e472–93. Available at: http://onlinelibrary.wiley.com/doi/10.1111/j.1467-789X.2010.00785.x/abstract;jsessionid=4F22BBBF93D401171846C42EDA076846.f03t01.

9. McAfee AJ, McSorley EM, Cuskelly GJ, et al. Red meat consumption: an overview of the risks and benefits. Meat Sci 2010;84(1):1–13. Available at: http://www.sciencedirect.com/science/article/pii/S0309174009002514.

10. Pericleous M, Mandair D, Caplin ME. Diet and supplements and their impact on colorectal cancer. J Gastrointest Oncol 2013;4(4):409–23. Available at: http://jgo.amegroups.com/article/view/868/html.

11. Baena R, Salinas P. Diet and colorectal cancer. Maturitas 2015;80(3):258–64. Available at: http://www.sciencedirect.com/science/article/pii/S0378512214004071.

12. Boada LD, Henriquez-Hernandez LA, Luzardo OP. The impact of red and processed meat consumption on cancer and other health outcomes: epidemiological evidences. Food Chem Toxicol 2016;92:236–44. Available at: http://www.sciencedirect.com/science/article/pii/S0278691516301144.

13. Carr PR, Walter V, Brenner H, et al. Meat subtypes and their association with colorectal cancer: systematic review and meta-analysis. Int J Cancer 2016; 138(2):293–302. Available at: http://onlinelibrary.wiley.com/doi/10.1002/ijc.29423/abstract.

14. Battaglia Richi E, Baumer B, Conrad B, et al. Health risks associated with meat consumption: a review of epidemiological studies. Int J Vitam Nutr Res 2015; 85(1–2):70–8. Available at: http://econtent.hogrefe.com/doi/pdf/10.1024/0300-9831/a000224.

15. Marshall JR. Prevention of colorectal cancer: diet, chemoprevention, and lifestyle. Gastroenterol Clin North Am 2008;37(1):73–82, vi. Available at: http://www.sciencedirect.com/science/article/pii/S088985530700132X?via%3Dihub.

16. Mehta M, Shike M. Diet and physical activity in the prevention of colorectal cancer. J Natl Compr Canc Netw 2014;12(12):1721–6. Available at: https://www.ncbi.nlm.nih.gov/pubmed/25505213.

17. Di Maso M, Talamini R, Bosetti C, et al. Red meat and cancer risk in a network of case-control studies focusing on cooking practices. Ann Oncol 2013;24(12):3107–12. Available at: https://academic.oup.com/annonc/article-lookup/doi/10.1093/annonc/mdt392.

18. Cross AJ, Leitzmann MF, Gail MH, et al. A prospective study of red and pro-
    cessed meat intake in relation to cancer risk. PLoS Med 2007;4(12):e325. Avail-
    able at: http://journals.plos.org/plosmedicine/article?id=10.1371/journal.pmed.
    0040325.

19. Cross AJ, Ferrucci LM, Risch A, et al. A large prospective study of meat con-
    sumption and colorectal cancer risk: an investigation of potential mechanisms
    underlying this association. Cancer Res 2010;70(6):2406–14. Available at:
    http://cancerres.aacrjournals.org/content/70/6/2406.long.

20. Ferrucci LM, Sinha R, Huang WY, et al. Meat consumption and the risk of inci-
    dent distal colon and rectal adenoma. Br J Cancer 2012;106(3):608–16. Avail-
    able at: https://www.nature.com/bjc/journal/v106/n3/full/bjc2011549a.html.

21. Bernstein AM, Song M, Zhang X, et al. Processed and unprocessed red meat
    and risk of colorectal cancer: analysis by tumor location and modification
    by time. PLoS One 2015;10(8):e0135959. Available at: http://journals.plos.org/
    plosone/article?id=10.1371/journal.pone.0135959.

22. Norat T, Bingham S, Ferrari P, et al. Meat, fish, and colorectal cancer risk: the
    European Prospective Investigation into cancer and nutrition. J Natl Cancer
    Inst 2005;97(12):906–16. Available at: https://academic.oup.com/jnci/article-
    lookup/doi/10.1093/jnci/dji164.

23. Takachi R, Tsubono Y, Baba K, et al. Red meat intake may increase the risk of
    colon cancer in Japanese, a population with relatively low red meat consump-
    tion. Asia Pac J Clin Nutr 2011;20(4):603–12. Available at: http://apjcn.nhri.
    org.tw/server/APJCN/20/4/603.pdf.

24. Lee SA, Shu XO, Yang G, et al. Animal origin foods and colorectal cancer risk: a
    report from the Shanghai Women's Health Study. Nutr Cancer 2009;61(2):
    194–205. Available at: https://www.ncbi.nlm.nih.gov/pmc/articles/PMC2810117/.

25. Egeberg R, Olsen A, Christensen J, et al. Associations between red meat and
    risks for colon and rectal cancer depend on the type of red meat consumed.
    J Nutr 2013;143(4):464–72. Available at: http://jn.nutrition.org/content/143/4/
    464.long.

26. Pietinen P, Malila N, Virtanen M, et al. Diet and risk of colorectal cancer
    in a cohort of Finnish men. Cancer Causes Control 1999;10(5):387–96.
    Available at: https://www.ncbi.nlm.nih.gov/pubmed/?term=Diet+and+risk+
    of+colorectal+cancer+in+a+cohort+of+Finnish+men.

27. English DR, MacInnis RJ, Hodge AM, et al. Red meat, chicken, and fish con-
    sumption and risk of colorectal cancer. Cancer Epidemiol Biomarkers Prev
    2004;13(9):1509–14. Available at: http://cebp.aacrjournals.org/content/13/9/
    1509.long.

28. Larsson SC, Rafter J, Holmberg L, et al. Red meat consumption and risk of can-
    cers of the proximal colon, distal colon and rectum: the Swedish Mammography
    Cohort. Int J Cancer 2005;113(5):829–34. Available at: http://onlinelibrary.wiley.
    com/doi/10.1002/ijc.20658/abstract.

29. Hu J, La Vecchia C, Morrison H, et al. Salt, processed meat and the risk of can-
    cer. Eur J Cancer Prev 2011;20(2):132–9. Available at: https://insights.ovid.com/
    pubmed?pmid=21160428.

30. Hu J, La Vecchia C, DesMeules M, et al. Meat and fish consumption and
    cancer in Canada. Nutr Cancer 2008;60(3):313–24. Available at: http://web.
    a.ebscohost.com/ehost/pdfviewer/pdfviewer?vid=1&sid=b9689530-fb78-4262-
    a6e4-99df636013b3%40sessionmgr4007.

31. Yu XF, Zou J, Dong J. Fish consumption and risk of gastrointestinal cancers: a meta-analysis of cohort studies. World J Gastroenterol 2014;20(41):15398–412. Available at: http://www.wjgnet.com/1007-9327/full/v20/i41/15398.htm.

32. Wu S, Feng B, Li K, et al. Fish consumption and colorectal cancer risk in humans: a systematic review and meta-analysis. Am J Med 2012;125(6): 551–9.e5. Available at: http://www.sciencedirect.com/science/article/pii/S0002934312001234.

33. Hall MN, Chavarro JE, Lee IM, et al. A 22-year prospective study of fish, n-3 fatty acid intake, and colorectal cancer risk in men. Cancer Epidemiol Biomarkers Prev 2008;17(5):1136–43. Available at: http://cebp.aacrjournals.org/content/17/5/1136.long.

34. Song M, Chan AT, Fuchs CS, et al. Dietary intake of fish, omega-3 and omega-6 fatty acids and risk of colorectal cancer: a prospective study in U.S. men and women. Int J Cancer 2014;135(10):2413–23. Available at: http://onlinelibrary.wiley.com/doi/10.1002/ijc.28878/abstract;jsessionid=0E04BD9AE738468AF1-B9623E4B782D24.f04t03.

35. Daniel CR, Cross AJ, Graubard BI, et al. Prospective investigation of poultry and fish intake in relation to cancer risk. Cancer Prev Res (Phila) 2011;4(11): 1903–11. Available at: http://cancerpreventionresearch.aacrjournals.org/content/4/11/1903.long.

36. Kojima M, Wakai K, Tamakoshi K, et al. Diet and colorectal cancer mortality: results from the Japan Collaborative Cohort Study. Nutr Cancer 2004;50(1): 23–32. Available at: https://www.ncbi.nlm.nih.gov/pubmed/?term=10.1207%2Fs15327914nc5001_4.

37. Sugawara Y, Kuriyama S, Kakizaki M, et al. Fish consumption and the risk of colorectal cancer: the Ohsaki Cohort Study. Br J Cancer 2009;101(5):849–54. Available at: https://www.nature.com/bjc/journal/v101/n5/full/6605217a.html.

38. Sanjoaquin MA, Appleby PN, Thorogood M, et al. Nutrition, lifestyle and colorectal cancer incidence: a prospective investigation of 10998 vegetarians and non-vegetarians in the United Kingdom. Br J Cancer 2004;90(1):118–21. Available at: https://www.nature.com/bjc/journal/v90/n1/full/6601441a.html.

39. Engeset D, Andersen V, Hjartaker A, et al. Consumption of fish and risk of colon cancer in the Norwegian Women and Cancer (NOWAC) study. Br J Nutr 2007; 98(3):576–82. Available at: https://www.cambridge.org/core/journals/british-journal-of-nutrition/article/consumption-of-fish-and-risk-of-colon-cancer-in-the-norwegian-women-and-cancer-nowac-study/F3956020F8E6E4F81FC59564F3AB9041.

40. Turunen AW, Suominen AL, Kiviranta H, et al. Cancer incidence in a cohort with high fish consumption. Cancer Causes Control 2014;25(12):1595–602. Available at: https://link.springer.com/article/10.1007%2Fs10552-014-0464-5.

41. Murff HJ, Shu XO, Li H, et al. A prospective study of dietary polyunsaturated fatty acids and colorectal cancer risk in Chinese women. Cancer Epidemiol Biomarkers Prev 2009;18(8):2283–91. Available at: http://cebp.aacrjournals.org/content/18/8/2283.long.

42. Vaughan VC, Hassing MR, Lewandowski PA. Marine polyunsaturated fatty acids and cancer therapy. Br J Cancer 2013;108(3):486–92. Available at: https://www.nature.com/bjc/journal/v108/n3/full/bjc2012586a.html.

43. Burkitt DP. Related disease–related cause? Lancet 1969;2(7632):1229–31. Available at: http://www.sciencedirect.com/science/article/pii/S0140673669907570?via%3Dihub.

44. De Filippo C, Cavalieri D, Di Paola M, et al. Impact of diet in shaping gut microbiota revealed by a comparative study in children from Europe and rural Africa. Proc Natl Acad Sci U S A 2010;107(33):14691–6. Available at: http://www.pnas.org/content/107/33/14691.long.

45. Duncan SH, Louis P, Thomson JM, et al. The role of pH in determining the species composition of the human colonic microbiota. Environ Microbiol 2009;11(8): 2112–22. Available at: http://onlinelibrary.wiley.com/doi/10.1111/j.1462-2920. 2009.01931.x/abstract;jsessionid=8D2C212C7348C08B18BAA234C74B27F7. f03t03.

46. Pan P, W Skaer C, Wang HT, et al. Loss of free fatty acid receptor 2 enhances colonic adenoma development and reduces the chemopreventive effects of black raspberries in ApcMin/+ mice. Carcinogenesis 2017;38(1):86–93. Available at: https://academic.oup.com/carcin/article-lookup/doi/10.1093/carcin/bgw122.

47. Pan P, Skaer CW, Stirdivant SM, et al. Beneficial regulation of metabolic profiles by black raspberries in human colorectal cancer patients. Cancer Prev Res (Phila) 2015;8(8):743–50. Available at: http://cancerpreventionresearch.aacr-journals.org/content/8/8/743.long.

48. Pan P, Lam V, Salzman N, et al. Black raspberries and their anthocyanin and fiber fractions alter the composition and diversity of gut microbiota in F-344 rats. Nutr Cancer 2017;69:943–51. Available at: https://www.ncbi.nlm.nih.gov/pubmed/28718724.

49. Pan P, Skaer CW, Wang HT, et al. Black raspberries suppress colonic adenoma development in ApcMin/+ mice: relation to metabolite profiles. Carcinogenesis 2015;36(10):1245–53. Available at: https://academic.oup.com/carcin/article-lookup/doi/10.1093/carcin/bgv117.

50. Pan P, Skaer CW, Wang HT, et al. Systemic metabolite changes in wild-type C57BL/6 mice fed black raspberries. Nutr Cancer 2017;69(2):299–306. Available at: https://www.ncbi.nlm.nih.gov/pubmed/28094560.

51. Howe GR, Benito E, Castelleto R, et al. Dietary intake of fiber and decreased risk of cancers of the colon and rectum: evidence from the combined analysis of 13 case-control studies. J Natl Cancer Inst 1992;84(24):1887–96. Available at: https://www.ncbi.nlm.nih.gov/pubmed/?term=Dietary+intake+of+fiber+and+decreased+risk+of+cancers+of+the+colon+and+rectum+evidence+from+the+combined+analysis+of+13+case-control+studies.

52. Aune D, Chan DS, Lau R, et al. Dietary fibre, whole grains, and risk of colorectal cancer: systematic review and dose-response meta-analysis of prospective studies. BMJ 2011;343:d6617. Available at: http://www.bmj.com/content/343/bmj.d6617.long.

53. Ben Q, Sun Y, Chai R, et al. Dietary fiber intake reduces risk for colorectal adenoma: a meta- analysis. Gastroenterology 2014;146(3):689–99.e6. Available at: http://www.sciencedirect.com/science/article/pii/S0016508513015862?via%3Dihub.

54. Park Y, Hunter DJ, Spiegelman D, et al. Dietary fiber intake and risk of colorectal cancer: a pooled analysis of prospective cohort studies. JAMA 2005;294(22): 2849–57. Available at: http://jamanetwork.com/journals/jama/fullarticle/202011.

55. Bradbury KE, Appleby PN, Key TJ. Fruit, vegetable, and fiber intake in relation to cancer risk: findings from the European Prospective Investigation into Cancer and Nutrition (EPIC). Am J Clin Nutr 2014;100(Suppl 1):394S–8S. Available at: http://ajcn.nutrition.org/content/100/Supplement_1/394S.long.

56. Murphy N, Norat T, Ferrari P, et al. Dietary fibre intake and risks of cancers of the colon and rectum in the European prospective investigation into cancer and

nutrition (EPIC). PLoS One 2012;7(6):e39361. Available at: http://journals.plos. org/plosone/article?id=10.1371/journal.pone.0039361.

57. Kunzmann AT, Coleman HG, Huang WY, et al. Dietary fiber intake and risk of colorectal cancer and incident and recurrent adenoma in the Prostate, Lung, Colorectal, and Ovarian Cancer Screening Trial. Am J Clin Nutr 2015;102(4): 881–90. Available at: http://ajcn.nutrition.org/content/102/4/881.long.

58. Michels KB, Fuchs CS, Giovannucci E, et al. Fiber intake and incidence of colorectal cancer among 76,947 women and 47,279 men. Cancer Epidemiol Biomarkers Prev 2005;14(4):842–9. Available at: http://cebp.aacrjournals.org/content/14/4/842.long.

59. Lin J, Zhang SM, Cook NR, et al. Dietary intakes of fruit, vegetables, and fiber, and risk of colorectal cancer in a prospective cohort of women (United States). Cancer Causes Control 2005;16(3):225–33. Available at: https://link.springer.com/article/10.1007%2Fs10552-004-4025-1.

60. Zhong X, Fang YJ, Pan ZZ, et al. Dietary fiber and fiber fraction intakes and colorectal cancer risk in Chinese adults. Nutr Cancer 2014;66(3):351–61. Available at: http://web.b.ebscohost.com/ehost/pdfviewer/pdfviewer?vid=1&sid=d0c9c12a-798c-40fb-a5f0-fad3ade540a2%40sessionmgr104.

61. Shin A, Li H, Shu XO, et al. Dietary intake of calcium, fiber and other micronutrients in relation to colorectal cancer risk: results from the Shanghai Women's Health Study. Int J Cancer 2006;119(12):2938–42. Available at: http://onlinelibrary.wiley.com/doi/10.1002/ijc.22196/abstract.

62. Wakai K, Date C, Fukui M, et al. Dietary fiber and risk of colorectal cancer in the Japan collaborative cohort study. Cancer Epidemiol Biomarkers Prev 2007; 16(4):668–75. Available at: http://cebp.aacrjournals.org/content/16/4/668.long.

63. Otani T, Iwasaki M, Ishihara J, et al. Dietary fiber intake and subsequent risk of colorectal cancer: the Japan Public Health Center-based prospective study. Int J Cancer 2006;119(6):1475–80. Available at: http://onlinelibrary.wiley.com/doi/10.1002/ijc.22007/abstract;jsessionid=77AF8D12EFADE-D621251AE93EA8090AE.f04t03.

64. Dahm CC, Keogh RH, Spencer EA, et al. Dietary fiber and colorectal cancer risk: a nested case- control study using food diaries. J Natl Cancer Inst 2010; 102(9):614–26. Available at: https://academic.oup.com/jnci/article-lookup/doi/10.1093/jnci/djq092.

65. Schatzkin A, Mouw T, Park Y, et al. Dietary fiber and whole-grain consumption in relation to colorectal cancer in the NIH-AARP Diet and Health Study. Am J Clin Nutr 2007;85(5):1353–60. Available at: http://ajcn.nutrition.org/content/85/5/1353.long.

66. Kyro C, Skeie G, Loft S, et al. Intake of whole grains from different cereal and food sources and incidence of colorectal cancer in the Scandinavian HELGA cohort. Cancer Causes Control 2013;24(7):1363–74. Available at: https://link.springer.com/article/10.1007%2Fs10552-013-0215-z.

67. Hansen L, Skeie G, Landberg R, et al. Intake of dietary fiber, especially from cereal foods, is associated with lower incidence of colon cancer in the HELGA cohort. Int J Cancer 2012;131(2):469–78. Available at: http://onlinelibrary.wiley.com/doi/10.1002/ijc.26381/abstract.

68. Egeberg R, Olsen A, Loft S, et al. Intake of wholegrain products and risk of colorectal cancers in the Diet, Cancer and Health cohort study. Br J Cancer 2010; 103(5):730–4. Available at: https://www.nature.com/bjc/journal/v103/n5/full/6605806a.html.

69. Bakken T, Braaten T, Olsen A, et al. Consumption of whole-grain bread and risk of colorectal cancer among Norwegian women (the NOWAC Study). Nutrients 2016;8(1) [pii:E40]. Available at: http://www.mdpi.com/2072-6643/8/1/40.
70. Knudsen MD, Kyro C, Olsen A, et al. Self-reported whole-grain intake and plasma alkylresorcinol concentrations in combination in relation to the incidence of colorectal cancer. Am J Epidemiol 2014;179(10):1188–96. Available at: https://academic.oup.com/aje/article-lookup/doi/10.1093/aje/kwu031.
71. van Duijnhoven FJ, Bueno-De-Mesquita HB, Ferrari P, et al. Fruit, vegetables, and colorectal cancer risk: the European Prospective Investigation into Cancer and Nutrition. Am J Clin Nutr 2009;89(5):1441–52. Available at: http://ajcn.nutrition.org/content/89/5/1441.long.
72. Zamora-Ros R, Barupal DK, Rothwell JA, et al. Dietary flavonoid intake and colorectal cancer risk in the European prospective investigation into cancer and nutrition (EPIC) cohort. Int J Cancer 2017;140(8):1836–44. Available at: http://onlinelibrary.wiley.com/doi/10.1002/ijc.30582/abstract.
73. Nimptsch K, Zhang X, Cassidy A, et al. Habitual intake of flavonoid subclasses and risk of colorectal cancer in 2 large prospective cohorts. Am J Clin Nutr 2016;103(1):184–91. Available at: http://ajcn.nutrition.org/content/103/1/184.long.
74. Park Y, Subar AF, Kipnis V, et al. Fruit and vegetable intakes and risk of colorectal cancer in the NIH-AARP diet and health study. Am J Epidemiol 2007;166(2):170–80. Available at: https://academic.oup.com/aje/article-lookup/doi/10.1093/aje/kwm067.
75. Simons CC, Hughes LA, Arts IC, et al. Dietary flavonol, flavone and catechin intake and risk of colorectal cancer in the Netherlands Cohort Study. Int J Cancer 2009;125(12):2945–52. Available at: http://onlinelibrary.wiley.com/doi/10.1002/ijc.24645/abstract.
76. Gilsing AM, Schouten LJ, Goldbohm RA, et al. Vegetarianism, low meat consumption and the risk of colorectal cancer in a population based cohort study. Sci Rep 2015;5:13484. Available at: https://www.nature.com/articles/srep13484.
77. Annema N, Heyworth JS, McNaughton SA, et al. Fruit and vegetable consumption and the risk of proximal colon, distal colon, and rectal cancers in a case-control study in Western Australia. J Am Diet Assoc 2011;111(10):1479–90. Available at: http://www.sciencedirect.com/science/article/pii/S0002822311012156.
78. Kashino I, Mizoue T, Tanaka K, et al. Vegetable consumption and colorectal cancer risk: an evaluation based on a systematic review and meta-analysis among the Japanese population. Jpn J Clin Oncol 2015;45(10):973–9. Available at: https://academic.oup.com/jjco/article-lookup/doi/10.1093/jjco/hyv111.
79. Aune D, Lau R, Chan DS, et al. Nonlinear reduction in risk for colorectal cancer by fruit and vegetable intake based on meta-analysis of prospective studies. Gastroenterology 2011;141(1):106–18. Available at: http://www.sciencedirect.com/science/article/pii/S0016508511005221.
80. Koushik A, Hunter DJ, Spiegelman D, et al. Fruits, vegetables, and colon cancer risk in a pooled analysis of 14 cohort studies. J Natl Cancer Inst 2007;99(19):1471–83. Available at: https://academic.oup.com/jnci/article-lookup/doi/10.1093/jnci/djm155.
81. Wu QJ, Yang Y, Vogtmann E, et al. Cruciferous vegetables intake and the risk of colorectal cancer: a meta-analysis of observational studies. Ann Oncol 2013;24(4):1079–87. Available at: https://academic.oup.com/annonc/article-lookup/doi/10.1093/annonc/mds601.

82. Orlich MJ, Singh PN, Sabate J, et al. Vegetarian dietary patterns and the risk of colorectal cancers. JAMA Intern Med 2015;175(5):767–76. Available at: http://jamanetwork.com/journals/jamainternalmedicine/fullarticle/2174939.

83. Godos J, Bella F, Sciacca S, et al. Vegetarianism and breast, colorectal and prostate cancer risk: an overview and meta-analysis of cohort studies. J Hum Nutr Diet 2017;30(3):349–59. Available at: http://onlinelibrary.wiley.com/doi/10.1111/jhn.12426/abstract.

84. Key TJ, Appleby PN, Spencer EA, et al. Cancer incidence in vegetarians: results from the European Prospective Investigation into Cancer and Nutrition (EPIC-Oxford). Am J Clin Nutr 2009;89(5):1620S–6S. Available at: http://ajcn.nutrition.org/content/89/5/1620S.long.

85. Hu J, Morrison H, Mery L, et al. Diet and vitamin or mineral supplementation and risk of colon cancer by subsite in Canada. Eur J Cancer Prev 2007;16(4):275–91. Available at: https://insights.ovid.com/pubmed?pmid=17554200.

86. Guallar E, Stranges S, Mulrow C, et al. Enough is enough: stop wasting money on vitamin and mineral supplements. Ann Intern Med 2013;159(12):850–1. Available at: http://annals.org/aim/article/1789253/enough-enough-stop-wasting-money-vitamin-mineral-supplements.

87. Bassett JK, Severi G, Hodge AM, et al. Dietary intake of B vitamins and methionine and colorectal cancer risk. Nutr Cancer 2013;65(5):659–67. Available at: http://web.a.ebscohost.com/ehost/pdfviewer/pdfviewer?vid=1&sid=cdfeb64f-2153-4d7d-9fb5-b11879c93b6b%40sessionmgr4008.

88. de Vogel S, Dindore V, van Engeland M, et al. Dietary folate, methionine, riboflavin, and vitamin B-6 and risk of sporadic colorectal cancer. J Nutr 2008;138(12):2372–8. Available at: http://jn.nutrition.org/content/138/12/2372.long.

89. Roswall N, Olsen A, Christensen J, et al. Micronutrient intake and risk of colon and rectal cancer in a Danish cohort. Cancer Epidemiol 2010;34(1):40–6. Available at: http://www.sciencedirect.com/science/article/pii/S187778210900191X?via%3Dihub.

90. Gorczyca AM, He K, Xun P, et al. Association between magnesium intake and risk of colorectal cancer among postmenopausal women. Cancer Causes Control 2015;26(12):1761–9. Available at: https://link.springer.com/article/10.1007%2Fs10552-015-0669-2.

91. Ma E, Sasazuki S, Inoue M, et al. High dietary intake of magnesium may decrease risk of colorectal cancer in Japanese men. J Nutr 2010;140(4):779–85. Available at: http://jn.nutrition.org/content/140/4/779.long.

92. Chen GC, Pang Z, Liu QF. Magnesium intake and risk of colorectal cancer: a meta-analysis of prospective studies. Eur J Clin Nutr 2012;66(11):1182–6. Available at: https://www.nature.com/ejcn/journal/v66/n11/full/ejcn2012135a.html.

93. Qu X, Jin F, Hao Y, et al. Nonlinear association between magnesium intake and the risk of colorectal cancer. Eur J Gastroenterol Hepatol 2013;25(3):309–18. Available at: https://insights.ovid.com/pubmed?pmid=23222473.

94. Jenab M, Bueno-de-Mesquita HB, Ferrari P, et al. Association between pre-diagnostic circulating vitamin D concentration and risk of colorectal cancer in European populations: a nested case- control study. BMJ 2010;340:b5500. Available at: http://www.bmj.com/content/340/bmj.b5500.long.

95. Han C, Shin A, Lee J, et al. Dietary calcium intake and the risk of colorectal cancer: a case control study. BMC Cancer 2015;15:966. Available at: https://bmccancer.biomedcentral.com/articles/10.1186/s12885-015-1963-9.

96. Lipworth L, Bender TJ, Rossi M, et al. Dietary vitamin D intake and cancers of the colon and rectum: a case-control study in Italy. Nutr Cancer 2009;61(1):

70–5. Available at: http://web.b.ebscohost.com/ehost/pdfviewer/pdfviewer?
vid=1&sid=e72b0afe-89ef-4caa-abd1-6991deda2a1f%40sessionmgr102.

97. Yu F, Jin Z, Jiang H, et al. Tea consumption and the risk of five major cancers: a
dose-response meta-analysis of prospective studies. BMC Cancer 2014;14:
197. Available at: https://bmccancer.biomedcentral.com/articles/10.1186/1471-
2407-14-197.

98. Zhang YF, Xu Q, Lu J, et al. Tea consumption and the incidence of cancer: a
systematic review and meta-analysis of prospective observational studies. Eur
J Cancer Prev 2015;24(4):353–62. Available at: https://insights.ovid.com/
pubmed?pmid=25370683.

99. Budhathoki S, Iwasaki M, Yamaji T, et al. Coffee intake and the risk of colorectal adenoma: the colorectal adenoma study in Tokyo. Int J Cancer 2015;
137(2):463–70. Available at: http://onlinelibrary.wiley.com/doi/10.1002/ijc.
29390/abstract;jsessionid=C3E326FFE6B568001D12F7D791A779CC.f04t01.

100. Nakamura T, Ishikawa H, Mutoh M, et al. Coffee prevents proximal colorectal adenomas in Japanese men: a prospective cohort study. Eur J Cancer Prev 2016;
25(5):388–94. Available at: https://insights.ovid.com/pubmed?pmid=26291025.

101. Kyle JA, Sharp L, Little J, et al. Dietary flavonoid intake and colorectal cancer: a
case-control study. Br J Nutr 2010;103(3):429–36. Available at: https://www.
cambridge.org/core/journals/british-journal-of-nutrition/article/dietary-flavonoid-
intake-and-colorectal-cancer-a-casecontrol-study/3F10583E013C401B6AE0CD
790867A092.

102. Sinha R, Cross AJ, Daniel CR, et al. Caffeinated and decaffeinated coffee and
tea intakes and risk of colorectal cancer in a large prospective study. Am J
Clin Nutr 2012;96(2):374–81. Available at: http://ajcn.nutrition.org/content/96/2/
374.long.

103. Yang G, Shu XO, Li H, et al. Prospective cohort study of green tea consumption and
colorectal cancer risk in women. Cancer Epidemiol Biomarkers Prev 2007;16(6):
1219–23. Available at: http://cebp.aacrjournals.org/content/16/6/1219.long.

104. Sun CL, Yuan JM, Koh WP, et al. Green tea and black tea consumption in relation to colorectal cancer risk: the Singapore Chinese Health Study. Carcinogenesis 2007;28(10):2143–8. Available at: https://academic.oup.com/carcin/article-
lookup/doi/10.1093/carcin/bgm171.

105. Nowak MA, Waclaw B. Genes, environment, and "bad luck". Science 2017;
355(6331):1266–7. Available at: http://science.sciencemag.org/content/355/
6331/1266.long.

106. Tomasetti C, Li L, Vogelstein B. Stem cell divisions, somatic mutations, cancer
etiology, and cancer prevention. Science 2017;355(6331):1330–4. Available
at: http://science.sciencemag.org/content/355/6331/1330.long.

Colon Cancer
Inflammation-Associated Cancer

Sherief Shawki, MD[a], Jean Ashburn, MD[a], Steven A. Signs, PhD[b],
Emina Huang, MD[a,c],*

KEYWORDS

- Colitis-associated cancer • Colitis cancer surveillance
- Colitis-associated cancer management • 3D human models

KEY POINTS

- Colitis-associated cancer is a complex disease process for which the pathogenesis is unclear.
- Advanced colonoscopic techniques are the standard of care for surveillance of those patients with colitis. Unique pathology mandates close surveillance and multidisciplinary discussion.
- When proctocolectomy is deemed necessary, specialized considerations for restorative procedures and surveillance are required.
- Novel model systems for providing personalized medicine and for understanding pathogenesis include colonic organoids.

INTRODUCTION

Although colitis-associated cancer constitutes less than 2% of all colon cancers,[1] the challenges associated with this type of this cancer have implications that relate to many other cancers, including disease progression, lack of clarity regarding pathogenesis, and a broader context for all inflammation-associated cancers.

Disclosure Statement: E. Huang is supported by a grant from the National Institutes of Health (NIH; R01 CA142808; R01 CA157663 and U01 CA214300). E. Huang and S. Signs receive support via the Cleveland Clinic Research Project Committees Award #47. This project was supported in part by the National Center for Advancing Translational Sciences, UL1TR000439. The content is solely the responsibility of the authors and does not necessarily represent the official views of the NIH, E. Huang is also the recipient of a Velosano Pilot Award and the Metastatic Colon Cancer Research Center of Excellence Award (Cleveland Clinic Digestive Disease and Surgery Institute, Lerner Research Institute, Taussig Cancer Center).
^a Department of Colorectal Surgery, Cleveland Clinic, A30, 9500 Euclid Avenue, Cleveland, OH 44195, USA; ^b Department of Stem Cell Biology and Regenerative Medicine, Cleveland Clinic, Cleveland Clinic Lerner Research Institute, NE3, 9500 Euclid Avenue, Cleveland, OH 44195, USA; ^c Department of Stem Cell Biology and Regenerative Medicine, Cleveland Clinic, NE3, 9500 Euclid Avenue, Cleveland, OH 44195, USA
* Corresponding author. Cleveland Clinic, 9500 Euclid Avenue, A307, Cleveland, OH 44195.
E-mail address: huange2@ccf.org

Inflammatory bowel disease (IBD), including ulcerative colitis (UC) and Crohn's disease (CD), is associated with an increased risk for developing colorectal cancer (CRC). Historically, some investigators advocated prophylactic colectomy for patients with longstanding UC to reduce CRC-related mortality.[2] Although the exact magnitude remains unknown, patients with IBD are known to have an increased risk of developing colorectal neoplasia. This discrepancy in incidence is due to the wide variability in reported results as a result of variations in sources of information, such as data from low-volume versus high-volume centers, population-based data versus case reporting, and other small series.[3] In a large metaanalysis of 116 studies, the risk of cancer in patients with mucosal UC after disease duration of 10, 20, and 30 years was estimated to be 2%, 8%, and 18%, respectively. The reported prevalence of CRC in this analysis was 3.7%.[1] Another report of a 30-year surveillance program calculated the risk of neoplasia (both dysplasia and carcinoma) to be 7.7% at 20 years. This risk increased to 15.8% at 30 years of disease duration.[3] In another analysis of a 30-year colonoscopic surveillance program in patients with UC, the cumulative incidence of CRC was 2.5%, 7.6%, and 10.8% at 20, 30, and 40 years of disease, respectively.[4] Comparable findings have been demonstrated in CD and the reported incidence was 8% at 22 years.[5] Similarly, the cumulative risk of CRC in CD was reported as 0.3%, 1.6%, and 2.4% at 5, 15, and 25 years after diagnosis, respectively.[6]

CRC is one of the most devastating complications of IBD. It is associated with significant morbidity, and a mortality rate of up to 15%.[7,8] To reduce the risk of CRC in these patients, endoscopic surveillance guidelines have been developed to allow for the detection and potential removal of precancerous lesions. Such strategies aim to decrease the incidence of CRC in patients with IBD and improve mortality rates.[7,9]

With the availability of colonoscopy to evaluate the extent of the disease related to IBD and obtaining tissue biopsies, and realizing the risk factors associated with developing CRC in patients with IBD, efforts have been made to limit and/or prevent CRC-related mortality, while maximizing organ preservation. The increased risk for IBD-associated CRC prompted the practice of surveillance colonoscopy in these patients.[10] Despite the lack of prospective, controlled trials to evaluate the risk, benefit, and cost effectiveness of this surveillance approach, sufficient evidence is available to support the broad adoption of these strategies. Subsequent reports showed less risk of CRC, which could be attributed to either more timely surgical intervention, or perhaps greater use of chemopreventive agents such as aminosalicylates, or possibly more implementation of surveillance colonoscopy.[3,7,10]

EPIDEMIOLOGY
Risk Factors for Developing Carcinoma in Patients with Inflammatory Bowel Disease

There are some factors that had been associated with increased risk of developing CRC in patients with IBD, including age at the onset of disease, duration of the disease, the anatomic extent of disease, histologic changes versus macroscopic changes, backwash ileitis, primary sclerosing cholangitis, and family history.

Age at onset of disease
Early age at the onset of IBD disease has not been shown consistently to represent an independent risk factor for CRC. However, it reflects a longer duration of disease with associated colitis-related burden of increased risk of malignancy. The cumulative risk of CRC in patients with extensive UC has been estimated to be 40% in patients who had the disease before 15 years of age and 25% in patients who developed the disease between 15 and 39 years of age.[11,12]

Duration of disease

The relationship between disease duration and the risk of neoplasia is proportional. It has been demonstrated that the longer the duration of the disease, the greater risk of developing CRC that is significant after 8 years of disease. Although CRC can arise before 8 years of disease, it happens in small proportions of patients and is sufficiently infrequent to justify commencing surveillance earlier than 8 years.[13]

Anatomic extent of disease

The risk of CRC has been attributed to the extent of disease in both UC and CD. Based on the anatomic extent in UC, patients are classified into 3 categories: extensive, with inflammation proximal to the splenic flexure; left sided, in which presence of disease is located in the descending colon up to (but not proximal to) the splenic flexure; and proctosigmoiditis, where disease is limited to the rectum with or without sigmoid colon involvement.[12] In UC, the risk for CRC is greatest in patients with extensive disease, and intermediate in those with left-sided disease, whereas patients with proctosigmoiditis are at no or minimal risk of CRC.[3]

Histologic changes versus macroscopic changes

A proportional relationship exists between the degree of histologic inflammation and the risk of CRC. Indeed, CRC can arise in endoscopically normal mucosa that shows histologic evidence of disease on pathology. Additionally, carcinoma may also arise in regions where active colitis has remitted, that is, areas with no active inflammation but with histologic findings of inactive colitis in areas where the mucosa had never been inflamed, the risk of neoplasia is not increased and remains comparable with the non-IBD population.[3]

Therefore, histologic abnormalities are a more reliable determinant of disease status and risk for carcinoma than are macroscopic changes. Thus, the anatomic extent of the disease should be determined based on both endoscopic and histologic evaluation, whichever reveals more substantial evidence of involvement and could be done either at time of diagnosis or screening. For surveillance purposes, microscopic evaluation should be included in the assessment rather than endoscopic images alone. For example, a patient with macroscopic evidence of disease only in the rectosigmoid junction, but who has histologic evidence of active inflammation in the descending colon, should undergo surveillance according to left-sided extent of the disease. Furthermore, patients with CD who have more than one-third of their colon involved are at an increased risk for CRC.

Backwash ileitis and the risk of colorectal cancer

Inflammation in the ileum associated with colitis in the ascending colon and cecum is known as backwash ileitis. There is no evidence to suggest that backwash ileitis is an independent risk factor for developing CRC.[3,12]

Primary sclerosing cholangitis

There is a strong association between PSC and CRC in patients with IBD. In a recent metaanalysis the risk of CRC in patients with UC with PSC increased 4-fold when compared with patients with UC without PSC. This intrinsic risk remained after liver transplant at a rate of 1% per patient per year. Patients with PSC may harbor a subclinical form of colitis (either UC or CD) for an extended duration before their diagnosis. Therefore, patients with PSC and IBD are recommended to commence annual colonoscopy from the time of diagnosis of PSC. In addition, they are recommended to continue surveillance after liver transplantation.[3,10,12,13]

Family history of colorectal cancer
A positive family history is regarded as an important independent risk factor with regard to CRC development. A patient with IBD and a positive family history for a sporadic CRC in a first-degree relative has double the risk of developing CRC. Furthermore, if that first-degree relative was younger than 50 years of age at time of diagnosis, this risk will increase to 9-fold in the patient with IBD. Although family history is regarded as independent risk factor for developing CRC in patients with IBD, it is unclear if it should independently influence the surveillance intervals.[3,12,13]

Other factors and special considerations
Colorectal strictures, especially in UC, are associated with increased risk of developing neoplasia.[14] Similarly, the presence of a foreshortened colon, as indicative of long-standing inflammation, raises the concern for developing malignancy. The presence of these features requires extra vigilance by the endoscopist during screening and surveillance, and warrants extra biopsies with potentially shorter intervals between surveillance colonoscopies.

PATHOGENESIS

The pathogenesis of UC is unclear and, subsequently, the progression of colitis to inflammation to cancer is similarly unclear. Some combination of genetic susceptibility, exposure to antigens in the microenvironment, and immune reactivity governs the range of clinical phenotypes.[15] However, the relationship between these elements is not clear and therefore, prevention and therapy are challenging.

First, the genetics are complex. Although there have been multiple genes that have been associated with IBD and less specifically with UC, the precise correlations are less robust than they are for sporadic colon cancer. Indeed, the adenoma to carcinoma sequence[16] is not so reliably reproduced. In fact, a variation of this sequence, known as the inflammation to dysplasia to carcinoma sequence, is believed to be operative. In this sequence, noted genetic mutations in p53, Kras, and APC occur in a sequence and with frequencies far different than in sporadic colon cancer. For example, the initiating mutation in colitis is believed to be in p53, where there may be a field effect in long-term, clinically quiescent, or minimal disease.[16–18] For example, sporadic CRCs are associated with *APC* mutations early in their pathogenesis. In contrast, colitis-associated cancer is believed to acquire p53 mutations or loss of heterozygosity early in its pathogenesis, with *APC* aberrations occurring later. In colitis-associated cancer, allelic deletion of p53 occurs in approximately 50% of cases.[19] More recent studies using next-generation sequencing indicate that genetic alterations occur in upwards of 89% of patients.[20,21] Indeed, such mutations were identified in nondysplastic, but chronically inflamed mucosa.[22] Overall, genome-wide messenger RNA and micro-RNA profiles are quite different when comparing sporadic CRC with colitis-associated cancer.[23]

Although genetics and epigenetic influences undoubtedly contribute to the propensity of the phenotype, the microenvironment and how the gut reacts to these challenges controls the phenotype. The microenvironment in this context has 2 major components: the cellular microenvironment and the microbiome (**Fig. 1**). Because UC and downstream dysplasia result from these interactions, they must be considered in the pathogenesis, and potentially as therapeutic targets. The cellular elements of the microenvironment include multiple cells types including neutrophils, monocytes, T cells, fibroblasts, and the endothelia. Because this process is driven by

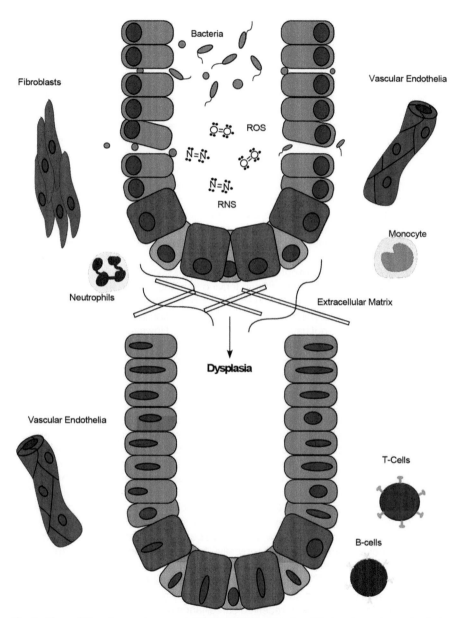

Fig. 1. The colitic microenvironment. The pathogenesis of colitis involves elements of the microenvironment, coopted in the progression to dysplasia and cancer. Interactions initiated by the inflammatory process result in the creation of reactive oxygen (ROS) and reactive nitrogen species (RNS). Early intravasation of neutrophils and vasculature give way to chronic influences of fibroblasts, myeloid cells, and T cells. During the acute phase, loss of intercellular adhesion results in leakiness that allows penetration of bacteria into the submucosa with immune responses. (*Courtesy of* Jennifer Stiene.)

inflammation, the inflammatory secretome of these cells and their functions in antigen presentation, wound healing, management of injured, and dead cells, as well as the interactions with gut bacteria and environmental exposures are the keys to reconciling the inflammatory process in a positive or a pathologic manner. In this process, the microenvironmental influences, including especially the influences of known inflammatory cells such as neutrophils, monocytes, and T cells with their secreted chemokines and cytokines, by the inflammatory and proliferative cascades that are initiated.[18,24] Dominant signaling pathways involved are WNT, STAT3, tumor necrosis factor-α, and nuclear factor κB.[25–28] The second aspect of the microenvironment, but constituting an increasingly more important contribution to this environment, are the bacteria. The load of bacteria in the colon is estimated to be 10^{11} per gram of tissue.[17] These bacteria have been noted to supply nutrients for the colon, provide a protective barrier from pathogens in the colon, and aid in the development of the gut immune system. The relationship between these bacteria and the host epithelia and microenvironment requires a symbiotic balance to remain in check.

Within the epithelia themselves, the mucus secreted by goblet cells is a barrier against infiltration by bacteria and pathogens. This sticky, gellike coating helps to maintain gut homeostasis. During attacks of colitis, the integrity of this coating is violated, thus, permitting contact of the pathogens with the underlying immune system that lies deep to the stroma. Other epithelial cells, including Paneth cells, constitute gut defenses. Here the secretion of antimicrobial peptides such as defensins and lysozyme also protective. Notably, Paneth cells are not usually present in the colon. However, after an acute attack, these cells, which constitute the regenerative niche of the colonic crypts, reappear, seemingly to prepare a bed for new colonic crypts to repopulate the mucosa.[29]

SURVEILLANCE

In the era of preemptive and preventive practice of medicine, at-risk patients with IBD should undergo surveillance colonoscopies at regular intervals, depending on level of risk. Although the efficacy of endoscopic surveillance has not been evaluated in prospective, randomized, controlled trials, evidence based on case series, case control studies, and population-based cohort studies had demonstrated some benefits suggesting earlier detection of cancer and possibly improved CRC-related survival.[13] The more long-standing duration and extensive expression of UC or CD colitis puts the patient with IBD at higher risk for developing dysplasia and CRC.[10] Further, as mentioned, the extent of the disease does not necessarily correspond with the visually inflamed mucosa examined endoscopically, because colonoscopic imaging can underestimate the extent of disease.

In a Cochrane analysis,[30] there was no clear evidence that surveillance colonoscopy prolongs survival, whereas a subsequent cohort study reported a 100% CRC-related 5-year survival in 23 patient who received surveillance compared with 74% in the non-surveillance group.[31] One analysis demonstrated that surveillance colonoscopy could be cost effective when performed in a high-risk group of patients with extensive colitis with moderate or severe active inflammation, PSC, a family history of CRC in a first-degree family member aged less than 50 years at diagnosis, and any degree of dysplasia encountered in previous 5 years.

According to the American Gastroenterological Association guidelines published in 2010, the recommendations were to obtain 4 quadrant biopsies every 10 cm summing for at least 33 "random" tissue specimens from all segments of the colon and rectum in an attempt to detect endoscopically invisible flat lesions as well as biopsy or resect all visible lesions.[3]

Visible Versus Invisible Lesions and White Light Endoscopy Versus Chromoendoscopy

The practice of random biopsies arose in early 1980s in the era of fiberoptic and early video endoscopy, where dysplasia was surprisingly found in a biopsy taken from unsuspected mucosa. Hence, the term "invisible dysplasia."[32] Subsequently, it was observed that patients who had biopsies from a lesion or a mass were found to have colorectal neoplasia; thus, the term "dysplasia-associated lesion or mass" was coined.[32,33] Random surveillance biopsies effectively samples about 1% of colonic mucosa.[34,35] Furthermore, it has been estimated that, to detect 1 colorectal neoplasia, 1266 random biopsies were needed.[36]

Image-enhanced endoscopy in IBD surveillance using high-definition chromoendoscopy enabled endoscopists to identify the previously deemed invisible dysplasia detected on random biopsy, and made them visible in the majority of patients.[13] Surface chromoendoscopy enhances areas of mucosal nodularity and highlights regions with topographic abnormalities, such as depressions and elevations that could be missed on standard white light endoscopy. Randomized and case control studies have shown a 2-to 3-fold improvement in per-patient dysplasia detection and a 4- to 5-fold increase in per-lesion dysplasia detection when chromoendoscopy was used.[37–41] A metaanalysis of prospective studies comparing chromoendoscopy with standard definition white light endoscopy showed that chromoendoscopy with targeted biopsies is associated with a 7% increase in detection yield, and the calculated the needed number to treat to detect 1 additional patient with neoplasia (dysplasia or cancer) is 14.3 (95% confidence interval [CI], 9.7-30.3).[42] Once the lesion is identified, chromoendoscopy will enable to delineate the lesion morphology, size, and border, in addition to evaluating for any endoscopic features of submucosal invasion.[13]

If deemed resectable, then the lesion should be tattooed and resected or referred to an endoscopist with expertise in endoscopic mucosal resection and/or endoscopic submucosal dissection. Additionally, targeted biopsies should be obtained from lesions thought to be unresectable as well as lesions of uncertain significance.[13] The mucosa surrounding lesions that underwent endoscopic resection should also be biopsied to ensure that margins are free from dysplasia. The benefit of surveillance may be compromised in the context of pseudopolyps. Because affected patients should be made aware of this fact, some will opt for prophylactic colectomy over continuing surveillance in this situation.[3]

Dysplasia in Inflammatory Bowel Disease

In patients with IBD, dysplasia is defined histologically as unequivocal neoplastic changes of the intestinal mucosa in the background of chronic inflammation. It can also be classified as an endoscopically visible dysplastic lesion that is detected via resection or targeted biopsy, or an endoscopically invisible lesion detected by random biopsies.[13] Although dysplasia is a good marker of developing CRC, there are limitations in predicting the natural history of dysplasia in patients with IBD. Dysplasia is present in 75% to 90% of patients with IBD-related cancer, although carcinoma may occur without a prior history of dysplasia.[3,12] Taylor and colleagues[43] found 26% of cancer in proctocolectomy specimens without any coexisting findings of dysplasia. Furthermore, patients with low-grade dysplasia (LGD) do not necessarily evolve into an antecedent phase of detectable high-grade dysplasia (HGD) before developing CRC.[3,12]

Type of Lesions Detected Endoscopically

The Paris classification[44] is a simplified method to describe endoscopically visible lesions, and has led to abandoning using the term "DALM" (dysplastic-associated lesion or mass).[44–46] In this classification, lesions are categorized into polyploid (where lesions are protruding ≥2.5 mm from mucosa into the lumen) and nonpolypoid (lesions with no or little protrusion [<2.5 mm] above the mucosa). Polyploid lesions can be described as pedunculated or sessile. Nonpolypoid lesions are further classified as slightly elevated, flat, or depressed. The location of the lesion should be identified as within or outside an area of known colitis. In addition, lesions borders should be described as distinct or indistinct. Furthermore, special attention should be given to evaluate for presence of overlying ulceration or any other signs indicative of submucosal invasion, including depressions and/or failure of mucosal lift upon attempting submucosal injection.[47,48]

Histologic Interpretation

The pathologic evaluation of surveillance biopsy specimens in patients with IBD should be undertaken in accordance to the recommendations of the IBD Dysplasia Morphology Working Group findings published in 1983.[12] Importantly, the pathologic interpretation of dysplasia had been notorious for interobserver variability in mucosal biopsy specimens. Thus, pathologists with expertise in gastrointestinal disorder should be able to review and confirm findings.[3]

Active inflammatory changes may impose some challenges on the pathologic evaluation of biopsy specimens for dysplasia. However, disease activity per se does not preclude accurate pathologic interpretation. Accordingly, endoscopic examination should not be deferred for lengthy time intervals in patients with active inflammation merely for the purpose of increasing diagnostic accuracy. Nonetheless, postponement for acceptable time interval for any intervention to reduce inflammation is reasonable.[12]

Surveillance for Colorectal Endoscopic Neoplasia Detection and Management in Inflammatory Bowel Disease Patients

International consensus recommendations: Surveillance for Colorectal Endoscopic Neoplasia Detection and Management in Inflammatory Bowel Disease Patients: International Consensus Recommendations

Despite the overall agreement on CRC neoplasia in patients with IBD, there has been a lack of consistency regarding surveillance, techniques, nomenclature, management, and follow-up.[48] Therefore, unifying consensus recommendations on the surveillance and management of dysplasia in patients with IBD were needed. The Surveillance for Colorectal Endoscopic Neoplasia Detection and Management in Inflammatory Bowel Disease Patients: International Consensus Recommendations (SCENIC) international consensus aimed to address methods for detection and management of colitic dysplasia. The consensus working group developed recommendations regarding the description of dysplasia and, ultimately, recommendations were made on how to implement the recommendations in clinical practice.[49]

Classification (nomenclature) of dysplasia in inflammatory bowel disease

The term DALM can be polypoid, nonpolypoid, or a masslike lesion; therefore, it is not specific and may cause confusion. To avoid confusion, a subgroup of panelists devised new set of terms based on the descriptive terms used in Paris classification[44] to describe the macroscopic appearance of dysplasia in IBD (see above). Therefore, The SCENIC panelists recommended abandoning the term DALM.[48] The term "endoscopically resectable" should be used, and indicates (i) clearly identified and distinct margin of the lesions, (ii) resectability seems feasible on endoscopic evaluation and seems to be completely removed upon evaluation after resection, and (iii) histopathologic examination confirms complete resection as well as the absence of dysplasia in biopsy specimens obtained from mucosa immediately adjacent to the resection site.[48]

Further, SCENIC recommended the use of chromoendoscopy when performing surveillance colonoscopy in patients with IBD rather than white light endoscopy. Thus, shifting the clinical practice from random toward targeted biopsy technique. The statistics of studies comparing chromoendoscopy with white light standard definition colonoscopy alone showed a significant increase in rate of identifying patients with dysplasia using chromoendoscopy (relative risk, 1.8; 95% CI, 1.2–2.6).[32,48] When surveillance is undertaken using white light endoscopy, high definition is recommended rather than standard definition. Image-enhanced narrow band imaging is not suggested in place of white light colonoscopy or chromoendoscopy.[48]

MANAGEMENT OF COLITIS-ASSOCIATED CANCER
Management of Endoscopically Visible Lesions

Lesions identified in a known segment of inflamed colon during surveillance colonoscopy and deemed resectable should undergo endoscopic resection aiming to achieve complete resection. Biopsies from the flat mucosa adjacent to the resection site should be obtained to ensure lateral margins are free of dysplasia.[13,47] The most important principle is to maximize the potential for complete eradication on first attempt. En bloc resection allows evaluating completeness of resection as well as margin status, which is crucial for subsequent decision making.[7]

Provided that there is no endoscopically invisible or flat dysplasia, a complete resection confirmed on histopathological evaluation prompts close monitoring and surveillance. According to the SCENIC recommendations, after histologic confirmation of complete resection for polypoid and nonpolypoid lesions, the SCENIC statement "suggested" surveillance colonoscopy for such lesions rather than colectomy after "complete" removal with an interval between 1 and 6 months from the index colonoscopy as an acceptable interval.[13,48]

An endoscopically invisible dysplastic lesion detected randomly during white light endoscopy, and confirmed by a second gastroenterology pathologist, should prompt referral to an expert endoscopist skilled in surveillance using chromoendoscopy.[12,48,50] In these examinations, in addition to targeted biopsies, random biopsies should be considered to rule out the presence of invisible dysplasia. Given the associated high risk of synchronous and metachronous CRC, an endoscopically invisible HGD, or multifocal LGD is an indication for colectomy.[13,51]

In all cases, colectomy remains an option, and the risks and benefits of endoscopic resection and surveillance and colon resection should be discussed carefully. Lesions detected in histologically proven noncolitic segments of colon can be treated as sporadic adenomas and follow the standard postpolypectomy surveillance recommendations.[3,12] Pathology that is indefinite for dysplasia should prompt aggressive treatment of underlying active inflammation, followed by repeat colonoscopy, ideally with surface chromoendoscopy.[13,52,53]

The presence of HGD in a completely resected dysplasia necessitates a discussion with the patient regarding risks and benefits of continuing surveillance and surgical intervention. Decisions should be made and fashioned on a case-by-case basis.[13] In patients with IBD who had dysplasia on 1 colonoscopy followed by the absence of dysplasia on a subsequent colonoscopy does not preclude or lessen the risk of carcinoma.[3,12]

Pouch Surveillance

In patients with IBD who underwent restorative proctocolectomy (RPC) ileal pouch-anal anastomosis (IPAA), the incidence of pouch carcinoma seems to be low. No consensus exists regarding optimal patient selection for surveillance, surveillance intervals, or preferred surveillance technique. Potential risk factors presumed to be associated with a higher risk of developing neoplasia after RPC and IPAA include a history of dysplasia or CRC, PSC, refractory pouchitis, and type C pouch mucosa (atrophic mucosa with severe inflammation).[13,54]

A case control, population-based study of 1200 patients with IBD and IPAA found that only a history of colorectal neoplasia was associated with pouch-related neoplasia, where the hazards ratio was 3.8 (95% CI, 1.4-10.2) for prior dysplasia, and 24.7 (95% CI, 9.6–63.4) for prior carcinoma.

In this cohort, 63% of pouch carcinoma occurred in the anal transition zone.[55] In a recent systematic review and metaanalysis including 8403 pouch patients with a variable duration of follow-up, the pooled prevalence of carcinoma in the IPAA was 0.5% (95% CI, 0.3%-0.6%). In another subset of 7647 patients in whom pouch dysplasia was reported, the pooled pouch dysplasia prevalence was 0.8% (95% CI, 0.5%-1.3%). This finding was similarly true in studies including only high-risk patients such as those with a history of prior CRC, pouchitis, longer duration of the disease (>8 years), or PSC (0.9%-4.6%).[7,56–58]

The cumulative incidences of pouch carcinoma was found to be 0.4%, 0.9%, 1.4%, 2.7%, and 3.4% after 5, 10, 15, 20, and 25 years, respectively, from IPAA construction.[7,55,59] Risk factors in this systematic review were similar to the previously mentioned factors.

Patients without a history of colorectal neoplasia before RPC and IPAA had a very low incidence of pouch-related neoplasia, accounting for about 2.2% after 15 years. Thus, patients with history of dysplasia or carcinoma before their pouch creation should undergo semiannual surveillance, whereas patients with history of Primary Sclerosing cholangitis and refractory pouchitis may be considered for a yearly examination. During each, surveillance biopsies should be obtained from the pouch as well as anal transition zone. There are no available data on the use and/or yield of image-enhanced endoscopy in pouch surveillance.

Surgical Management

A dysplastic lesion that is not resectable endoscopically is an indication for colectomy. Endoscopic features suggesting unresectability include ill-defined margins, features of submucosal invasion, asymmetrical lift upon submucosal injection not attributed to inflammation-induced fibrosis, overlying ulceration, large depressions, and flat neoplastic changes adjacent to the lesion. Technically challenging locations may also prompt surgery. Surgery is also indicated for endoscopically invisible HGD, or multifocal LGD, recurrence after resection, or lesions removed but that do not meet resectability criteria by the SCENIC guidelines.

In patients with UC, colonic stricture should considered a malignancy until proved otherwise, especially if thorough endoscopic evaluation cannot be performed and obtaining proper tissue samples is not feasible; in such situations, surgery is also indicated.

SPECIAL CONSIDERATIONS

Mucosectomy Versus Stapled Anastomosis and Keeping the Anal Transitional Zone

The decision to choose mucosectomy with hand-sewn anastomosis versus stapled pouch-anal anastomosis with anal transitional zone (ATZ) preservation is a challenging and highly debated topic. Proponents of the former advocate that mucosectomy ensures eradication of at-risk colorectal mucosa, eliminating the risk of cancer. With this technique, there is significant manipulation of the anal canal during retraction with removal of the distal rectal "sampling" zone. These variations often result in postoperative functional problems, with higher rates of fecal seepage and incontinence.[60]

In contrast, stapled IPAA is technically more feasible, less time consuming, and less likely to be associated with untoward functional outcomes.[61] Stapled IPAA is performed by preserving the most distal portion of the rectum called the rectal cuff. Studies have shown that islands of columnar epithelial cells are retained after mucosectomy in 20% of cases.[62] Indeed, many of the described cases of pouch adenocarcinoma occur despite mucosectomy.

In our practice, if no dysplasia was noted in the pathologic colorectal specimen and the patient exhibits no other risk factors (PSC, history of family CRC) then stapled IPAA is performed, followed by annual ileal pouch and ATZ biopsies with pathologic evaluation. This surveillance period may be extended to every 2 to 3 years if ATZ remains negative for dysplasia. Patients with dysplasia confined to the colon and upper rectum without other risk factors may still be candidates for stapled IPAA after careful counseling and discussion regarding oncologic risks and benefits. Before determination, the rectum is extensively biopsied throughout, and if no dysplasia exists in the lower rectum, a stapled IPAA may be offered without significant increased oncologic risk. ATZ evaluation with biopsies are done on annual basis. The presence of CRC and dysplasia in the lower two-thirds of the rectum prompts mucosectomy and handsewn anastomosis.[60] The risk of dysplastic transformation within the ileal pouch itself for patients with IBD is low.[60,63]

A proposed algorithm for the management of ATZ dysplasia after IPAA was recommended. For HGD in the ATZ, careful ATZ biopsies should be performed at 3- to 6-month intervals. If no further dysplasia is detected, then annual biopsies can be carried out. However, should dysplasia persist on 2 consecutive biopsies, then transperineal mucosectomy and pouch advancement, or a transabdominal approach could be considered for removal of the rectal cuff, or anal canal stripping for control of retained mucosa. For LGD, similar biopsies intervals are preferred. If apparent regression of dysplasia is proved, then yearly biopsies done thereafter. However, the presence of LGD for 3 (instead of 2 as in HGD) occurrences should prompt surgical intervention, as described.[60]

Rectal Cancer in Patients with Colitis

The treatment of stages II and III rectal cancer must involve a multidisciplinary approach for the best oncologic outcomes. Neoadjuvant chemoradiotherapy has become a cornerstone in the multidisciplinary protocols, and subsequent studies have validated the benefits of preoperative radiation therapy in patients who do not have IBD.[64] All patients with or without IBD should have neoadjuvant therapy considered in certain circumstances, but especially those patients in whom a restorative procedure is considered. Adherence to strict oncologic surgical principles regarding circumferential radial margins and total mesorectal excision must be obeyed.[65] As with any type of restorative procedure, preoperative radiation avoids potentially devastating functional complications associated with radiation exposure to the newly created ileal J-pouch, if appropriate for the patient's disease.

Gastrointestinal toxicity remains a challenge and occasionally results in unplanned delays and interruptions in treatment, negatively influencing local control and survival.[66] Acute gastrointestinal toxicity could be partially due to the large amount of normal small bowel that is in the standard pelvic radiation field. A dose–the volume relationship between amount of small bowel exposed to and receiving low and intermittent doses of radiation and the rate of severe diarrhea have been reported.[67,68] However, such short-term toxicities do not outweigh the increase in survival benefit.[69]

In a retrospective analysis of 161 patients with IBD who had rectal cancer, 66 patients (41%) received preoperative radiotherapy, including short course (32 patients), long course (13 patients), and chemoradiotherapy (21 patients). Grade 3 or higher gastrointestinal toxicity was encountered in 0%, 7.7%, and 28.6% of cases, respectively. Grade 3 or higher toxicity was overall 28% and not associated with the type of preoperative therapy. The authors concluded that radiotherapy does not impose excessive rates of toxicity preoperatively or postoperatively in patients with IBD with rectal cancer, supporting the use of standard radiotherapy protocols in patients with IBD with rectal cancer.[70]

Risk of Cancer After Colectomy

The cumulative risk of bowel surgery in patients with UC is 25% to 30%, and is estimated to be 70% to 80% in patients with CD.[7,71,72] RPC with IPAA is considered the standard procedure of choice for UC and selected patients with indeterminate colitis. However, this procedure is usually performed over multiple operations, with the first stage being a total abdominal colectomy and end ileostomy. Patient and clinician concerns about comorbidities such as sexual and urinary function or fertility may lead to choosing a total proctocolectomy with permanent ileostomy.[7]

It has been reported that total abdominal colectomy and ileorectal anastomosis (IRA) may be a consideration in certain patients with UC.[63] Alternatively, total abdominal colectomy and IRA may be the first restorative option for patients with extensive CD.[63,73] The benefits of such an approach include preserved continence, as well as urinary and sexual function. Furthermore, when fecundity is of concern, this procedure, particularly when performed laparoscopically, may decrease postoperative adhesions, thereby increasing the probability of spontaneous pregnancy.[63,74,75]

A systematic review and metaanalysis recently studied the risk of neoplasia after colectomy in patients with IBD. A pooled analysis of 1011 patients with IBD with a variable follow-up ranging from 0.25 to 40 years demonstrated a 2.1% prevalence of carcinoma in the retained rectal stump (95% CI, 1.3–3.0). However, the cumulative rectal cancer incidence in patients with UC with a rectal stump or IRA was evaluated in 1 study and shown to be 12.6% after 24 years from surgery.[76] This analysis detected no difference in carcinoma of rectal stump prevalence between UC and CD (2.2% [95% CI, 1.3%-3.4%] vs 2.1% [95% CI, 0.6%-4.4%]).[7]

For IRA, the calculated pooled rectal carcinoma prevalence was 2.4% (95% CI, 1.7%-3.3%), and the pooled prevalence of dysplasia was 2.5% (95% CI, 1.2%-4.2%). The duration of follow-up varied from 1 to 35 years. There was a lesser prevalence of carcinoma in studies published after 1990. Three studies in this review reported on the cumulative incidence of rectal carcinoma in patients with IBD who underwent IRA[7,77–79] The pooled analysis showed cumulative incidence of 0%, 5%, and 10% after 10, 20, and 25 years from IBD onset, respectively.[7] One study estimated 0%, 2%, 5%, and 14% cumulative incidences of rectal carcinoma after 5, 10, 15, and 20 years from IRA construction, and 7%, 9%, 20%, and 25% for rectal dysplasia, respectively.[80]

Regardless, in all situations, a detailed discussion regarding functional outcomes, risks of neoplasia, and fertility should be undertaken with the patient. Final decisions should be individually tailored.

PERSONALIZED MEDICINE FOR COLITIS-ASSOCIATED CANCER: 3-DIMENSIONAL HUMAN MODELS

The heterogeneity of human disease and the relative absence of in vitro models, and advances in stem cell biology have promoted the acquisition of new human based 3-dimensional models. In 2011, Sato developed long-term in vitro cultures from murine bowel and from human colon. The cultures involved an air interface, and were able to be propagated indefinitely. These techniques have been modified, and Sato and colleaguees [81,82], Li and Yan[83,84] now use Matrigel pillows for embedding the organoids and growth is maintained by a rich media containing R-spondin, Wnt3A, and Noggin to support the crypt units. However, these techniques were used for disease states, especially cancer. Although the terminal state of colitis might be cancer, there are other manifestations of the disease state that might be modeled and interrogated using such a system.

In 2015, Van Dussen and associates[85] reported the capacity to isolate and propagate primary epithelial organoids from patients with IBD. Like the techniques reported by Sato, Clevers, and Kuo, they were maintained in a Matrigel pillow, and sustained in a media rich in Wnt 3A, Noggin, and R-spondin. These organoids were able to demonstrate biological activity in the face of a challenge, including an *Escherichia coli* bacterial interface where differential adhesion was examined. Further studies by Mokry and coworkers[86] on IBD used these techniques to query for risk coding by non–protein-coding epigenetic elements. These investigators queried a small number of organoids from patients with both CD and UC, finding that some single nucleotide polymorphisms correlated with active promoting regions of the DNA, correlating with transcriptional regulation.

Our own experience with such techniques indicates that these models may be used to generate highly reproducible individualized models of patients with these diseases (**Fig. 2**). Not only will a limited view of personalized medicine be available, but also

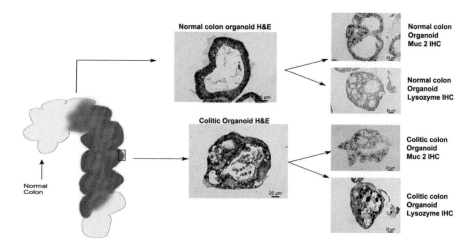

Fig. 2. A new model to interrogate colitis: the colitic organoid. Recent advances in stem cell biology have resulted in methodology to isolate and propagate primary colonic tissues in vitro. **Normal colon organoid** with simple epithelia, mucin secretion (MUC2), and lack of lysozyme, a marker for the niche initiator cell, the Paneth cell. **Colitic colon organoid**, bearing a stratified epithelium, relative lack of MUC2 and increased lysozyme. In this case, the colitic process initiates a regenerative cue, and the niche initiating cells, Paneth cells, are marked by the stain for lysozyme. H&E, hematoxylin and eosin; IHC, immunohistochemistry. (*Courtesy of* Jennifer Stiene.)

mechanisms of in vitro and in vivo investigation will be possible using these technologies.

Research Summary

The advent of personalized medicine has arrived for multiple disease states, including cancer. Recent advances in technology now have the potential to generate rapid models, allowing in vitro and in silico functional data to not only better understand the disease, but to potential test preventive and therapeutic strategies on individual avatars. The models presented here are just the beginning of a new phase of investigation.

FUTURE TREATMENT STRATEGIES

Current therapy is targeted nonspecifically against the inflammatory condition, which initiates these diseases and their malignant sequelae. Surgery to prevent the development of oncogenesis has its own set of complications. Future initiatives include personalizing treatment, perhaps using organoids from individual patients to test therapies ex vivo or, even better, as targets of gene therapy to convert the colitic and oncogenetic processes to those that result in the regeneration of normal bowel. As more sophisticated strategies are available, one could indeed envision using gut flora to effect such therapeutic strategies, resulting in the recreation of a normal colon.

ACKNOWLEDGMENTS

The authors are grateful for the artwork provided by Jennifer Stiene for this article.

REFERENCES

1. Eaden JA, Abrams KR, Mayberry JF. The risk of colorectal cancer in ulcerative colitis: a meta-analysis. Gut 2001;48(4):526–35.
2. Itzkowitz SH, Harpaz N. Diagnosis and management of dysplasia in patients with inflammatory bowel diseases. Gastroenterology 2004;126(6):1634–48.
3. Farraye FA, Odze RD, Eaden J, et al. AGA medical position statement on the diagnosis and management of colorectal neoplasia in inflammatory bowel disease. Gastroenterology 2010;138(2):738–45.
4. Rutter MD, Saunders BP, Wilkinson KH, et al. Thirty-year analysis of a colonoscopic surveillance program for neoplasia in ulcerative colitis. Gastroenterology 2006;130(4):1030–8.
5. Gillen CD, Walmsley RS, Prior P, et al. Ulcerative colitis and Crohn's disease: a comparison of the colorectal cancer risk in extensive colitis. Gut 1994;35(11):1590–2.
6. Jess T, Loftus EV Jr, Velayos FS, et al. Risk of intestinal cancer in inflammatory bowel disease: a population-based study from Olmsted County, Minnesota. Gastroenterology 2006;130(4):1039–46.
7. Derikx LA, Nissen LH, Smits LJ, et al. Risk of neoplasia after colectomy in patients with inflammatory bowel disease: a systematic review and meta-analysis. Clin Gastroenterol Hepatol 2016;14(6):798–806.e20.
8. Connelly TM, Koltun WA. The surgical treatment of inflammatory bowel disease-associated dysplasia. Expert Rev Gastroenterol Hepatol 2013;7(4):307–21 [quiz: 322].

9. Ananthakrishnan AN, Cagan A, Cai T, et al. Colonoscopy is associated with a reduced risk for colon cancer and mortality in patients with inflammatory bowel diseases. Clin Gastroenterol Hepatol 2015;13(2):322–9.e1.
10. Huang LC, Merchea A. Dysplasia and cancer in inflammatory bowel disease. Surg Clin North Am 2017;97(3):627–39.
11. Baars JE, Kuipers EJ, van Haastert M, et al. Age at diagnosis of inflammatory bowel disease influences early development of colorectal cancer in inflammatory bowel disease patients: a nationwide, long-term survey. J Gastroenterol 2012; 47(12):1308–22.
12. Itzkowitz SH, Present DH. Consensus conference: colorectal cancer screening and surveillance in inflammatory bowel disease. Inflamm Bowel Dis 2005;11(3): 314–21.
13. American Society for Gastrointestinal Endoscopy Standards of Practice Committee, Shergill AK, Lightdale JR, Bruining DH, et al. The role of endoscopy in inflammatory bowel disease. Gastrointest Endosc 2015;81(5):1101–21.e1-13.
14. Lashner BA, Turner BC, Bostwick DG, et al. Dysplasia and cancer complicating strictures in ulcerative colitis. Dig Dis Sci 1990;35(3):349–52.
15. Sartor RB. Mechanisms of disease: pathogenesis of Crohn's disease and ulcerative colitis. Nat Clin Pract Gastroenterol Hepatol 2006;3(7):390–407.
16. Fearon ER, Vogelstein B. A genetic model for colorectal tumorigenesis. Cell 1990; 61(5):759–67.
17. Baumler AJ, Sperandio V. Interactions between the microbiota and pathogenic bacteria in the gut. Nature 2016;535(7610):85–93.
18. Chen S, Huang EH. The colon cancer stem cell microenvironment holds keys to future cancer therapy. J Gastrointest Surg 2014;18(5):1040–8.
19. Burmer GC, Rabinovitch PS, Haggitt RC, et al. Neoplastic progression in ulcerative colitis: histology, DNA content, and loss of a p53 allele. Gastroenterology 1992;103(5):1602–10.
20. Yaeger R, Shah MA, Miller VA, et al. Genomic alterations observed in colitis-associated cancers are distinct from those found in sporadic colorectal cancers and vary by type of inflammatory bowel disease. Gastroenterology 2016;151(2): 278–87.e6.
21. Robles AI, Traverso G, Zhang M, et al. Whole-exome sequencing analyses of inflammatory bowel disease-associated colorectal cancers. Gastroenterology 2016;150(4):931–43.
22. Hussain SP, Amstad P, Raja K, et al. Increased p53 mutation load in noncancerous colon tissue from ulcerative colitis: a cancer-prone chronic inflammatory disease. Cancer Res 2000;60(13):3333–7.
23. Colliver DW, Crawford NP, Eichenberger MR, et al. Molecular profiling of ulcerative colitis-associated neoplastic progression. Exp Mol Pathol 2006;80(1):1–10.
24. Romano M, DE Francesco F, Zarantonello L, et al. From inflammation to cancer in inflammatory bowel disease: molecular perspectives. Anticancer Res 2016;36(4): 1447–60.
25. Grivennikov S, Karin E, Terzic J, et al. IL-6 and Stat3 are required for survival of intestinal epithelial cells and development of colitis-associated cancer. Cancer Cell 2009;15(2):103–13.
26. Grivennikov SI, Karin M. Dangerous liaisons: STAT3 and NF-kappaB collaboration and crosstalk in cancer. Cytokine Growth Factor Rev 2010;21(1):11–9.
27. Xiao H, Gulen MF, Qin J, et al. The Toll-interleukin-1 receptor member SIGIRR regulates colonic epithelial homeostasis, inflammation, and tumorigenesis. Immunity 2007;26(4):461–75.

28. Yang J, Liao X, Agarwal MK, et al. Unphosphorylated STAT3 accumulates in response to IL-6 and activates transcription by binding to NFkappaB. Genes Dev 2007;21(11):1396–408.

29. Clevers H. The Paneth cell, caloric restriction, and intestinal integrity. N Engl J Med 2012;367(16):1560–1.

30. Collins PD, Mpofu C, Watson AJ, et al. Strategies for detecting colon cancer and/ or dysplasia in patients with inflammatory bowel disease. Cochrane Database Syst Rev 2006;(2):CD000279.

31. Lutgens MW, Oldenburg B, Siersema PD, et al. Colonoscopic surveillance improves survival after colorectal cancer diagnosis in inflammatory bowel disease. Br J Cancer 2009;101(10):1671–5.

32. Soetikno R, Kaltenbach T, McQuaid KR, et al. Paradigm shift in the surveillance and management of dysplasia in inflammatory bowel disease (west). Dig Endosc 2016;28(3):266–73.

33. Blackstone MO, Riddell RH, Rogers BH, et al. Dysplasia-associated lesion or mass (DALM) detected by colonoscopy in long-standing ulcerative colitis: an indication for colectomy. Gastroenterology 1981;80(2):366–74.

34. East JE. Colonoscopic cancer surveillance in inflammatory bowel disease: what's new beyond random biopsy? Clin Endosc 2012;45(3):274–7.

35. Guagnozzi D, Lucendo AJ. Colorectal cancer surveillance in patients with inflammatory bowel disease: what is new? World J Gastrointest Endosc 2012;4(4):108–16.

36. Rutter MD. Surveillance programmes for neoplasia in colitis. J Gastroenterol 2011;46(Suppl 1):1–5.

37. Kiesslich R, Fritsch J, Holtmann M, et al. Methylene blue-aided chromoendoscopy for the detection of intraepithelial neoplasia and colon cancer in ulcerative colitis. Gastroenterology 2003;124(4):880–8.

38. Kiesslich R, Neurath MF. Magnifying chromoendoscopy: effective diagnostic tool for screening colonoscopy. J Gastroenterol Hepatol 2007;22(11):1700–1.

39. Marion JF, Waye JD, Present DH, et al. Chromoendoscopy-targeted biopsies are superior to standard colonoscopic surveillance for detecting dysplasia in inflammatory bowel disease patients: a prospective endoscopic trial. Am J Gastroenterol 2008;103(9):2342–9.

40. Rutter MD, Saunders BP, Schofield G, et al. Pancolonic indigo carmine dye spraying for the detection of dysplasia in ulcerative colitis. Gut 2004;53(2):256–60.

41. Hurlstone DP, Sanders DS, Lobo AJ, et al. Indigo carmine-assisted high-magnification chromoscopic colonoscopy for the detection and characterisation of intraepithelial neoplasia in ulcerative colitis: a prospective evaluation. Endoscopy 2005;37(12):1186–92.

42. Soetikno R, Subramanian V, Kaltenbach T, et al. The detection of nonpolypoid (flat and depressed) colorectal neoplasms in patients with inflammatory bowel disease. Gastroenterology 2013;144(7):1349–52, 1352.e1–6.

43. Taylor BA, Pemberton JH, Carpenter HA, et al. Dysplasia in chronic ulcerative colitis: implications for colonoscopic surveillance. Dis Colon Rectum 1992;35(10):950–6.

44. The Paris endoscopic classification of superficial neoplastic lesions: esophagus, stomach, and colon: November 30 to December 1, 2002. Gastrointest Endosc 2003;58(6 Suppl):S3–43.

45. Murthy SK, Kiesslich R. Evolving endoscopic strategies for detection and treatment of neoplastic lesions in inflammatory bowel disease. Gastrointest Endosc 2013;77(3):351–9.

46. Allen PB, Kamm MA, De Cruz P, et al. Dysplastic lesions in ulcerative colitis: changing paradigms. Inflamm Bowel Dis 2010;16(11):1978–83.
47. Rutter MD, Riddell RH. Colorectal dysplasia in inflammatory bowel disease: a clinicopathologic perspective. Clin Gastroenterol Hepatol 2014;12(3):359–67.
48. Laine L, Kaltenbach T, Barkun A, et al. SCENIC international consensus statement on surveillance and management of dysplasia in inflammatory bowel disease. Gastroenterology 2015;148(3):639–51.e28.
49. Guyatt GH, Oxman AD, Vist GE, et al. GRADE: an emerging consensus on rating quality of evidence and strength of recommendations. BMJ 2008;336(7650):924–6.
50. Annese V, Daperno M, Rutter MD, et al. European evidence based consensus for endoscopy in inflammatory bowel disease. J Crohns Colitis 2013;7(12):982–1018.
51. Zisman TL, Bronner MP, Rulyak S, et al. Prospective study of the progression of low-grade dysplasia in ulcerative colitis using current cancer surveillance guidelines. Inflamm Bowel Dis 2012;18(12):2240–6.
52. Pekow JR, Hetzel JT, Rothe JA, et al. Outcome after surveillance of low-grade and indefinite dysplasia in patients with ulcerative colitis. Inflamm Bowel Dis 2010;16(8):1352–6.
53. van Schaik FD, ten Kate FJ, Offerhaus GJ, et al. Misclassification of dysplasia in patients with inflammatory bowel disease: consequences for progression rates to advanced neoplasia. Inflamm Bowel Dis 2011;17(5):1108–16.
54. Liu ZX, Kiran RP, Bennett AE, et al. Diagnosis and management of dysplasia and cancer of the ileal pouch in patients with underlying inflammatory bowel disease. Cancer 2011;117(14):3081–92.
55. Derikx LA, Kievit W, Drenth JP, et al. Prior colorectal neoplasia is associated with increased risk of ileoanal pouch neoplasia in patients with inflammatory bowel disease. Gastroenterology 2014;146(1):119–28.e1.
56. Imam MH, Eaton JE, Puckett JS, et al. Neoplasia in the ileoanal pouch following colectomy in patients with ulcerative colitis and primary sclerosing cholangitis. J Crohns Colitis 2014;8(10):1294–9.
57. Kuiper T, Vlug MS, van den Broek FJ, et al. The prevalence of dysplasia in the ileoanal pouch following restorative proctocolectomy for ulcerative colitis with associated dysplasia. Colorectal Dis 2012;14(4):469–73.
58. Vento P, Lepisto A, Karkkainen P, et al. Risk of cancer in patients with chronic pouchitis after restorative proctocolectomy for ulcerative colitis. Colorectal Dis 2011;13(1):58–66.
59. Kariv R, Remzi FH, Lian L, et al. Preoperative colorectal neoplasia increases risk for pouch neoplasia in patients with restorative proctocolectomy. Gastroenterology 2010;139(3):806–12, 812.e1–2.
60. Remzi FH, Fazio VW, Delaney CP, et al. Dysplasia of the anal transitional zone after ileal pouch-anal anastomosis: results of prospective evaluation after a minimum of ten years. Dis Colon Rectum 2003;46(1):6–13.
61. Tuckson W, Lavery I, Fazio V, et al. Manometric and functional comparison of ileal pouch anal anastomosis with and without anal manipulation. Am J Surg 1991;161(1):90–5 [discussion: 95–6].
62. O'Connell PR, Pemberton JH, Weiland LH, et al. Does rectal mucosa regenerate after ileoanal anastomosis? Dis Colon Rectum 1987;30(1):1–5.
63. Borjesson L, Willen R, Haboubi N, et al. The risk of dysplasia and cancer in the ileal pouch mucosa after restorative proctocolectomy for ulcerative proctocolitis is low: a long-term term follow-up study. Colorectal Dis 2004;6(6):494–8.

64. Swedish Rectal Cancer Trial, Cedermark B, Dahlberg M, Glimelius B, et al. Improved survival with preoperative radiotherapy in resectable rectal cancer. N Engl J Med 1997;336(14):980–7.

65. MacFarlane JK, Ryall RD, Heald RJ. Mesorectal excision for rectal cancer. Lancet 1993;341(8843):457–60.

66. Fietkau R, Rodel C, Hohenberger W, et al. Rectal cancer delivery of radiotherapy in adequate time and with adequate dose is influenced by treatment center, treatment schedule, and gender and is prognostic parameter for local control: results of study CAO/ARO/AIO-94. Int J Radiat Oncol Biol Phys 2007;67(4):1008–19.

67. Robertson JM, Lockman D, Yan D, et al. The dose-volume relationship of small bowel irradiation and acute grade 3 diarrhea during chemoradiotherapy for rectal cancer. Int J Radiat Oncol Biol Phys 2008;70(2):413–8.

68. Tho LM, Glegg M, Paterson J, et al. Acute small bowel toxicity and preoperative chemoradiotherapy for rectal cancer: investigating dose-volume relationships and role for inverse planning. Int J Radiat Oncol Biol Phys 2006;66(2):505–13.

69. Chang BW, Kumar AM, Koyfman SA, et al. Radiation therapy in patients with inflammatory bowel disease and colorectal cancer: risks and benefits. Int J Colorectal Dis 2015;30(3):403–8.

70. Bosch SL, van Rooijen SJ, Bokkerink GM, et al. Acute toxicity and surgical complications after preoperative (chemo)radiation therapy for rectal cancer in patients with inflammatory bowel disease. Radiother Oncol 2017;123(1):147–53.

71. Andersson P, Soderholm JD. Surgery in ulcerative colitis: indication and timing. Dig Dis 2009;27(3):335–40.

72. Martin ST, Vogel JD. Restorative procedures in colonic Crohn disease. Clin Colon Rectal Surg 2013;26(2):100–5.

73. Lofberg R, Liljeqvist L, Lindquist K, et al. Dysplasia and DNA aneuploidy in a pelvic pouch. Report of a case. Dis Colon Rectum 1991;34(3):280–3 [discussion: 283–4].

74. Gullberg K, Stahlberg D, Liljeqvist L, et al. Neoplastic transformation of the pelvic pouch mucosa in patients with ulcerative colitis. Gastroenterology 1997;112(5): 1487–92.

75. Sarigol S, Wyllie R, Gramlich T, et al. Incidence of dysplasia in pelvic pouches in pediatric patients after ileal pouch-anal anastomosis for ulcerative colitis. J Pediatr Gastroenterol Nutr 1999;28(4):429–34.

76. Johnson WR, Hughes ES, McDermott FT, et al. The outcome of patients with ulcerative colitis managed by subtotal colectomy. Surg Gynecol Obstet 1986; 162(5):421–5.

77. Andersson P, Norblad R, Soderholm JD, et al. Ileorectal anastomosis in comparison with ileal pouch anal anastomosis in reconstructive surgery for ulcerative colitis–a single institution experience. J Crohns Colitis 2014;8(7):582–9.

78. Grundfest SF, Fazio V, Weiss RA, et al. The risk of cancer following colectomy and ileorectal anastomosis for extensive mucosal ulcerative colitis. Ann Surg 1981; 193(1):9–14.

79. Baker WN, Glass RE, Ritchie JK, et al. Cancer of the rectum following colectomy and ileorectal anastomosis for ulcerative colitis. Br J Surg 1978;65(12):862–8.

80. da Luz Moreira A, Kiran RP, Lavery I. Clinical outcomes of ileorectal anastomosis for ulcerative colitis. Br J Surg 2010;97(1):65–9.

81. Sato T, Stange DE, Ferrante M, et al. Long-term expansion of epithelial organoids from human colon, adenoma, adenocarcinoma, and Barrett's epithelium. Gastroenterology 2011;141(5):1762–72.

82. Sugimoto S, Sato T. Establishment of 3D intestinal organoid cultures from intestinal stem cells. Methods Mol Biol 2017;1612:97–105.
83. Li X, Nadauld L, Ootani A, et al. Oncogenic transformation of diverse gastrointestinal tissues in primary organoid culture. Nat Med 2014;20(7):769–77.
84. Yan KS, Janda CY, Chang J, et al. Non-equivalence of Wnt and R-spondin ligands during Lgr5+ intestinal stem-cell self-renewal. Nature 2017;545(7653):238–42.
85. VanDussen KL, Marinshaw JM, Shaikh N, et al. Development of an enhanced human gastrointestinal epithelial culture system to facilitate patient-based assays. Gut 2015;64(6):911–20.
86. Mokry M, Middendorp S, Wiegerinck CL, et al. Many inflammatory bowel disease risk loci include regions that regulate gene expression in immune cells and the intestinal epithelium. Gastroenterology 2014;146(4):1040–7.

Colorectal Cancer:
Imaging Conundrums

Nathan C. Hall, MD, PhD[a,b,c],*, Alexander T. Ruutiainen, MD[d]

KEYWORDS

- Computed tomography • PET • TNM staging • Colorectal cancer • Surgery • Liver
- Metastases • Lymph nodes

KEY POINTS

- At some sensitivity threshold, preoperative imaging technologies detect cancer-containing tissue too small for standard surgical identification and extirpation.
- FDG PET/CT improves sensitivity for detecting extrahepatic metastases at the cost of specificity, possibly resulting in erroneous disease overstaging.
- Resolving these imaging conundrums may be possible by the widespread adoption of real-time imaging guidance during operative procedures.

INTRODUCTION

Despite its decreasing incidence over the last four decades, colon cancer remains the third leading cause of new cancers in the United States.[1–3] In part, this trend toward diminishing incidence may be attributable to the success and use of colorectal cancer screening programs, resulting in earlier diagnoses, along with trends toward generally healthier lifestyle choices.[2] Likely partially as a result, colon cancer survival rates have continued to improve over this timeframe, albeit with logarithmic growth at ever-diminishing rates. This trend may also be partly attributable to improvements in accuracy of preoperative disease staging, which result in

Disclosure: N.C. Hall is the Service Chief of Diagnostic Imaging and the Acting Section Chief of Nuclear Medicine for the Corporal Michael J. Crescenz VA Medical Center in Philadelphia, PA. A.T. Ruutiainen is the Section Chief of Diagnostic Radiology for the Corporal Michael J. Crescenz VA Medical Center in Philadelphia, PA. The contents of this article do not represent the views of the US Department of Veterans Affairs or the United States Government.
[a] Department of Radiology, Hospital of the University of Pennsylvania, 3400 Spruce Street, Philadelphia, PA 19104, USA; [b] Diagnostic Imaging, Nuclear Medicine, Corporal Michael J. Crescenz VA Medical Center, 3900 Woodland Avenue, Philadelphia, PA 19104, USA; [c] Department of Surgery, Division of Surgical Oncology, The Ohio State University Wexner Medical Center, 410 West 10th Avenue, Columbus, OH 43210, USA; [d] Diagnostic Radiology, Corporal Michael J. Crescenz VA Medical Center, 3900 Woodland Avenue, Philadelphia, PA 19104, USA
* Corresponding author. Hospital of the University of Pennsylvania, 3400 Spruce Street, Philadelphia, PA 19104.
E-mail address: nathan.hall@uphs.upenn.edu

surgonc.theclinics.com

progressively more complete surgical resections along with more common and appropriate use of chemotherapy in a larger percentage of patients with colorectal cancer.[2,3]

Surgical resection with curative intent remains the therapeutic approach for most patients, even those with limited metastatic disease.[4,5] When such surgery is undertaken, resecting all areas of disease is critically important. To accomplish such a complete resection, the surgeon needs two things: highly accurate preoperative staging information; and the ability to use this information intraoperatively to localize and resect all areas of tumor. Recent advancements in imaging capabilities have afforded surgeons progressively more accurate preoperative staging information: these advances have likely also contributed to the improving survival rates.[6,7]

Among the substantial technological improvements in imaging instrumentation has been the increasing resolution of multidetector computed tomography (CT), which has improved sensitivity for the detection of ever-smaller foci of abnormal tissue. In addition, the development and use of combined functional/metabolic and morphologic fused cross-sectional imaging, [18]fluorodeoxyglucose (FDG) PET combined with CT (FDG PET/CT), has improved the detection of extrahepatic metastatic disease well beyond the capabilities of other available imaging modalities.[8,9] Unfortunately, the radioactive sugar (FDG) is metabolized nonspecifically, demonstrating increased uptake in tumor cells and areas of infection, inflammation, trauma, and even normal physiologic background metabolism. Thus, the increase in sensitivity for the detection of extrahepatic metastases has been largely offset by the nonspecificity of FDG PET/CT, resulting in the potential for incorrectly overstaging patients because of false-positive findings.

Although these improvements in the preoperative staging of colon cancer are exciting, they have focused attention on confounding imaging conundrums. The first of these is a conundrum of sensitivity: the challenge of translating the improved detectability of disease from the radiology reading room to the operating room. That is, the resolution of CT may now be so exquisite that the sensitivity for detecting small foci of disease has exceeded the current limitations of intraoperative localization using conventional methods. This challenge is even more acute when the considering the even-higher sensitivity of FDG PET/CT.

A contrasting problem is the conundrum of specificity: ever-improving lesion detectability and the ever-increasing staging sensitivity may result in a lack of staging specificity. That is, the benefits of increased sensitivity from the use of PET/CT may be offset by the false-positive findings that can result from the nonspecificity of tracer uptake into nonmalignant tissues with increased glucose metabolism caused by inflammation or other benign processes.

In this article we argue that a potential solution to these interrelated imaging conundrums is to improve the translation of information from the radiologist to the surgeon. Namely, if imaging has improved to such a degree that the surgeon may not be able to identify and resect all malignant tissue that has been preoperatively identified, then additional tools are needed to bridge this gap. In particular, real-time intraoperative imaging technology is needed to help surgeons use the imaging information in the operating room. Similarly, to overcome issues with the nonspecificity of preoperative imaging, more specific intraoperative tools are needed to help differentiate FDG avid tissues as being either benign or malignant. Ultimately, if these conundrums can be appropriately resolved, the benefits to improved treatment efficacy, lack of toxicity, and ultimately overall patient survival could be substantial.

THE CONUNDRUM OF SENSITIVITY: TRANSLATING LESION DETECTABILITY FROM THE READING ROOM INTO THE OPERATING ROOM

Surgery remains the primary treatment of colorectal cancer.[10] This is because surgical intervention provides the only curative therapy for early stages of disease, and many cases with isolated liver and/or lung metastases.[11,12] The last few decades have witnessed significant advancements in chemotherapy and radiation therapy; nevertheless, surgery remains the gold standard therapeutic intervention. As such, accurate preoperative staging of disease extent with identification of all tissue containing tumor cells remains essential; in fact, its success directly impacts patient survival.[10,13–17] This is because complete excision of all areas of disease provides the only curative treatment of all stages of localized disease (stage I-III), and stage IV disease with limited liver and/or lung metastases.[5,18–20] The goal of complete resection is the rationale for the incorporation of more extensive lymphadenectomy into the standard therapeutic surgical procedure.[21,22]

For a surgeon to successfully target resection of all areas of disease, the areas of malignancy must be detectable. Most disease is detected preoperatively, although the preoperative information must ultimately be translated into surgical decisions. Such preoperative staging is typically performed with imaging. CT has been the mainstay of imaging for the staging of colorectal cancer, particularly over the past few decades. More recently, PET/CT has begun to emerge as a modality potentially carrying additional benefit in the preoperative staging process.[6,9,23–26]

Nevertheless, although patient survival has continued to improve, recently the survival gains have not been directly proportional to the improved sensitivity and accuracy of preoperative staging. One potential explanation for this is that the detailed preoperative information is valuable only if it is effectively translated for use in making real-time surgical decisions. If the sensitivity of the preoperative staging examinations surpasses the sensitivity of the surgeon in identifying and resecting the lesions during the operative procedure, then further improvements in overall survival are unlikely to occur. This is the conundrum of sensitivity: the challenge of translating the continued gains in the sensitivity of preoperative imaging into further gains in patient survival.

In traditional practice, the surgeon has been tasked with "mentally fusing" the preoperative information with the appearance of the living patient. In some operating rooms, this task has been partly aided by intraoperative review of imaging studies. Nevertheless, even then, it has ultimately been the surgeon's eyes and hands that have been responsible for localizing the sites of disease. However, there are fundamental limitations to the sensitivity of intraoperative human sensation. With the ever-increasing sensitivity of preoperative imaging, at some point, the sensitivity of the surgeon's sensation will be surpassed by the sensitivity of preoperative imaging. Based on a comparison of the sensitivity of CT for the detection of lymph node metastases and the 5-year survival curve of colon cancer, we believe that this inflection point has already occurred.

Table 1 demonstrates that the sensitivity of preoperative imaging with CT has steadily improved between 1986 and 2017. Nevertheless, the overall 5-year survival of patients with colon cancer has demonstrated only logarithmic improvement. This relationship is illustrated in **Fig. 1** as a simplified model of the conundrum of sensitivity: if the surgical removal of all malignant nodes provides patients with a better chance of a definitive cure, and all preoperatively detected nodes can be technically removed, then logically, the ever-increasing sensitivity in the detection of such malignant nodes should translate to continued improvements in patient survival. However, because this linearly proportionate improvement is not supported by the observed data, it suggests

Table 1
Sensitivity of computed tomography for lymph node metastases

First Author & Publication Year	Sensitivity for Lymph Node Metastases (%)	Average Sensitivity for 5-Year Block (%)
Freeny et al,[68] 1986	26	31
Thompson et al,[69] 1986	22	
Balthazar et al,[28] 1988	73	
Holdsworth et al,[71] 1988	25	
Keeney et al,[73] 1989	13	
Rifkin et al,[75] 1989	27	
Acunas et al,[76] 1990	75	54
Fujita et al,[78] 1990	50	
Karl et al,[79] 1993	73	
McAndrew & Saba,[81] 1994*	19	
Gazelle et al,[83] 1995	90	63
Okizuka et al,[85] 1995	60	
Zerhouni et al,[45] 1996	49	
Dux et al,[88] 1996	69	
Thoeni,[90] 1997	45	
Harvey et al,[91] 1998	55	
Gomille et al,[92] 1998	71	
Hundt et al,[94] 1999	84	
Cademartiri et al,[96] 2002	58	68
Filippone et al,[98] 2004	90	
Chung et al,[100] 2004	66	
Wiering et al,[9] 2005	55	74
Chung et al,[70] 2005	85	
Chamadol et al,[44] 2005	92	
Sun et al,[72] 2005	71	
Ashraf et al,[74] 2006	66	
Dighe et al,[39] 2010	70	76
Stabile Ianora (Air) et al,[77] 2012	78	
Stabile Ianora (Water) et al,[77] 2012	81	
Haji et al,[80] 2012	80	
Lim et al,[82] 2013	83	
Lao et al,[84] 2013	54	
Rollven et al,[86] 2013	72	
Flor et al,[87] 2013	94	
Norgaard et al,[89] 2014	81	
Engelman et al,[25] 2014	33	
Lee & Lee,[26] 2014	99	
Sibileau et al,[93] 2014	91	
de Vries et al,[95] 2014	71	
Choi et al,[97] 2015	88	87
Wiegering et al,[99] 2015	77	
Stagnitti et al,[101] 2015	90	
Elibol et al,[102] 2016	84	
Singla et al,[103] 2017	90	
Koh et al,[104] 2017	85	
Malmstrøm et al,[31] 2017	96	

* Indicates that data from the publication came from that timeframe (1990-94) although the publication date is from 1999. 1999 is the actual publication year.

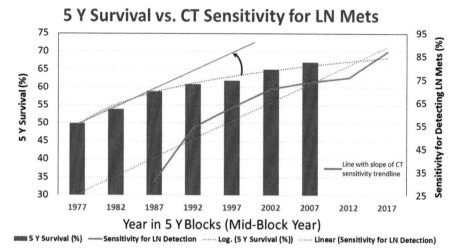

Fig. 1. A graphical model demonstrating the trends of 5-year overall colon cancer survival and sensitivity of CT for detecting lymph node metastases over time. Overall 5-year survival increases over time at a logarithmically decreasing rate of improvement. Dotted blue line shows divergence between the improvements in the detectability of malignant lymph nodes and observed 5-year patient survival. Improvements in sensitivity of CT for the detection of malignant lymph nodes occur linearly with a constant rate of improvement over time. Solid orange line shows averaged sensitivity from publications during the specific 5-year time periods. Dotted orange line shows linear trendline derived from averaged CT sensitivities from publications. The blue line has the same slope as that of the CT sensitivity trendline and is superimposed over the 5-year survival bar graph to compare these rates with each other. Initially, the rate of improvement in overall 5-year survival approximates the rate of improvement of CT sensitivity for detecting malignant lymph nodes. Over time the two rates of improvement diverge with CT sensitivity continuing at the same rate and survival improving at a slower rate. The divergence of these rates (*purple arrow*) may be at least partially explained by the increasing difficulty of identifying and resecting all malignant lymph nodes because CT technology continues to improve sensitivity for detecting smaller and smaller malignant lymph nodes that may appear normal to the naked eye. LN, lymph node.

that at least one of the basic assumptions of such a hypothesis is incorrect. In particular, it might be either that the removal of all malignant nodes ultimately does not matter to patient survival, or that there is disconnect between the preoperative detectability of such nodes and the surgeon's capacity to identify and remove them.

Conceptually, it may be possible that at some point, the removal of ever-more malignant tissue might have diminishing-returns on patient survival. Once most disease has been surgically removed, such adjuvant therapies as chemotherapy and radiation therapy may be sufficient to eradicate any remaining disease. If true, then a heroic search for the last remaining cancer cell in the operating room may be pointless. Although this concept seems to hold true for many cancer types with effective chemotherapy regimens, effective therapy for colorectal cancer continues to depend proportionally more heavily on completeness of surgical resection than effectiveness of adjuvant chemotherapy.

Therefore, we believe that the alternative explanation for the data is more probable: that is, that the divergence of the nodal-detectability and patient survival curves may be attributable to the surgeon's inability to intraoperatively localize all the tissue that has been identified preoperatively. This explanation, although difficult to empirically separate from the former possibility, is a plausible explanation for the observed data.

THE CONUNDRUM OF SPECIFICITY: THE CONFLICT BETWEEN LESION DETECTABILITY AND SENSITIVITY

In the past, double-contrast barium enema was used for the evaluation of patients with suspected colorectal cancer.[27–29] However, that modality provided only a limited picture of the colon, being confined to the evaluation of luminal contours and mucosal detail. At the same time, ultrasound had also been used to evaluate patients with colorectal cancer, but its utility was primarily limited to the detection of conspicuous liver metastases.[30,31] Ultrasound technology does excel in intraoperative guidance: in that role it has been shown to be superior to preoperative transabdominal ultrasound for the detection of liver metastases.[32–34] Ultimately, however, the sensitivity of CT for detecting hepatic and extrahepatic metastases has largely obviated the use of ultrasound for the staging of colon cancer.[24] Even so, conventional CT can occasionally struggle with specificity in the differentiation of some benign versus malignant liver lesions. Both multiphase CT and multiphase MRI have improved specificities in making these distinctions, partly because of their ability in assessing the dynamic enhancement of liver lesions.[35] For the assessment of nodal disease, all anatomic modalities struggle with the characterization of small nonnecrotic nodes, which may nevertheless harbor malignant cells, and occasionally with nodes that are enlarged on a reactive basis. Routine CT may also have difficulty in assessing the depth of tumor involvement in the colonic wall, although at least for many rectal cancers, this can now be performed with MRI.[36]

Despite some isolated limitations, CT has emerged to be the primary imaging modality for the preoperative staging of colorectal cancer.[37–39] This is partly attributable to the significant technological advancements in CT hardware and post-processing software, which have led to dramatic improvements in resolution and lesion detectability.[40,41] Multiring detector spiral CT, now the standard of care, has improved sensitivity in the detection of liver metastases to 70% to 90% and has provided surgeons with a more accurate roadmap for each surgical procedure.[35,42–45] CT is able to detect more than 90% of metastatic liver lesions measuring more than 1 cm.[46] Finally, with its capacity to scan large portions of the body quickly, CT holds potential to excel in the detection of distant metastases.[38]

FDG PET/CT has been shown to have sensitivity and specificity for detection of liver metastases similar to that of CT (78%–95%).[24,47] In addition, other studies have shown that PET/CT has superior sensitivity and accuracy than anatomic imaging modalities for the detection of extrahepatic occult metastatic disease.[19,25] As such, the addition of FDG PET/CT imaging to the preoperative staging of patients with hepatic metastatic disease leads to a change in therapeutic management in up to 20% of patients.[19] Despite this evidence supporting PET/CT as a superior staging modality for patients with metastatic disease, current National Comprehensive Cancer Network guidelines for colorectal cancer do not recommend the use of FDG PET/CT in the initial staging of patients.[5] Thus far, FDG PET/CT has found only a niche role in the evaluation of patients with an unexplained rise in their carcinoembryonic antigen who have indeterminate extrahepatic lesions on conventional cross-sectional imaging that are suspected to represent a tumor recurrence.[47,48]

However, the addition of FDG PET/CT to the preoperative diagnostic armamentarium carries potential for further improving the sensitivity of preoperative staging. FDG PET/CT has been shown to significantly improve staging with respect to colorectal liver metastases.[23] Additionally, adding FDG PET/CT to the preoperative staging work-up improves the sensitivity for detecting extrahepatic metastases over contrast-enhanced CT alone.[23]

FDG PET/CT has poor sensitivity for detecting lymph node metastases, which can result in an unacceptably high false-negative rate.[8,24,35,43,48–50] However, when positive, FDG PET/CT has good specificity for the detection of nodal metastases.[51]

Importantly, however, FDG PET/CT imaging has been shown to detect extrahepatic disease in 25% of patients who are otherwise thought to have had isolated liver metastases. The additional information gained from the addition of FDG PET/CT imaging changed treatment strategy approximately 20% to 25% of the time.[23,52] Crucially, an improvement in 5-year survival has been demonstrated for patients receiving a staging PET/CT before resection of known liver metastases, likely attributable to the improved sensitivity for the detection of extrahepatic metastases.[23,35,52,53]

Even so, adding FDG PET/CT imaging to the preoperative staging work-up does have a major potential limitation. Although sensitivity for detecting areas of nonnodal metastatic disease is improved over CT alone, positive FDG PET/CT findings are nonspecific and can lead to the inappropriate up-staging of disease extent caused by false-positive findings.[54,55] This is the conundrum of specificity: how can the improved sensitivity offered by PET/CT be effectively translated into the preoperative assessment and operative management with the confounding complication of poor specificity? Until this challenge is resolved, FDG PET/CT is unlikely to find a recommended role in the initial staging of colon cancer.

For any given test, there is always a theoretical conflict between sensitivity and specificity. For a given receiver operating curve (which is set by the intrinsic properties of the test), improved sensitivity can only be obtained at the cost of decreased specificity, and vice versa. Medical work-up, however, is not confined to single tests: improving sensitivity and specificity together is also possible by combining a series of tests into a process of Bayesian reasoning. This is commonly performed in screening scenarios, where a highly sensitive (but nonspecific) test is followed by a more specific study for confirmation.

If the staging work-up of colon cancer is reframed in this way, it becomes clear that the role of preoperative imaging can focus on improving sensitivity, even if that improvement comes at the cost of somewhat-reduced specificity. This is only possible, however, if there is another test, either preoperatively or perhaps intraoperatively, that can ensure optimum specificity.

A SOLUTION TO BOTH CONUNDRUMS: INTRAOPERATIVE GUIDANCE

The preoperative imaging of colon cancer has steadily improved over the past two decades. Improvements in technology have provided ever-increasing lesion detectability, thereby increasing the sensitivity for the detection of occult metastatic disease. However, these gains in sensitivity have not translated into sustained gains in patient survival: the conundrum of sensitivity. At the same time, this ever-increasing sensitivity has created pressure to maintain or improve the specificity of the preoperative imaging: the conundrum of specificity. These combined conundrums are likely a major reason why FDG PET/CT has not yet found a recommended role in the routine staging of newly diagnosed colon cancer.

A potential solution to both of these conundrums is the adoption of real-time intraoperative guidance. Such guidance might include, but is not limited to, the use of fluorescent probes, radioactive tracers, intraoperative imaging procedures (CT, gamma camera, ultrasound), and spectroscopy.[56–62] Much of this technology has already been developed and simply needs to be incorporated into the operative environment.[63–66] For example, FDG, in combination with preoperative diagnostic FDG PET/CT, has been used intraoperatively with the assistance of a handheld gamma probe to assist the surgeon in accurately locating and determining the extent of FDG-avid tissue during an operative procedure in colorectal cancer and many other cancer types.[63–65,67]

Intraoperative guidance has the potential to resolve the conundrum of sensitivity. If the divergence between the improving nodal detectability and the observed 5-year survival is in fact attributable to the sensitivity of preoperative imaging surpassing the surgeon's sensitivity for localizing lesions using conventional methods, then the incorporation of intraoperative guidance may result in substantial gains in patient survival. Similarly, intraoperative guidance can also resolve the conundrum of specificity. If intraoperative imaging technologies can provide optimized specificity in differentiating benign from malignant tissue, then the staging work-up could tolerate a somewhat-diminished preoperative specificity to ensure the highest-possible sensitivity.

Indeed, the synergies between the reconciliation of the interlinked conundrums of sensitivity and specificity could be substantial. Of course, ways to facilitate the use of existing techniques for intraoperative guidance need to be explored further. Even so, the time has arrived for the widespread incorporation of real-time intraoperative imaging guidance into the management of colon cancer.

REFERENCES

1. Ries LAG, Melbert D, Krapcho M, et al. SEER cancer statistics review, 1975-2005. Bethesda (MD): U.S. National Institutes of Health, National Cancer Institute; 2008.

2. Siegel RL, Miller KD, Fedewa SA, et al. Colorectal cancer statistics, 2017. CA Cancer J Clin 2017;67(3):177–93.

3. Siegel RL, Miller KD, Jemal A. Cancer Statistics, 2017. CA Cancer J Clin 2017; 67(1):7–30.

4. Surveillance, epidemiology and end results program of the National Cancer Institute. 2017. Available at: https://seer.cancer.gov/statfacts/html/colorect. html. Accessed October 15, 2017.

5. Benson AB 3rd, Venook AP, Cederquist L, et al. Colon cancer, version 1.2017, NCCN clinical practice guidelines in oncology. J Natl Compr Canc Netw 2017;15(3):370–98.

6. Kijima S, Sasaki T, Nagata K, et al. Preoperative evaluation of colorectal cancer using CT colonography, MRI, and PET/CT. World J Gastroenterol 2014;20(45): 16964–75.

7. Van Cutsem E, Verheul HM, Flamen P, et al. Imaging in colorectal cancer: progress and challenges for the clinicians. Cancers (Basel) 2016;8(9) [pii:E81].

8. Delbeke D, Vitola JV, Sandler MP, et al. Staging recurrent metastatic colorectal carcinoma with PET. J Nucl Med 1997;38(8):1196–201.

9. Wiering B, Krabbe PF, Jager GJ, et al. The impact of fluor-18-deoxyglucose-positron emission tomography in the management of colorectal liver metastases. Cancer 2005;104(12):2658–70.

10. Killeen S, Mannion M, Devaney A, et al. Complete mesocolic resection and extended lymphadenectomy for colon cancer: a systematic review. Colorectal Dis 2014;16(8):577–94.

11. Ito K, Govindarajan A, Ito H, et al. Surgical treatment of hepatic colorectal metastasis: evolving role in the setting of improving systemic therapies and ablative treatments in the 21st century. Cancer J 2010;16(2):103–10.

12. Koppe MJ, Boerman OC, Oyen WJ, et al. Peritoneal carcinomatosis of colorectal origin: incidence and current treatment strategies. Ann Surg 2006;243(2): 212–22.

13. Carloss H, Huang B, Cohen A, et al. The impact of number of lymph nodes removed on five-year survival in stage II colon and rectal cancer. J Ky Med Assoc 2004;102(8):345–7.

14. Goldstein NS. Lymph node recoveries from 2427 pT3 colorectal resection specimens spanning 45 years: recommendations for a minimum number of recovered lymph nodes based on predictive probabilities. Am J Surg Pathol 2002; 26(2):179–89.

15. Hohenberger W, Weber K, Matzel K, et al. Standardized surgery for colonic cancer: complete mesocolic excision and central ligation–technical notes and outcome. Colorectal Dis 2009;11(4):354–64 [discussion: 364–5].

16. Swanson RS, Compton CC, Stewart AK, et al. The prognosis of T3N0 colon cancer is dependent on the number of lymph nodes examined. Ann Surg Oncol 2003;10(1):65–71.

17. Bokey EL, Chapuis PH, Dent OF, et al. Surgical technique and survival in patients having a curative resection for colon cancer. Dis Colon Rectum 2003; 46(7):860–6.

18. Moran B, Cunningham C, Singh T, et al. Association of Coloproctology of Great Britain & Ireland (ACPGBI): guidelines for the management of cancer of the colon, rectum and anus (2017) - surgical management. Colorectal Dis 2017; 19(Suppl 1):18–36.

19. Vogel JD, Eskicioglu C, Weiser MR, et al. The American Society of Colon and Rectal Surgeons clinical practice guidelines for the treatment of colon cancer. Dis Colon Rectum 2017;60(10):999–1017.

20. Watanabe T, Muro K, Ajioka Y, et al. Japanese Society for Cancer of the Colon and Rectum (JSCCR) guidelines 2016 for the treatment of colorectal cancer. Int J Clin Oncol 2017. [Epub ahead of print].

21. Chang GJ, Rodriguez-Bigas MA, Skibber JM, et al. Lymph node evaluation and survival after curative resection of colon cancer: systematic review. J Natl Cancer Inst 2007;99(6):433–41.

22. Nissan A, Protic M, Bilchik AJ, et al. United States Military Cancer Institute Clinical Trials Group (USMCI GI-01) randomized controlled trial comparing targeted nodal assessment and ultrastaging with standard pathological evaluation for colon cancer. Ann Surg 2012;256(3):412–27.

23. Selzner M, Hany TF, Wildbrett P, et al. Does the novel PET/CT imaging modality impact on the treatment of patients with metastatic colorectal cancer of the liver? Ann Surg 2004;240(6):1027–34 [discussion:1035–6].

24. Niekel MC, Bipat S, Stoker J. Diagnostic imaging of colorectal liver metastases with CT, MR imaging, FDG PET, and/or FDG PET/CT: a meta-analysis of prospective studies including patients who have not previously undergone treatment. Radiology 2010;257(3):674–84.

25. Engelmann BE, Loft A, Kjaer A, et al. Positron emission tomography/computed tomography for optimized colon cancer staging and follow up. Scand J Gastroenterol 2014;49(2):191–201.

26. Lee JH, Lee MR. Positron emission tomography/computed tomography in the staging of colon cancer. Ann Coloproctol 2014;30(1):23–7.

27. Hough DM, Malone DE, Rawlinson J, et al. Colon cancer detection: an algorithm using endoscopy and barium enema. Clin Radiol 1994;49(3):170–5.

28. Balthazar EJ, Megibow AJ, Hulnick D, et al. Carcinoma of the colon: detection and preoperative staging by CT. AJR Am J Roentgenol 1988;150(2): 301–6.
29. Johnson CD, Carlson HC, Taylor WF, et al. Barium enemas of carcinoma of the colon: sensitivity of double- and single-contrast studies. AJR Am J Roentgenol 1983;140(6):1143–9.
30. Limberg B. Diagnosis of large bowel tumours by colonic sonography. Lancet 1990;335(8682):144–6.
31. Malmstrom ML, Gogenur I, Riis LB, et al. Endoscopic ultrasonography and computed tomography scanning for preoperative staging of colonic cancer. Int J Colorectal Dis 2017;32(6):813–20.
32. Kulig J, Popiela T, Klek S, et al. Intraoperative ultrasonography in detecting and assessment of colorectal liver metastases. Scand J Surg 2007;96(1):51–5.
33. Ong KO, Leen E. Radiological staging of colorectal liver metastases. Surg Oncol 2007;16(1):7–14.
34. Rafaelsen SR, Jakobsen A. Contrast-enhanced ultrasound vs multidetector-computed tomography for detecting liver metastases in colorectal cancer: a prospective, blinded, patient-by-patient analysis. Colorectal Dis 2011;13(4): 420–5.
35. Floriani I, Torri V, Rulli E, et al. Performance of imaging modalities in diagnosis of liver metastases from colorectal cancer: a systematic review and meta-analysis. J Magn Reson Imaging 2010;31(1):19–31.
36. Horton KM, Abrams RA, Fishman EK. Spiral CT of colon cancer: imaging features and role in management. Radiographics 2000;20(2):419–30.
37. Nerad E, Lahaye MJ, Maas M, et al. Diagnostic accuracy of CT for local staging of colon cancer: a systematic review and meta-analysis. AJR Am J Roentgenol 2016;207(5):984–95.
38. Leufkens AM, van den Bosch MA, van Leeuwen MS, et al. Diagnostic accuracy of computed tomography for colon cancer staging: a systematic review. Scand J Gastroenterol 2011;46(7–8):887–94.
39. Dighe S, Purkayastha S, Swift I, et al. Diagnostic precision of CT in local staging of colon cancers: a meta-analysis. Clin Radiol 2010;65(9):708–19.
40. Ginat DT, Gupta R. Advances in computed tomography imaging technology. Annu Rev Biomed Eng 2014;16:431–53.
41. Runge VM, Marquez H, Andreisek G, et al. Recent technological advances in computed tomography and the clinical impact therein. Invest Radiol 2015; 50(2):119–27.
42. Akgul O, Cetinkaya E, Ersoz S, et al. Role of surgery in colorectal cancer liver metastases. World J Gastroenterol 2014;20(20):6113–22.
43. Bipat S, van Leeuwen MS, Comans EF, et al. Colorectal liver metastases: CT, MR imaging, and PET for diagnosis–meta-analysis. Radiology 2005;237(1):123–31.
44. Chamadol N, Ninpiethoon T, Bhudhisawasd V, et al. The role of CT scan in preoperative staging of colorectal carcinoma. J Med Assoc Thai 2005;88(12): 1847–53.
45. Zerhouni EA, Rutter C, Hamilton SR, et al. CT and MR imaging in the staging of colorectal carcinoma: report of the radiology diagnostic oncology group II. Radiology 1996;200(2):443–51.
46. Kuszyk BS, Bluemke DA, Urban BA, et al. Portal-phase contrast-enhanced helical CT for the detection of malignant hepatic tumors: sensitivity based on comparison with intraoperative and pathologic findings. AJR Am J Roentgenol 1996; 166(1):91–5.

47. Expert Panel on Gastrointestinal Imaging, Fowler KJ, Kaur H, et al. ACR appropriateness criteria(R) pretreatment staging of colorectal cancer. J Am Coll Radiol 2017;14(5S):S234–244.

48. Briggs RH, Chowdhury FU, Lodge JP, et al. Clinical impact of FDG PET-CT in patients with potentially operable metastatic colorectal cancer. Clin Radiol 2011;66(12):1167–74.

49. Matthews R, Choi M. Clinical utility of positron emission tomography magnetic resonance imaging (PET-MRI) in gastrointestinal cancers. Diagnostics (Basel) 2016;6(3) [pii:E35].

50. Metser U, Even-Sapir E. Increased (18)F-fluorodeoxyglucose uptake in benign, nonphysiologic lesions found on whole-body positron emission tomography/computed tomography (PET/CT): accumulated data from four years of experience with PET/CT. Semin Nucl Med 2007;37(3):206–22.

51. Kantorova I, Lipska L, Belohlavek O, et al. Routine (18)F-FDG PET preoperative staging of colorectal cancer: comparison with conventional staging and its impact on treatment decision making. J Nucl Med 2003;44(11):1784–8.

52. Schussler-Fiorenza CM, Mahvi DM, Niederhuber J, et al. Clinical risk score correlates with yield of PET scan in patients with colorectal hepatic metastases. J Gastrointest Surg 2004;8(2):150–7 [discussion:157–8].

53. Fernandez FG, Drebin JA, Linehan DC, et al. Five-year survival after resection of hepatic metastases from colorectal cancer in patients screened by positron emission tomography with F-18 fluorodeoxyglucose (FDG-PET). Ann Surg 2004;240(3):438–47 [discussion:447–50].

54. Audollent R, Eveno C, Dohan A, et al. Pitfalls and mimickers on (18)F-FDG-PET/CT in peritoneal carcinomatosis from colorectal cancer: An analysis from 37 patients. J Visc Surg 2015;152(5):285–91.

55. Culverwell AD, Scarsbrook AF, Chowdhury FU. False-positive uptake on 2-[(1)(8) F]-fluoro-2-deoxy-D-glucose (FDG) positron-emission tomography/computed tomography (PET/CT) in oncological imaging. Clin Radiol 2011;66(4):366–82.

56. Azhdarinia A, Ghosh P, Ghosh S, et al. Dual-labeling strategies for nuclear and fluorescence molecular imaging: a review and analysis. Mol Imaging Biol 2012; 14(3):261–76.

57. de Boer E, Harlaar NJ, Taruttis A, et al. Optical innovations in surgery. Br J Surg 2015;102(2):e56–72.

58. DeLong JC, Hoffman RM, Bouvet M. Current status and future perspectives of fluorescence-guided surgery for cancer. Expert Rev Anticancer Ther 2016; 16(1):71–81.

59. Koch M, Ntziachristos V. Advancing surgical vision with fluorescence imaging. Annu Rev Med 2016;67:153–64.

60. Liberale G, Bourgeois P, Larsimont D, et al. Indocyanine green fluorescence-guided surgery after IV injection in metastatic colorectal cancer: a systematic review. Eur J Surg Oncol 2017;43(9):1656–67.

61. Orbay H, Bean J, Zhang Y, et al. Intraoperative targeted optical imaging: a guide towards tumor-free margins in cancer surgery. Curr Pharm Biotechnol 2013;14(8):733–42.

62. Rosenthal EL, Warram JM, Bland KI, et al. The status of contemporary image-guided modalities in oncologic surgery. Ann Surg 2015;261(1):46–55.

63. Povoski SP, Hall NC, Martin EW Jr, et al. Multimodality approach of perioperative 18F-FDG PET/CT imaging, intraoperative 18F-FDG handheld gamma probe detection, and intraoperative ultrasound for tumor localization and verification

of resection of all sites of hypermetabolic activity in a case of occult recurrent metastatic melanoma. World J Surg Oncol 2008;6:1.

64. Povoski SP, Hall NC, Murrey DA Jr, et al. Multimodal imaging and detection approach to 18F-FDG-directed surgery for patients with known or suspected malignancies: a comprehensive description of the specific methodology utilized in a single-institution cumulative retrospective experience. World J Surg Oncol 2011;9:152.

65. Povoski SP, Neff RL, Mojzisik CM, et al. A comprehensive overview of radio-guided surgery using gamma detection probe technology. World J Surg Oncol 2009;7:11.

66. Sun D, Bloomston M, Hinkle G, et al. Radioimmunoguided surgery (RIGS), PET/CT image-guided surgery, and fluorescence image-guided surgery: past, present, and future. J Surg Oncol 2007;96(4):297–308.

67. Sarikaya I, Povoski SP, Al-Saif OH, et al. Combined use of preoperative 18F FDG-PET imaging and intraoperative gamma probe detection for accurate assessment of tumor recurrence in patients with colorectal cancer. World J Surg Oncol 2007;5:80.

68. Freeny PC, Marks WM, Ryan JA, et al. Colorectal carcinoma evaluation with CT: preoperative staging and detection of postoperative recurrence. Radiology 1986;158(2):347–53.

69. Thompson WM, Halvorsen RA, Foster WL Jr, et al. Preoperative and postoperative CT staging of rectosigmoid carcinoma. AJR Am J Roentgenol 1986;146(4): 703–10.

70. Chung DJ, Huh KC, Choi WJ, et al. CT colonography using 16-MDCT in the evaluation of colorectal cancer. AJR Am J Roentgenol 2005;184(1):98–103.

71. Holdsworth PJ, Johnston D, Chalmers AG, et al. Endoluminal ultrasound and computed tomography in the staging of rectal cancer. Br J Surg 1988;75(10): 1019–22.

72. Sun CH, Li ZP, Meng QF, et al. Assessment of spiral CT pneumocolon in preoperative colorectal carcinoma. World J Gastroenterol 2005;11(25):3866–70.

73. Keeney G, Jafri SZ, Mezwa DG. Computed tomographic evaluation and staging of cecal carcinoma. Gastrointest Radiol 1989;14(1):65–9.

74. Ashraf K, Ashraf O, Haider Z, et al. Colorectal carcinoma, preoperative evaluation by spiral computed tomography. J Pak Med Assoc 2006;56(4):149–53.

75. Rifkin MD, Ehrlich SM, Marks G. Staging of rectal carcinoma: prospective comparison of endorectal US and CT. Radiology 1989;170(2):319–22.

76. Acunas B, Rozanes I, Acunas G, et al. Preoperative CT staging of colon carcinoma (excluding the recto-sigmoid region). Eur J Radiol 1990;11(2):150–3.

77. Stabile Ianora AA, Moschetta M, Pedote P, et al. Preoperative local staging of colosigmoideal cancer: air versus water multidetector-row CT colonography. Radiol Med 2012;117(2):254–67.

78. Fujita N, Hasegawa T, Kubo K, et al. CT in colon cancer. Rinsho Hoshasen 1990; 35(8):915–21 [in Japanese].

79. Karl RC, Morse SS, Halpert RD, et al. Preoperative evaluation of patients for liver resection. Appropriate CT imaging. Ann Surg 1993;217(3):226–32.

80. Haji A, Ryan S, Bjarnason I, et al. Colonoscopic high frequency mini-probe ultrasound is more accurate than conventional computed tomography in the local staging of colonic cancer. Colorectal Dis 2012;14(8):953–9.

81. McAndrew MR, Saba AK. Efficacy of routine preoperative computed tomography scans in colon cancer. Am Surg 1999;65(3):205–8.

82. Lim M, Hussain Z, Howe A, et al. The oncological outcome after right hemicolectomy and accuracy of CT scan as a preoperative tool for staging in right sided colonic cancers. Colorectal Dis 2013;15(5):536–43.
83. Gazelle GS, Gaa J, Saini S, et al. Staging of colon carcinoma using water enema CT. J Comput Assist Tomogr 1995;19(1):87–91.
84. Lao IH, Chao H, Wang YJ, et al. Computed tomography has low sensitivity for the diagnosis of early colon cancer. Colorectal Dis 2013;15(7):807–11.
85. Okizuka H, Sugimura K, Shinozaki N, et al. Colorectal carcinoma: evaluation with ultrafast CT. Clin Imaging 1995;19(4):247–51.
86. Rollven E, Holm T, Glimelius B, et al. Potentials of high resolution magnetic resonance imaging versus computed tomography for preoperative local staging of colon cancer. Acta Radiol 2013;54(7):722–30.
87. Flor N, Mezzanzanica M, Rigamonti P, et al. Contrast-enhanced computed tomography colonography in preoperative distinction between T1-T2 and T3-T4 staging of colon cancer. Acad Radiol 2013;20(5):590–5.
88. Dux M, Richter GM, Roeren T, et al. Gastrointestinal imaging with hydrosonography and hydro-CT. Rofo 1996;164(5):359–67 [in German].
89. Norgaard A, Dam C, Jakobsen A, et al. Selection of colon cancer patients for neoadjuvant chemotherapy by preoperative CT scan. Scand J Gastroenterol 2014;49(2):202–8.
90. Thoeni RF. Colorectal cancer. Radiologic staging. Radiol Clin N Am 1997;35(2):457–85.
91. Harvey CJ, Amin Z, Hare CM, et al. Helical CT pneumocolon to assess colonic tumors: radiologic-pathologic correlation. AJR Am J Roentgenol 1998;170(6):1439–43.
92. Gomille T, Aleksic M, Ulrich B, et al. [Significance of CT in the detection of regional lymph node metastases in colorectal carcinoma]. Radiologe 1998;38(12):1077–82 [in German].
93. Sibileau E, Ridereau-Zins C, Vanel D, et al. Accuracy of water-enema multidetector computed tomography (WE-MDCT) in colon cancer staging: a prospective study. Abdom Imaging 2014;39(5):941–8.
94. Hundt W, Braunschweig R, Reiser M. Evaluation of spiral CT in staging of colon and rectum carcinoma. Eur Radiol 1999;9(1):78–84.
95. de Vries FE, da Costa DW, van der Mooren K, et al. The value of pre-operative computed tomography scanning for the assessment of lymph node status in patients with colon cancer. Eur J Surg Oncol 2014;40(12):1777–81.
96. Cademartiri F, Luccichenti G, Rossi A, et al. Spiral hydro-CT in the evaluation of colo-sigmoideal cancer. Radiol Med 2002;104(4):295–306.
97. Choi AH, Nelson RA, Schoellhammer HF, et al. Accuracy of computed tomography in nodal staging of colon cancer patients. World J Gastrointest Surg 2015;7(7):116–22.
98. Filippone A, Ambrosini R, Fuschi M, et al. Preoperative T and N staging of colorectal cancer: accuracy of contrast-enhanced multi-detector row CT colonography–initial experience. Radiology 2004;231(1):83–90.
99. Wiegering A, Kunz M, Hussein M, et al. Diagnostic value of preoperative CT scan to stratify colon cancer for neoadjuvant therapy. Int J Colorectal Dis 2015;30(8):1067–73.
100. Chung HW, Chung JB, Park SW, et al. Comparison of hydrocolonic sonograpy accuracy in preoperative staging between colon and rectal cancer. World J Gastroenterol 2004;10(8):1157–61.

101. Stagnitti A, Barchetti F, Barchetti G, et al. Preoperative staging of colorectal cancer using virtual colonoscopy: correlation with surgical results. Eur Rev Med Pharmacol Sci 2015;19(9):1645–51.
102. Elibol FD, Obuz F, Sokmen S, et al. The role of multidetector CT in local staging and evaluation of retroperitoneal surgical margin involvement in colon cancer. Diagn Interv Radiol 2016;22(1):5–12.
103. Singla SC, Kaushal D, Sagoo HS, et al. Comparative analysis of colorectal carcinoma staging using operative, histopathology and computed tomography findings. Int J Appl Basic Med Res 2017;7(1):10–4.
104. Koh FHX, Tan KK, Teo LLS, et al. Prospective comparison between magnetic resonance imaging and computed tomography in colorectal cancer staging. ANZ J Surg 2017. [Epub ahead of print].

Minimally Invasive Surgical Approaches to Colon Cancer

Jean F. Salem, MD, Sriharsha Gummadi, MD, John H. Marks, MD*

KEYWORDS

- Colon cancer • Minimally invasive surgery • Laparoscopic colectomy
- Single incision laparoscopic surgery • Robotic colectomy

KEY POINTS

- Colon cancer remains the most common abdominal visceral malignancy affecting both men and women in America.
- Open colectomy has been the standard of care for colon cancer patients the past 100 years; however, although highly effective, the major trauma associated with it has a significant morbidity rate and represents a large operation for patients to recover from.
- Minimally invasive colon surgery is an option, and surgeons aim to continue to make it simpler, more reproducible, and easier to teach and learn.
- Juxtaposing the current state of minimally invasive colorectal surgery for colon cancer with open surgery offers insights to future directions.

INTRODUCTION

Colon cancer remains the most common abdominal visceral malignancy affecting both men and women in America. It remains one of the top 3 carcinomas for both new diagnosis and mortality in the United States. More than a million Americans are estimated to be living with colon cancer.[1] Over the past several decades, national statistics revealed a reduction in both the incidence and death rates with improved 5-year survival.[1] These outcomes can be attributed in large part to better screening methods but also to advancements in care.

The mainstay treatment of colon cancer patients remains surgery. Open colectomy has been the standard of care for the past 100 years. Although highly effective, the major trauma associated with it has a significant morbidity rate and represents a large operation for patients to recover from. The laparoscopic revolution started in 1987 with the first report of a laparoscopic cholecystectomy. The patient benefits were

Disclosure: The authors have nothing to disclose.
Division of Colorectal Surgery, Lankenau Medical Center, 100 East Lancaster Avenue, Wynnewood, PA 19096, USA
* Corresponding author. Lankenau Medical Center, Medical Science Building, Suite 375, 100 East Lancaster Avenue, Wynnewood, PA 19096.
E-mail address: marksj@mlhs.org

immediately obvious. Patients recover quicker, have less postoperative pain, are in the hospital for shorter periods of time, and are back to their normal quality of life much sooner. Due to the obvious success of laparoscopic cholecystectomy, a flood of intra-abdominal procedures were performed laparoscopically. The first laparoscopic colectomy was performed in November 1991, in the same month by Jacobs and colleagues[2] and by Fowler and White.[3] At that time, based on the experience of adoption of laparoscopic cholecystectomy, the common belief was that more than 70% of colon procedures would be done in a laparoscopic fashion by the mid-1990s. The real challenges with minimally invasive surgery (MIS) in a multiquadrant approach, however, represented serious difficulties for surgeons. On top of this, rather than operating for a benign disease, a majority of colon surgeries were done for cancer and mishaps in this regard could prove fatal to patients. This fear was born from early reports of port site recurrences. Although this ultimately proved a technical issue based on poor operative technique, it resulted in the quick initiation of a moratorium on laparoscopy for colon cancer outside of the trial period. It took more than a decade for these trials to be completed. This significantly retarded the growth of laparoscopic colorectal surgery. To this day, the adoption of minimally invasive colorectal surgery, although improving, has remained low. In 2007, 3 years after the report of the major Clinical Outcomes of Surgical Therapy (COST) trial, still less than 15% of elective colectomies were performed laparoscopically in the United States.[4] The last largely published data in 2012 showed the best adoption at 59%, but in many areas it is still in the 40% range.[5] In contrast, in the authors' unit, 95% of the cases are performed in a minimally invasive fashion.

The learning curve for laparoscopic colectomy remains steep. The need to retract multiple organs, identify complex anatomy, and control large vessels makes the operation a difficult one. As understanding of the problems and challenges of laparoscopic colectomy have improved, however, the ability to teach this has also improved. A focus on the key principles of the steps of the operation, the anatomy, and the ability to retract and expose proper tissue planes has facilitated the performance and adoption of this approach. This should make minimally invasive colon surgery simpler, more reproducible, and easier to teach and learn. The purpose of this review is to describe the current state of minimally invasive colorectal surgery for colon cancer and to compare this with open surgery and offer insights to future directions.

EVOLUTION OF MINIMALLY INVASIVE SURGICAL TECHNIQUES IN COLON CANCER

Over the past 25 years, new options and challenges have presented themselves to general and colorectal surgeons in addressing colon cancer in a minimally invasive fashion. In the early 1990s, multiport laparoscopic colectomy was introduced. Advantages of MIS were realized and patients had shorter hospital stays, less postoperative pain, and lower infection rates. The obvious decrease in abdominal wall trauma led to improved patient recovery. In the mid-2000s, single port surgery was first introduced. As an offshoot notes, technology improved to allow for development of an operation with minimal visible scar and parietal trauma. The first single-incision laparoscopic surgery (SILS) colectomy was performed in 2008 by Geisler and colleagues at the Cleveland Clinic.[6] Their experience suggested that this was safe and could be performed with improved cosmesis, pain control, and recovery.[6,7] The challenge of this approach was due to all the instrumentation run through the abdominal incision in parallel, causing a great number of collisions at the operative field. The development of both flexible-tip laparoscopes and angled instrumentation addressed these problems, as shown in many studies, with excellent results. A major criticism for this technique, however, came from the fact that it is more technically challenging and it has never been shown in any trials to offer any real advantages. Nonetheless, the cosmetic advantages are readily apparent. Although feasible in proper hands, widespread application of this approach has been slow. This leads to the next iteration of MIS for treatment of colon cancer in the form of robotic surgery.

The first report of robotic-assisted colectomy was published in 2002.[8] The development of a multiquadrant operating robot in the form of the da Vinci Xi system (Intuitive Surgical, Sunnyvale, CA, USA) in 2014 has ushered in a wave of adoption of a robotic approach. There has been a multitude of criticisms about robotic surgery adding cost and time to operations without demonstrating clear oncologic and clinical benefits. The major counterargument has been that, to date, even 25 years after the first performance of the laparoscopic colectomy, still less than 50% of cases are done in a minimally invasive fashion in America.

The goal of this article is to outline the methods of minimally invasive approach, in one of these forms, so it can be better offered to more colon cancer patients in the United States and around the world.

PATIENT SELECTION IN MINIMALLY INVASIVE SURGERY FOR COLON CANCER

Any operation with good outcomes is dependent on careful patient selection. Historic contraindications to a minimally invasive approach included elderly patients, high-risk patients, patients with multiple abdominal operations, patients who need complex surgery, and those with serious comorbidities. All these factors can add a level of difficulty to the technical performance of an operation and are associated with increased morbidity and mortality rates. Clearly none of these is a hard contraindication but rather a relative contraindication. A surgeon's main goal is and must always be performance of the operation in as safe and perfect a fashion as possible. If this can be done in a minimally invasive fashion, with a single-port or multiport laparoscopic approach or a robotic approach, all the better for patients. Of paramount importance, however, is that no core principles of the oncologic operation should be sacrificed to accomplish the operation in a minimally invasive fashion. To this end, in the authors' hands, the only 2 absolute contraindications to laparoscopic surgery are (1) a tumor of a large enough size that the extraction site to remove it would be large enough to perform the entirety of the operation and (2) a high-grade large bowel obstruction that leads to a reduced intraabdominal domain. The impaired visibility coupled with the friability of the tissue in the setting of a cancer make a MIS approach in this setting ill advised.

Patients with major comorbidities are often denied laparoscopic colorectal resection because they are at a "high risk to tolerate it." Concerns regarding abdominal insufflation and the possibility of extended operative time cause surgeons to shy away from this approach. Paradoxically, these patients have the most to gain from a minimally invasive approach. Small incisions are related to less need for narcotics, limited respiratory effort, and shorter intubation time. The authors published data regarding this high-risk patient population to conclude that in an experienced hand, laparoscopic colorectal surgery can be performed safer in high-risk surgical patients.[9] The most dramatic results found were in laparoscopic resections in groups 80 years of age or older with no mortality and a decreased length of stay to 6 days.[9] The better-than-expected outcomes in this patient population reinforce the benefits of MIS for this patient group and argue against using a parameter of exclusion based on age, morbid obesity, and American Society of Anesthesiologists classifications to offer complex laparoscopic procedures to patients. This decision has to be fluid, however, based on surgeons' honest appraisal of both their skill set and a patient's tolerance of any setback.

ADVANTAGES OF MINIMALLY INVASIVE SURGERY IN COLON CANCER

A multitude of studies have been conducted in looking at open compared with laparoscopic colon cancer resection. This is probably the most intensely studied procedure ever scrutinized. In none of these studies has there ever been shown to be a negative impact for laparoscopic surgery. The benefits have ranged from decreased length of stay, smaller incisions, less narcotic usage, less blood loss, lower transfusion rates, and improved pulmonary function after surgery. Although short-term advantages have been shown, there have not been demonstrated long-term differences in oncologic outcomes.

In 2002, Lacy and colleagues[10] randomized patients with adenocarcinoma undergoing colonic resection to open surgery and laparoscopic surgery. They showed a decreased number of morbidities (31 vs 12; P = .001; open vs laparoscopic), decreased time until detection of peristalsis (55 hours vs 36 hours; P = .001; open vs laparoscopic), and a shorter hospital stay (7.9 days vs 5.2 days; open vs laparoscopic; P = .005).[10]

The 2004 COST randomized 872 patients with adenocarcinoma of the colon to open colectomy or laparoscopic colectomy and reported their results in *The New England Journal of Medicine*.[11] Perioperative recovery was faster in the laparoscopic group as reflected by a shorter hospital stay (5.6 vs 6.4; $P<.001$), less postoperative pain, and briefer use of narcotics.[11]

Similarly, the 2005 Colon Cancer Laparoscopic or Open Resection (COLOR) trial, randomized 627 patients to laparoscopic colectomy and 621 patients to open colectomy.[12] Again, they noted that patients assigned to laparoscopic resection had earlier recovery of bowel function, need for fewer analgesics, and shorter hospital stay compared with those assigned to open resection.[12] They also found a decreased in intraoperative blood loss in the laparoscopic group (175 mL vs 100 mL; $P<.0001$; open vs laparoscopic).

As discussed previously, several smaller studies have also shown a variety other benefits of laparoscopic surgery. Schwenk and colleagues[13] showed that pulmonary function, as measured by recovery of forced vital capacity and forced expiratory volume in 1 second, is less impaired by laparoscopic surgery.

It has also been postulated that decreased trauma from laparoscopic surgery results in less immune suppression of colon cancer patients and potentially improved oncologic outcome. The most common parallel has been the worse outcome in colon cancer patients who have been transfused. This has been postulated to be due to immune suppression by transfusion. It has been suggested that survival could be improved if the immunosuppression from the trauma from surgery could be reduced.[14] Larry Whelan's group has demonstrated lower interleukin 6 levels after laparoscopic colorectal resection compared with open conventional surgery.[15] Although Lacy's group showed an improved survival in stage III colon cancer patients who had laparoscopic resection, this has not been shown in any of the larger multi-institutional studies.[10] As data and experience accrue with the MIS procedures, it is unquestionable that this approach will continue to expand to treat colon cancer. The complexity of the operations and the steep learning curve are only temporary hurdles and are being addressed to help the practicing and learning surgeons. The authors provide a well-developed and reproducible approach for tackling the challenges of multiquadrant minimally invasive colon cancer surgery.

RIGHT COLON CANCER
Surgical Techniques

Laparoscopic right colectomy
The patient is put in a split leg supine or modified lithotomy position. The patient is secured to the table with chest wrap. No supports are ever placed above the shoulders,

to avoid brachial plexus injury. The patient has to be securely attached to the table because Trendelenburg is often used to retract the bowel out of the way. The room is set up with the surgeon and assistant standing to the patient's left side and the scrub nurse in-between the patient's legs. The monitor is placed on the patient's right side.

The authors advocate a 3-trocar technique with a 12-mm umbilical port, 5-mm port at the left lower quadrant 2 fingerbreadths medial to the left anterior superior iliac spine, and a third 5-mm port to the left midline at the level of the infraumbilical fat mound. The 12-mm port is then expanded and used as the wound extraction site and a place for an extracorporeal anastomosis. Conversely if a patient has a diastasis or an umbilical hernia, in an effort to avoid a hernia in this region, a 5-mm port is placed supraumbilically and a 5-mm camera is used. In this instance, the specimen is extracted through a muscle-splitting incision in the right upper quadrant and the anastomosis is performed there.

The procedure begins once ports are in place by a thorough exploration of the abdomen to rule out metastatic disease. The liver, the peritoneal cavity, and the pelvis are inspected to make sure there is no metastasis or carcinomatosis. The operation is generally performed with the table in a flat position. Sometimes there is a gentle Trendelenburg and the left side is tilted slightly down to allow the small bowel to be passed out of the way; however, a more extreme Trendelenburg places the small bowel into the operative field and more steep left side down causes the ascending colon to sometimes fall toward the camera and obscure the view. The first step is positioning of the small bowel into the patient's left side to the left of the superior mesenteric artery (SMA). The greater omentum is then lifted up and over the transverse colon. The operative field is then fully visualized.

The second step is identification and ligation of the ileocolic artery. The best way to identify the artery is to lift up on the cecum and retract it to the right. This puts the ileocolic artery on stretch and reliably allows its identification. The ileocolic artery is then dissected free and the retroperitoneal embryologic fusion plane between the mesentery of the transverse and ascending colon and the retroperitoneum identified. This retroperitoneum is swept posteriorly. Immediately cephalad to the ileocolic artery there is the bare area of the mesentery of the ascending colon and immediately behind this is the third portion of the duodenum. Care must be taken not to injure the duodenum, because it is close here while dissecting out the vessels. The ileocolic artery is then transected leaving 1 cm to 2 cm remnant so that if any bleeding is encountered, the vessel can be readily grasped and controlled without risk of endangering the SMA. The authors generally transect the vessels with LigaSure (Medtronic, Minneapolis, MN, USA); however, this can be done with any form of vessel sealer, clip, or stapler. Endo-Tie (Ethicon, Bridgewater, NJ, USA) can be placed on the vessel if needed. The authors do not do this routinely except in patients with high risk of arterial calcification. Once the vessel is transected, the dissection is taken out in a medial-to-lateral fashion beneath the retroperitoneum out to the line of Toldt and cephalad up over the duodenum and the head of the pancreas to the root of the mesentery. The greater omentum is then taken off of the transverse colon and the dissection is met from inferiorly to superiorly. The colon is then transected with a GIA (Medtronic, Minneapolis, MN, USA) 60 blue load stapler. The mesentery of the ileum is transected with some form of energy sealing device and the ileum is transected with a GIA blue load stapler. At this point, the lateral attachment along the line of Toldt is then fully mobilized. It is important to make sure that the mesentery and loops of the small bowel are not adhering in the pelvis because this can greatly impede the ability to do a tension-free ileocolic anastomosis. It is better to discover and address these not infrequently encountered adhesions, before attempting to exteriorize the bowel. To assess this, it is helpful at this point to put the patient in a steep Trendelenburg and the left side down and take the mesenteric veil of the ileum off the right pelvic brim. Once this is done, the patient is ready for anastomosis. The anastomosis can be performed in an extracorporeal fashion. This should always be done through a wound protector. Care should be taken to make sure the bowel is not twisted. It is the author's habit to always put a seromuscular stitch between the ileum to the transverse colon to assure proper orientation. Earlier in his career, the author John H. Marks preferred to simply mobilize the mesentery, take the blood supply intracorporeally but transect the bowel proximally, and distally extracorporeally with stapler. The authors now find it easier to do this intracorporeally as the authors had become more comfortable. Once the anastomosis is performed, it is mandatory to go back in abdominally, reassess matters, confirm that there is no twisting of the bowel or the mesentery, irrigate the abdomen, and confirm there is no bleeding.

Laparoscopic right colectomy with intracorporeal anastomosis was first popularized by Morris Franklin[16] and is readily accomplishable. An enterotomy and colotomy are made in the antimesenteric corner and an Endo GIA 60 load stapler is fired from the right upper quadrant, with the resultant defect closed either with a stapler or running sutures. Although typically challenging initially, this can be done safely and reproducibly. The major benefit of this approach is in patients with morbid obesity and it can result in fewer postoperative complications and surgical site infections as well as the ability to extract the specimen anywhere in the abdomen as the surgeon chooses.[17]

Single-incision surgery for right colon cancer

Single-incision surgery rapidly evolved since its first introduction in 2008.[7] It can be performed using a series of available access devices (not discussed in this article). The operative steps are identical to those of multiport laparoscopic right colectomy. Several studies on SILS right hemicolectomy were published, with postoperative cosmesis reported as the most apparent benefit.[7,18] Other reported benefits, including low morbidity rates and reduced incisional pain, have been suggested[19] but not shown in multi-institutional trials. In a case-match study the authors performed, the major difference demonstrated was that of decreased blood loss compared with multiport laparoscopic surgery.[20] Although statistically significant, the small volume difference probably has little clinical relevance. It is the authors' opinion that the major difference is that of cosmesis.

Robotic right colectomy

The major argument for incorporating robotics for a right colectomy has to do with the facility of intracorporeal anastomosis. The proposed benefit and ease of suturing robotically have increased its application in this field. In a multicenter study, Trastulli and colleagues[21] showed that robotic right colectomy with intracorporeal anastomosis (RRCIA) had better recovery outcomes, such as shorter length of hospital stay compared with laparoscopic right colectomy with extracorporeal anastomosis. Compared with laparoscopic right colectomy with intracorporeal anastomosis, RRCIA had a shorter time to first flatus. This has never been shown in large multi-institutional studies, however, and although theoretically beneficial in the hands of some surgeons, it is unlikely to show an advantage over expert laparoscopic surgeons. That said, the proposed use of the robot to lower the barrier of adoption represents a major potential benefit of this approach.

Extent of Resection

The extent of lymphadenectomy during laparoscopic right colectomy can affect the oncological outcome. The principle of complete mesocolic excision (CME), first introduced in the West in 2008, has been gradually accepted and increasingly applied by colorectal surgeons.[22] The main differences between the classic and CME dissection include the extent of lymphadenectomy (D2 vs D3) and whether or not to dissect the lymphoadipose tissues at the root of the mesocolon, which cover the anterior surface of the SMA and superior mesenteric vein, and the tissues surrounding the root of the middle colic artery. The technique is based on the principle that dissection in the mesocolic plane produces an intact fascial-lined specimen, which contains all the blood vessels and lymphatics through which the tumor may disseminate. This idea is an extrapolation of the total mesorectal excision principle.

Compared with D2 dissection, however, laparoscopic CME imposes a longer learning curve for surgeons and a higher surgery-related risk for patients due to the complicated surgical anatomy involved in the laparoscopic approach, especially the dissection in the vicinity of the superior mesenteric vessels. Neither the National Comprehensive Cancer Network guidelines nor the European Society for Medical Oncology guidelines have clearly defined the extent of lymphadenectomy of the radical right hemicolectomy.

Retrospective studies from Erlangen, Germany, and Leeds, United Kingdom, suggested a survival benefit of 7% to 15% for those adhering to a CME with central ligation for colon cancer.[23,24] In a recent retrospective population study from Denmark, 364 patients who underwent CME were compared with 1031 patients who were treated with non-CME colectomies.[25] For all patients, the 4-year disease-free survival rate was 85.5% after CME and 75.9% after non-CME surgery ($P = .001$). Overall survival, however, was not significantly higher in the CME group. To date there are no published prospective randomized studies to suggest the superiority of the CME. The Radical Extent of lympadenectomy: D2 dissection versus complete mesocolic excision of LAparoscopic Right Colectomy for right-sided colon cancer (RELARC) trial is under way comparing in a randomized trial D2 and CME for right colon cancer.[26] Although this is an area to remain attuned to, the widespread adoption of this approach is not advocated as yet.

LEFT COLON CANCER
Surgical Techniques

Multiport laparoscopic left colectomy
Laparoscopic left colectomy is carried out in a 3-trochar technique. For optimal organization, the operation is performed in a systematic 9-step format (**Box 1**). Port positions are shown in **Fig. 1**.

After full exploration of the abdominal cavity to make sure there is no evidence of metastatic disease or carcinomatosis, the operation is started.

Releasing the splenic flexure The splenic flexure is released with the patient in reverse Trendelenburg right side down. This is done as the first step of the operation to avoid the need to reposition the table and the small bowel more than 1 time. With the patient in moderate reverse Trendelenburg, full right side down, the authors place the camera in the number 1 port, a Babcock in the number 2 port, and the LigaSure vessel sealer in the number 3 port.

The left hand in port 2 is used to lift up the gastrocolic ligament. Gravity pulls the transverse colon down. A vessel sealer is used to transect the gastrocolic ligament and enter into the lesser sac. The dissection is taken to the splenic flexure where the upper portion of the line of Toldt is incised. The upper portion of the descending colon is then pulled medially (through the left hand in the number 2 port) and the attachments of the colon and descending mesentery to the retroperitoneum are mobilized. The vessel sealer is then switched to the left hand, through the number 2 port, and the right

> **Box 1**
> **Nine steps of left colectomy**
>
> 1. Splenic flexure mobilization
> 2. Positioning of small bowel
> 3. Dissection of IMA/IMV
> 4. Mobilization of left colon
> 5. Transection of the mesorectum
> 6. Transection of the rectum
> 7. Exteriorization of the specimen
> 8. Anastomosis
> 9. Closing

hand, in the number 3 port, is used to retract the mesentery to the descending colon toward the right hip. The mesentery of the descending colon is incised 1 cm inferior to the inferior border of the pancreas and once this is incised, the embryologic fusion plane is entered and the mesentery of the colon is lifted off the retroperitoneum. Care must be taken here to avoid going too lateral toward the colon and injuring the blood vessel within the mesentery, because the entirety of the blood supply to the left colon is coming off the left branch of the middle colic once the inferior mesenteric artery (IMA)is taken. Once the mesentery has been fully mobilized, step 1 is completed.

Positioning the small bowel The patient is then put in steep Trendelenburg right side down. The greater omentum is lifted up over the transverse colon. The small bowel is swept out of the pelvis. The small bowel in the area above the inferior mesenteric vein (IMV) is swept to the right upper quadrant. If necessary, additional ports can be placed to retract the small bowel out of the way. This is generally not necessary.

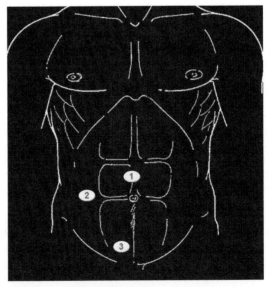

Fig. 1. Port positions for laparoscopic left colectomy.

Transection of the inferior mesenteric artery and the inferior mesenteric vein The camera is changed to the 10-mm scope and is moved to the number 2 port. The left hand is used to retract the sigmoid colon and to put the Gruber ligament on stretch. The sacral promontory is identified and incised. The retroperitoneum is opened 3 cm down into the pelvis and superiorly to the duodenojejunal junction. The hypogastric nerves are identified and swept posteriorly. This allows the proper plane between the retroperitoneum and mesentery to be identified, while simultaneously protecting the nerves and leading to rapid identification of the left ureter. This is generally done inferior to the IMA. Sometimes it is necessary, however, to go above the IMA to find the ureter in a cephalad fashion. Dissecting more fully underneath the IMV, sweeping the retroperitoneum down, and carrying the dissection from superior and inferior to the IMA to create an M-shaped sign (**Fig. 2**), a safe dissection is assured. The IMA is then transected with the vessel sealer. If a patient has bleeding, calcification of vessels, or atherosclerotic disease or is a smoker or a diabetic, the authors also place an Endo-Tie. Otherwise, the vessel sealer serves well enough as it is. The authors then transect the IMV with the vessel sealer. That said, control of the major vessels can be achieved in any number of ways: tying, clipping, and stapling as well as using an energy device.

Mobilization of the colon The dissection that has been carried out mediolaterally is entered by incising the line of Toldt and then fully mobilizing the colon up to the splenic flexure. This is generally the rapidest step in the dissection and is an ideal portion of the operation to start training less experienced assistants.

Transection of the mesorectum The authors incise the right and left perirectal sulcus, dissect the posterior wall of the rectum, and then transect the mesorectum with the vessel sealer, making sure not to corkscrew the mesentery. This means that the mesorectum is scored and transected at the same height on the right and left side of the mesorectum. Once this is done, the rectum is irrigated.

Transection of the rectum Transection of the rectum is done through the number 3 port, taking great care to transect perpendicular to the axis of the rectum. After the first firing of the Endo GIA purple load stapler (some may prefer a blue or green load stapler), the cut edge is retracted up to the left shoulder creating a little bit of a V-shape

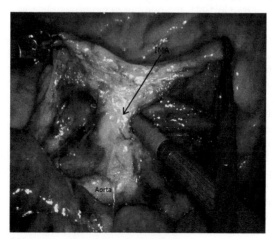

Fig. 2. Dissection of the IMA creating an M-shaped sign.

and then the rectum is transected with a second firing of the GIA stapler. In general, this is accomplished in 2 staplings.

Exteriorization of the specimen Exteriorization of the specimen is done by desufflating the abdomen and always using a wound protector. The specimen is passed from the left hand and grasped from the number 1 port by a Babcock through the wound protector. The specimen is exteriorized. The mesentery is stepped-up to the sigmoido-colic junction and the colon is transected. A purse-string is then placed. This is either done with 2-0 polydioxanone suture or an automatic purse-string. The EEA anvil is then inserted. In general, the authors use an EEA28 or EEA29 (Medtronic, Minneapolis, MN, USA) anvil. A larger diameter anvil is often not well accepted through the anal canal. Conversely, a EEA 25 anvil stapler is also not used, because this generally indicates a technical problem—the dissection not being low enough into the rectum or having the anastomosis in the rectosigmoid—or problems with spasm of the descending colon. Once the anvil is placed, gowns and gloves are changed and the specimen is dropped back into the abdominal cavity.

The anastomosis The abdomen is reinsufflated under direct vision. The EEA stapler is inserted through the anus and brought out generally immediately posterior to the staple line. The anvil is brought down with the left and right hands in ports 1 and 3, making sure the bowel is properly oriented and the mesentery is not twisted. The bowel is mated and closed and the line of the taeniae coli is inspected to make sure it is straight. The authors also inspect the mesentery to make sure there is no small bowel hernia underneath it. If using indocyanine green, this is the time the authors inject it and check for good vascularization. Once this is done, the stapler is closed and fired. Both donuts are inspected to make sure they are intact. An air leak test is routinely done to make sure there is no leak. This having been completed, the operation is concluded. The abdomen is irrigated and aspirated. The abdomen is closed.

Closing At this point, generally there is a muscle-splitting incision in the right lower quadrant where the specimen has been removed. This is closed with no. 1 polydioxanone suture. The single 12 mm port is closed with the 1-0 Vicryl. The skin is primary closed Vicryl and Steri-Strips are applied.

Hand-assisted laparoscopic left colectomy

Since it was first reported in 1991, the number of laparoscopic colectomy procedures remained low due to the technical challenges and the long steep learning curve of the new procedure. To overcome such difficulties, a surgical alternative in the form of hand-assisted laparoscopic colectomy (HALC) was introduced. It allows introduction of a surgeon's nondominant hand into the abdomen through a special hand port while maintaining pneumoperitoneum. A hand inside the abdomen helps to restore the tactile sensation, which is lacking in laparoscopic surgery, and allows safe finger dissection and retraction. Furthermore, in laparoscopic colonic resection, an incision is needed at the end of the operation to retrieve the specimen; such an incision may well be used at the beginning of the operation.

Studies showed that HALC has shorter operative time, lower conversion rate, and comparable complication rate and length of hospital stay.[27,28] Long-term complications of HALC, however, have been the center of recent debate. It has been shown that HALC increases the risk of postoperative ileus and development of intra-abdominal adhesions with future risk of small bowel obstruction.[29] Originally offered as a bridge to fully laparoscopic surgery, HALC, for most surgeons who have adopted it, has been an endpoint. Although reasonable outcomes have been reported, the authors advise surgeons to invest the time and mental energy in becoming fully proficient in purely laparoscopic approaches.

Single-incision laparoscopic left colectomy

SILS left colectomy is generally carried out in a similar order of steps. The port is placed in the umbilical area using a flexible-tip endoscope. This allows the surgeon to carry out the operation with straight graspers. If there is a periumbilical hernia or diastasis recti, the incision is made in a muscle-sparing fashion in the right lower quadrant and this becomes the extraction site. This avoids potential hernia sites.

Although there are fewer data on SILS left colectomy than right colectomy, the authors have found it highly accomplishable and easily extrapolate from a 3-trochar multiport laparoscopic approach. The authors pulled data comparing SILS and multiport laparoscopic surgery on 190 patients[20] and found that for left colectomies, SILS had less blood loss and smaller incisions and surprisingly was quicker than a multiport laparoscopic case.

The SILS is a safe and oncologically adequate procedure.[30] It provides a cosmetic benefit to patients It remains to be seen over a large series if this holds true for benefits of blood loss and time of surgery. The ultimate role for this approach in a time when full-spread laparoscopic surgery is not used for a left colectomy in more than 50% of patients raises questions as to what the future of this approach will be. Although the fewer incisions made to perform an operation safely is of benefit to patients, this approach may or may not be seen widespread in the future.

Robotic left colectomy

As discussed previously, the robot has been postulated as a mechanism to overcome limitations of laparoscopic surgery. It has been postulated that use of this technology will improve adoption rates and push MIS to greater than 50% across the United States. That said, the real goal should be an MIS rate in colorectal cancer in the 80% to 90% range.

The introduction of the daVinci Xi robot launched the era of multiquadrant robotic surgery. The improved docking and movability of the equipment has led to increased utilization of this technology. Additionally, as new robotic systems are poised to come into the operating room in the next 12 months to 24 months, it is safe to assume that utilization of robotics for MIS will continue to climb. A recent meta-analysis showed that in comparison with laparoscopic surgery, robotic colorectal surgery has faster recovery of bowel function, a shorter hospital stay, less blood loss, and lower rates of both overall postoperative complications and wound infections.[31] Although interesting information, it remains to be seen in any trial if there is any statistically significant benefit. Intellectually, it seems unlikely that there would be a marked difference in wound infections or length of hospital stay if both procedures are carried out by expert surgeons. It is the authors' opinion that the major benefit for robotic surgery will be in improving the quality of surgery for surgeons who either are not performing laparoscopic surgery to date or are having challenges in doing laparoscopic surgery.

The authors believe the natural evolution of this would be a robotic single-port surgery. The authors recently published the first cadaveric feasibility study of a robotic transanal surgery using a next-generation single-port system.[32] The authors should first perform, however, a definite feasibility study of transanal surgery using the new-generation single-port system. It is the authors' belief that once this system is available on the market, this generation of robots will overcome many of the challenges of single-port surgery and, combined with robotic surgery, usher in a new, even less invasive approach for left-sided colon cancers.

Special Considerations

Splenic flexure mobilization can be accomplished via 3 different approaches: inframesocolic, supramesocolic and lateral to medial.

Inframesocolic release of the splenic flexure is mainly used in robotic cases. It is an extension of the dissection cephalad after taking the IMV. Using blunt and sharp dissection, the plane underneath the mesentery of the transverse colon is entered above the pancreas, with care not to come beneath the pancreas. Having entered the lesser sac from below, the greater omentum is taken off of the transverse colon, in a fashion to assure adequate length. The remaining of the retroperitoneal attachments are incised, taking care not to injure the pancreas. This method is practical in robotic cases because it does not require any changes in patient position or docking of the robot.

The supramesocolic approach is used mostly in laparoscopic cases. The dissection starts medially by dissecting the gastrocolic ligament and entering the lesser sac. The dissection continues from a medial to lateral approach by taking all the retroperitoneal and splenic attachments.

The lateral-to-medial approach is rarely used in MIS. It is mostly used in open colectomies.

OUTCOMES

As discussed previously, concerns with obtaining an adequate oncologic resection historically served as a barrier to the early adoption of minimally invasive techniques in colorectal surgery. This, however, has not borne out in the literature. Laparoscopic surgery has been found equal to open surgery on principles of oncologic outcome: margins, lymph node interrogation, recurrence, and disease-free survival.

The ability to obtain an R0 resection with tumor-free margins is a keystone of oncologic colectomy. In 2004, the COST, one of the first major study groups, published resection margins as part of their oncologic analysis of laparoscopic colectomy compared with open colectomy.[11] They found proximal resection margins of 12 cm (open) versus 13 cm (laparoscopic). Similarly, they noted distal resection margins of 11 cm (open) versus 10 cm (laparoscopic). Subsequent evaluation by the 2005 COLOR also showed no difference in the distribution of resection margin positivity between the open and laparoscopic groups.[12] Hewett and colleagues[33] (ALCCaS Trial), however, did publish a significant difference in the distal margin of open versus laparoscopic cases (9 cm vs 7 cm; $P = .0004$). However the investigators noted that this is of unclear clinical significance and suggest that this may have been due to inadequate mobilization of the hepatic flexure during right colectomies (ad hoc analysis showed the difference to only exist in the right colectomy group). There was no statistical significant difference, however, in proximal margins or overall margin positivity.

Surgical colon cancer guidelines widely cite consensus for a goal of at least 12 lymph nodes for an adequate lymph node staging.[34] Similarly, Chang and colleagues[35] showed a positive correlation between the number of lymph nodes examined and survival in patients with stage II and stage III colon cancer. The 2004 COST study showed no difference in the median number of lymph nodes examined between the open and the laparoscopic groups (12 vs 12, open vs laparoscopic).[11] The 2005 COLOR trial was no different in its statement either (10 vs 10, open vs laparoscopic).[12] Lacy and colleagues[10] similarly showed no difference in the number of lymph nodes in the resected specimen of open versus laparoscopic colectomies (11.1 vs 11.1). The investigators of the ALCCaS Trial noted a median of 13 nodes in their specimens between open and laparoscopic groups.[33]

Recurrence rates and disease-free 5 year survival rates, however, must dominate any discussion of the adequacy of an oncologic operation. Fleshman and colleagues[36] published a 2-year extension on the COST trial (examining data 5 years after the index procedure) and noted no significant difference in disease-free 5 year survival rates (68.4% vs 69.2%; $P = .94$, open vs laparoscopic, respectively), local recurrence rates (2.6% vs 2.3%; $P = .79$, open vs laparoscopic, respectively), or overall recurrence rates (21.8% vs 19.4%, open vs laparoscopic, respectively). The 2005 COLOR Study Group published a long-term follow-up in 2009 that similarly showed no significant difference in the disease-free 5-year survival rates between open and laparoscopic colectomies.[37] The United Kingdom Medical Research Council Conventional versus Laparoscopi -Assisted Surgery in Colorectal Carcinoma Group (CLASICC) examined 639 patients undergoing surgery (open vs laparoscopic) for colon or rectal cancer. Again, they found no difference in local or distant recurrence rates.[38] The group reexamined the cohort 2 years later, finding no difference in the disease-free 5-year survival rate (58.6% vs 55.3%, open vs laparoscopic; $P = .483$).[39] Lacy and colleagues[10] showed lower cancer-related mortality in the laparoscopic group (21% vs 10%, open vs laparoscopic; $P = .03$). The investigators noted that this effect was predominantly in stage III tumors and suggested a role for surgical stress; however, a concession was made with the power of the study (N = 102 vs 106).

There is a historical concern for port site recurrence. Early reports of tumor recurrence rates of as high as 21% at trocar sites (3 of 14) provided some cause for concern.[40] No significant increase, however, in wound site recurrence rate was noted in any of the much larger multicenter randomized control trials. Specifically, the COST Study Group showed a 0.5% (open) versus 0.9% (laparoscopic) wound recurrence rate ($P = .43$).[36] The COLOR trial noted 0.3% (open) versus 1.3% (laparoscopic) wound recurrence rate ($P = .09$).[37] Finally, the CLASICC Trial Group published 0.6% (open) versus 2.5% (laparoscopic) wound recurrence rate ($P = .12$).[38] It is believed that both laparoscopic and open colorectal cancer resection can both achieve wound recurrence rates of less than 1%.[41] The Society of American Gastrointestinal and Endoscopic Surgeons published guidelines on minimally invasive colorectal surgery and made a strong recommendation for the use of a wound protector at the extraction site along with irrigation of the port sites, although acknowledging the current body of literature on its use is of low quality.[41]

SUMMARY

The COST trial represents one of the most important articles in the treatment of colon cancer of this generation. This study validated the use of minimally invasive surgical techniques in the surgical treatment of colon cancer. This is critical because surgery is the mainstay of colon cancer treatment and the sole therapy for patients with stage I and stage II disease.

MIS for colon cancer is a step forward. When properly performed, there is no additional danger to patients; on the contrary, short-term outcomes are improved compared with open surgery. It is the authors' opinion that as training and comfort levels with MIS in the form of laparoscopic and robotic surgery improve, penetrance will continue to increase and patient outcomes continue to improve. Every effort should be made by the surgical community to hasten this eventuality and make well performed minimally invasive colorectal cancer surgery the norm in America and around the world.

REFERENCES

1. Marley AR, Nan H. Epidemiology of colorectal cancer. Int J Mol Epidemiol Genet 2016;7(3):105–14.

2. Jacobs M, Verdeja JC, Goldstein HS. Minimally invasive colon resection (laparoscopic colectomy). Surg Laparosc Endosc 1991;1:144–50.
3. Fowler DL, White SA. Laparoscopy-assisted sigmoid resection. Surg Laparosc Endosc 1991;1:183–8.
4. Kang CY, Halabi WJ, Luo R, et al. Laparoscopic colorectal surgery: a better look into the latest trends. Arch Surg 2012;147:724–31.
5. Moghadamyeghaneh Z, Carmichael JC, Mills S, et al. Variations in laparoscopic colectomy utilization in the United States. Dis Colon Rectum 2015;58:950–6.
6. Remzi FH, Kirat HT, Kaouk JH, et al. Single-port laparoscopy in colorectal surgery. Colorectal Dis 2008;10(8):823–6.
7. Buscher P, Pugin F, Morel P. Single port access laparoscopic right hemicolectomy. Int J Colorectal Dis 2008;23(10):1013–6.
8. Weber PA, Merola S, Wasielewski A, et al. Telerobotic-assisted laparoscopic right and sigmoid colectomies for benign disease. Dis Colon Rectum 2002;45:1689–94.
9. Marks JH, Kawun UB, Hamdan W, et al. Redefining contraindications to laparoscopic colorectal resection for high-risk patients. Surg Endosc 2008;22(8):1899–904.
10. Lacy AM, Garcia-Valdecasas JC, Delgado S, et al. Laparoscopy-assisted colectomy versus open colectomy for treatment of non-metastatic colon cancer: a randomized trial. Lancet 2002;359(9325):2224–9.
11. Clinical Outcomes of Surgical Therapy Study Group. A comparison of laparoscopically assisted and open colectomy for colon cancer. N Engl J Med 2004;340:2050–9.
12. Colon Cancer Laparoscopic or Open Resection Study Group. Laparoscopic surgery versus open surgery for colon cancer: short-term outcomes of a randomized trial. Lancet Oncol 2005;6(7):477–84.
13. Schwenk W, Bohm B, Witt C. Pulmonary function following laparoscopic or conventional colorectal resection: a randomized controlled evaluation. Arch Surg 1999;134:6–12.
14. Eggermont AM, Steller EP, Sugarbaker PH. Laparotomy enhaces intraperitoneal tumor growth and abrogates the anti-tumor effects of interleukin-2 and lymphokine-activated killer cells. Surgery 1987;102:71–8.
15. Veldkamp R, Gholghesaei M, Bonjer HJ, et al. Laparoscopic resection of colon cancer: consensus of the European Association of Endoscopic Surgery (EAES). Surg Endosc 2004;18:1163–85.
16. Franklin ME, Gonzalez JJ, Miter DB, et al. Laparoscopic right hemicolectomy for cancer: 11-year experience. Rev Gastroenterol Mex 2004;69 Suppl 1:65–72.
17. Shapiro R, Keler U, Segev L, et al. Laparoscopic right hemicolectomy with intracorporeal anastomosis: short and long-term benefits in comparison with extracorporeal anastomosis. Surg Endosc 2016;30(9):3823–9.
18. Rieger NA, Lam FF. Single-incision laparoscopically assisted colectomy using standard laparoscopic instrumentation. Surg Endosc 2009;24:888–90.
19. Ramos-Valadez DI, Patel CB, Ragupathi M, et al. Single-incision laparoscopic right hemicolectomy : safety and feasibility in a series of consecutive cases. Surg Endosc 2010;24(10):2613–6.
20. Marks JH, Montenegro GA, Shields MV, et al. Single-port laparoscopic colorectal surgery shows equivalent or better outcomes to standard laparoscopic surgery: results of a 190-patient, 7-criterion case-match study. Surg Endosc 2015;29(6):1492–9.

21. Trastulli S, Coratti A, Guarino S, et al. Robotic right colectomy with intracorporeal anastomosis compared with laparoscopic right colectomy with extracorporeal and intracorporeal anastomosis: a retrospective multicenter study. Surg Endosc 2015;29(6):1512–21.

22. Dimitriou N, Griniatsos J. Complete mesocolic excision: techniques and outcomes. World J Gastrointest Oncol 2015;7(12):383–8.

23. Hohenberger W, Weber L, Matzel K, et al. Standadized surgery for colonic cancer: complete mesocolic excision and central ligation-technical notes and outcome. Colorectal Dis 2009;11:354–64.

24. West NP, Morris EJ, Rotimi O, et al. Pathology grading of colon cancer surgical resection and its association with survival: a retrospective observational study. Lancet Oncol 2008;9:857–65.

25. Bertelsen CA, Neuenschwander AU, Jansen JE, et al. Disease-free survival after complete mesocolic excision compared with conventional colon cancer surgery: a retrospective, population-based study. Lancet Oncol 2015;16:161–8.

26. Lu JY, Xu L, Xue HD, et al. The radical extent of lymphadenectomy – D2 dissection versus complete mesocolic excision of laparoscopic right colectomy for right-sided colon cancer (RELARC) trial: study protocol for a randomized controlled trial. Trials 2016;17(1):582.

27. HALS Study Group. Hand-assisted laparoscopic surgery vs standard laparoscopic surgery for colorectal disease. Surg Endosc 2000;14:896–901.

28. Marcello PW, Fleshman JW, Milsom JW, et al. Hand access vs laparoscopic colectomy: a multicenter prospective randomized study. Dis Colon Rectum 2008; 51:818–26.

29. Sonoda T, Pandey S, Trencheva K, et al. Long term complications of hand-assisted versus laparoscopic colectomy. J Am Coll Surg 2009;208:62–6.

30. Poon JT, Cheung CW, Fan JK, et al. Single-incision versus conventional laparoscopic colectomy for colonic neoplasm: a randomized, controlled trial. Surg Endosc 2012;26:2729–34.

31. Trastulli S, Cirocchi R, Desiderio J, et al. Robotic versus laparoscopic approach in colonic resections for cancer and benign diseases: systematic review and meta-analysis. PLoS One 2015;10(7):e0134062.

32. Marks J, Ng S, Mak T. Robotic transanal surgery (RTAS) with utilization of a next-generation single-port system: a cadaveric feasibility study. Tech Coloproctol 2017. [Epub ahead of print].

33. Hewett PJ, Allardyce RA, Bagshaw PF, et al. Short-term outcomes of the Australian randomized clinical study comparing laparoscopic and conventional open surgical treatments for colon cancer. The ALCCaS Trial. Ann Surg 2008;248(5): 728–38.

34. Nelson HP, Petrelli N, Carlin A, et al. Guidelines 2000 for colon and rectal cancer surgery. J Natl Cancer Inst 2001;93:583.

35. Chang GJ, Rodriguez-Bigas MA, Skibber JM, et al. Lymph node evaluation and survival after curative resection of colon cancer: systematic review. J Natl Cancer Inst 2007;99:433.

36. Fleshman J, Sargent DJ, Green E, et al. Laparoscopic colectomy for cancer is not inferior to open surgery based on 5-year data from the COST Study Group Trial. Ann Surg 2007;246(4):655–62.

37. Colon Cancer Laparoscopic or Open Resection Study Group. Survival after laparoscopic surgery versus open surgery for colon cancer: long-term outcome of a randomized clinical trial. Lancet Oncol 2009;10(1):44–52.

38. Jayne DG, Guillou PJ, Thorpe H, et al. Randomized trial of laparoscopic-assisted resection of colorectal carcinoma: 3-year results of the UK MRC CLASSICC Trial Group. J Clin Oncol 2007;25:3061.

39. Jayne DG, Thorpe HC, Copeland J, et al. Five-year follow-up of the Medical Research Council CLASICC trial of laparoscopically assisted versus open surgery for colorectal cancer. Br J Surg 2010;97:1638.

40. Berends FJ, Kazemier G, Bonjer HJ, et al. Subcutaneous metastases after laparoscopic colectomy. Lancet 1994;344:58.

41. Guidelines for Laparoscopic Resection of Curable Colon and Rectal Cancer. Available at: http://www.sages.org/publications/guidelines/guidelines-for-laparoscopic-resection-of-curable-colon-and-rectal-cancer/htm.

Population Screening for Hereditary Colorectal Cancer

Heather Hampel, MS, LGC

KEYWORDS

- Lynch syndrome • Cancer genetics • Hereditary • Colon cancer • Screening

KEY POINTS

- Hereditary colorectal cancer is common, with Lynch syndrome accounting for 4% of all colorectal cancer cases.
- All colorectal cancers should be screened for Lynch syndrome at the time of diagnosis.
- Other hereditary cancer syndromes can be identified in colorectal cancer patients at an appreciable frequency.
- It may be time to consider offering genetic counseling and testing to all colorectal cancer patients.

INTRODUCTION

Approximately 136,000 Americans will be diagnosed with colorectal cancer (CRC) this year.[1] Population studies have shown that 4% of these CRC cases are due to Lynch syndrome (LS).[2–4] Tumor screening for Lynch syndrome among all newly diagnosed CRC patients using either the microsatellite instability test or immunohistochemical staining for the 4 mismatch repair genes has been recommended by several professional organizations.[5–7] In addition, it has been recently shown that patients with microsatellite unstable colorectal cancer can benefit from immunotherapy using anti-PD1 and anti-PDL1 inhibitors.[8] Unfortunately, universal tumor screening for Lynch syndrome has not been implemented at all hospitals yet.[9] More recent studies have found that the prevalence of all hereditary cancer syndromes among unselected colorectal cancers is around 10%, and for those diagnosed under age 50, it closer to 16%.[10] At these levels of risk, it may be time to consider offering genetic counseling and testing to all colorectal cancer patients.

Disclosure: Ms. Hampel is on the scientific advisory board for InVitae Genetics and Genome Medical. She has stock in Genome Medical. She was the PI of a study which received donated genetic testing from Myriad Genetic Laboratories, Inc. She has consulted for Beacon LBS.
Division of Human Genetics, Department of Internal Medicine, The Ohio State University Comprehensive Cancer Center, 2012 Kenny Road, Room 257, Columbus, OH 43221, USA
E-mail address: Heather.Hampel@osumc.edu

LYNCH SYNDROME

Lynch syndrome is an autosomal dominant condition that leads to increased risks for CRC, as well as endometrial, ovarian, gastric, and several other cancers (**Table 1**). Lynch syndrome is caused by mutations in the mismatch repair (MMR) genes *MLH1*, *MSH2* (including deletions involving the upstream gene *EPCAM*, *MSH6*, and *PMS2*). When one of these genes is mutated in the germline, there is a high chance that the individual will acquire a second somatic mutation in the other copy of that gene in an at-risk cell during his or her lifetime. When that occurs, there will be no more MMR protein in the cell, so it will no longer be able to repair mismatch mutations in the DNA. This leads to both characteristics of Lynch syndrome that can be screened for in tumors to identify patients who are more likely to have this condition. The first is absence of an MMR protein(s) as demonstrated by immunohistochemical (IHC) staining (**Fig. 1**). If the MMR genes are functioning, the MMR proteins should be present in the tumor. If an MMR gene is not working because of a germline mutation plus a second somatic mutation, then the protein (and possibly its partner protein) will be absent in the tumor. The second characteristic that can help identify patients who are more likely to have Lynch syndrome is microsatellite instability (MSI). This is the result of defective MMR (dMMR), whereby the microsatellites, which are repetitive elements in human DNA such as the famous long tracts of 25 and 26 adenines in a row found in the BAT-25 and BAT-26 markers, become unstable. It is difficult for the DNA replication mechanism to copy these repeats exactly during mitosis. As a result, a few of the repeats might be lost or gained in a cell. If the MMR genes are working, they would repair these errors and continue to have the same number of repeats. If the MMR genes are not working, which is the case in tumors with mutations in both copies of the gene, these errors cannot be repaired, and the tumor will have a different number of repeats than the normal adjacent tissue or blood from that individual in which MMR is working properly. These tumors are called MSI-high tumors and are more likely to be caused by Lynch syndrome.

UNIVERSAL TUMOR SCREENING FOR LYNCH SYNDROME

MSI and IHC tests can be performed in the pathology department at the time of diagnosis of CRC. These tests can identify patients who are more likely to have Lynch syndrome; however, they are not diagnostic, because one can have a dMMR tumor because of either inherited mutations of the MMR genes (Lynch syndrome) or acquired mutations of the MMR genes (*MLH1* promoter methylation or double somatic MMR gene mutations). To reduce the number of patients requiring follow-up genetic counseling and testing for Lynch syndrome, most hospitals perform follow-up testing

Table 1
Lifetime cancer risks associated with Lynch syndrome

Cancer Type	General Public (%)	MLH1 & MSH2 (%)	MSH6 (%)	PMS2 (%)
Colon cancer	5.5	40–80	10–22	15–20
Endometrial cancer	2.7	25–60	16–26	15
Stomach	<1	1–13	≤3	6
Ovarian	1.6	4–24	1–11	6

Data from Bonadona V, Bonaiti B, Olschwang S, et al. Cancer risks associated with germline mutations in MLH1, MSH2, and MSH6 genes in Lynch syndrome. JAMA 2011;305:2304–10; and Senter L, Clendenning M, Sotamaa K, et al. The clinical phenotype of Lynch syndrome due to germ-line PMS2 mutations. Gastroenterology 2008;135:419–28.

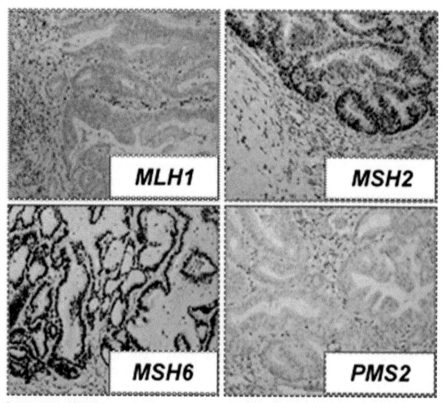

Fig. 1. Immunohistochemical staining of the 4 mismatch repair proteins in a colorectal cancer. Images showing the same tumor stained with antibodies to the *MLH1*, *MSH2*, *MSH6*, and *PMS2* proteins. The lack of nuclear staining for *MLH1* and *PMS2* indicates that these 2 proteins are missing in the tumor. This can either be due to an inherited *MLH1* mutation (Lynch syndrome) or acquired *MLH1* mutations (*MLH1* promoter methylation or double somatic *MLH1* gene mutations in the tumor). Additional testing would be necessary to confirm the diagnosis.

on either all microsatellite unstable cancers or those with MLH1 and PMS2 absent on IHC to assess whether the tumor has acquired *MLH1* methylation. This can be done either by directly assessing methylation of the *MLH1* promoter or by testing for the somatic *BRAF* V600E mutation, which is seen in 69% of methylated CRCs and has only rarely been reported in tumors from patients with Lynch syndrome.[11] The remaining patients who have MSI-high tumors or abnormal IHC not due to *MLH1* methylation should be referred for cancer genetic counseling and offered germline genetic testing to confirm their Lynch syndrome diagnosis. Studies have shown that this is feasible[2,3] and cost-effective.[12–14] Multiple professional organizations have recommended that universal tumor screening for Lynch syndrome be performed for all newly diagnosed CRC patients.[5–7] However, a survey performed in 2012 found that only 71% of National Cancer Institute (NCI)-designated comprehensive cancer centers, and only 15% to 36% of community cancer hospitals, were performing this testing.[9] This is becoming more important with the finding that dMMR tumors can benefit from immunotherapy.[8] Now that there is a treatment change associated with this finding, it is likely that more hospitals will begin to adopt this screening.

CANCER GENETIC TESTING IN UNSELECTED COLORECTAL CANCER PATIENTS

Next-generation sequencing has ushered in a new era of cancer genetics where one can test for multiple genes at the same time for far less cost than in the past.[15] There are laboratories performing large panels of common hereditary cancer genes including all of the Lynch syndrome genes for as little as $249 to $475 (www.color.com and www.invitae.com). This is making genetic testing much more accessible and is helping to define the prevalence and spectrum of cancer gene mutations among all cancer patients. Recent studies have shown that although Lynch syndrome is the most common cause of hereditary colorectal cancer, there are many other hereditary cancer syndromes among patients with CRC.[4,10] The first study included 450 CRC patients who were diagnosed under age 50.[10] All of these patients underwent tumor screening for Lynch syndrome, but they all also received germline genetic testing using a panel of hereditary cancer genes regardless of their tumor screening results. Sixteen percent of these early onset patients were found to have a mutation in an actionable cancer susceptibility gene. Half (8%) had Lynch syndrome, as expected, but the other half included mutations in other high risk CRC genes, moderate risk CRC genes, and genes that have not traditionally been associated with CRC (**Table 2**). Among the patients with dMMR tumors, 83% tested positive, and these cases were almost all accounted for by Lynch syndrome. Among the patients with proficient MMR tumors, 8% tested positive, and this group had a wider variety of cancer susceptibility gene mutations. The second study included 1058 unselected CRC patients of all ages who all received testing using a panel of cancer susceptibility genes.[4] Nearly 10% of these patients were found to have a mutation in an actionable cancer susceptibility gene; with 3.1% having Lynch syndrome and 7.0% have mutations in other genes (**Table 3**). At this level of risk (10%–16%), genetic counseling and testing should be considered for all patients with CRC, or at least those with early onset disease. For comparison, it is generally accepted that all ovarian cancer patients should be referred for genetic counseling and panel genetic testing due to an 18% prevalence of hereditary cancer syndromes.[16]

IMPLICATIONS

Making a diagnosis of a hereditary cancer syndrome can have important implications for the patient and for his/her family members. As seen in **Table 1**, for Lynch syndrome, individuals with a hereditary cancer syndrome have increased risks for the development of multiple cancers during their lifetime. The cancer risks are known for most of the inherited cancer predisposition conditions, and there are accepted intensive cancer surveillance and prevention recommendations for affected individuals. As a result, a CRC patient found to have a hereditary cancer syndrome will need different cancer surveillance (eg, annual colonoscopy) or prevention (eg, risk-reducing hysterectomy and bilateral salpingo-oophorectomy) options to reduce the risk of future cancers or catch them early when they are treatable. In addition, test results may affect the CRC patient's personal cancer treatment. In the case of Lynch syndrome, patients may be offered immunotherapy, which works in dMMR CRCs. Breast and ovarian cancers caused by BRCA1 or BRCA2 gene mutations are increasingly being treated with PARP inhibitors. Although there are no data on PARP inhibitors in CRC, it is possible that this therapy would be effective in a CRC patient with a germline BRCA mutation. Finally, and perhaps most importantly, these test results can have tremendous implications for these individuals' family members. Most hereditary cancer syndromes are autosomal dominant, meaning that half of the patient's children and siblings along with 1 of the patient's parents will also be affected. Furthermore, they will have aunts, uncles, and cousins at risk for the mutation on 1 side of the family. The end result of this

Table 2
Prevalence and spectrum of cancer gene mutations among early onset colorectal cancer patients

Gene	Associated Syndrome or Cancer(s)	Overall Penetrance	Patients with Mutation, Number (%)	(95% CI)
Any pathogenic or likely pathogenic mutation			72 (16)	(12.8–19.8)
Genes associated with colon cancer			59 (13.1)	(10.2–16.7)
MLH1	Lynch syndrome	High	13 (2.9)	(1.6–5.0)
MSH2	Lynch syndrome	High	16 (3.6)	(2.1–5.8)
MSH2/monoallelic MUTYH	Lynch syndrome/colon cancer	High/low	1 (0.2)	(0.01–1.4)
MSH6	Lynch syndrome	Moderate	2 (0.4)	(0.08–1.8)
PMS2	Lynch syndrome	Moderate	5 (1.1)	(0.4–2.7)
APC	Familial adenomatous polyposis (FAP)	High	5(1–1)	(0.4–2.7)
APC p. I1307K	Colon cancer	Low	4 (0.9)	(0.3–2.4)
MUTYH				
Biallelic	MUTYH-associated polyposis (MAP)	High	4 (0.9)	(0.3–2.4)
Monoallelic	Colon cancer	Low	7 (1.6)	(0.7–3.3)
SMAD4	Juvenile polyposis syndrome	High	1 (0.2)	(0.01–1.4)
APC/PMS2	FAP/Lynch syndrome	High/moderate	1 (0.2)	(0.01–1.4)
Genes not traditionally associated with colon cancer			13 (2.9)	(1.6–5.0)
BRCA1	Hereditary breast-ovarian cancer syndrome	High	2 (0.4)	(0.08–1.8)
BRCA2	Hereditary breast-ovarian cancer syndrome	High	4 (0.9)	(0.3–2.4)
ATM	Breast cancer, pancreatic cancer	Moderate	3 (0.7)	(0.2–2.1)
ATM/CHEK2	Breast cancer, pancreatic cancer	Moderate	1 (0.7)	(0.01–1.4)
PALB2	Breast cancer, pancreatic cancer	Moderate	2 (0.4)	(0.08–1.8)
CDKN2A	Melanoma, pancreatic cancer	High	1 (0.2)	(0.01–1.4)

From Pearlman R, Frankel WL, Swanson B, et al. Prevalence and spectrum of germline cancer susceptibility gene mutations among patients with early-onset colorectal cancer. JAMA Oncol 2017;3:464–71; with permission.

Table 3
Multigene panel test results among unselected colorectal cancer patients

Result	Syndrome/Gene	Frequency (%)
No germline mutation	Negative	90.1
High-penetrance mutations	Lynch syndrome (13 *MLH1*, 7 *MSH2*, 6 *MSH6*, 7 *PMS2*)	3.1
	Adenomatous polyposis (5 *APC*, 3 Biallellic *MUTYH*)	0.8
	Hereditary breast-ovarian cancer (3 *BRCA1*, 8 *BRCA2*)	1.0
	Other (*PALB2, CDKN2A, TP53*)	0.4
Moderate-penetrance mutations	Known moderate-risk CRC genes (18 monoallelic *MUTYH*, 14 *APC* I1307K, 2 *CHEK2*)	3.2
	Other moderate-risk (10 *ATM*, 1 *BARD1*, 3 *BRIP1*, 2 *NBN*)	1.5

Data from Yurgelun MB, Kulke MH, Fuchs CS, et al. Cancer susceptibility gene mutations in individuals with colorectal cancer. J Clin Oncol 2017;35(10):1086–95; with permission.

is that by diagnosing a cancer patient with a hereditary cancer syndrome, multiple family members are provided the opportunity to also learn whether or not they have the hereditary cancer syndrome that is running in the family. Most of these relatives will be still unaffected with cancer, affording an opportunity to keep them from getting cancer in the first place (primary prevention). This is a unique opportunity and multiplies the effects of any attempts at diagnosing cancer patients with a hereditary cancer syndrome.

SUMMARY

CRC is a common cancer. Most cases are not caused by hereditary cancer syndromes. However, it appears that 4% to 5% are due to Lynch syndrome, and perhaps another 6% are caused by various other hereditary cancer syndromes.[2,3,10] These results are critical to the patients and their family members, as they can direct treatment and cancer surveillance and prevention options. It is clear that all CRC patients should be screened for dMMR at the time of diagnosis for 2 reasons: (1) to identify patients who are more likely to have Lynch syndrome, and (2) to identify patients who may benefit from immunotherapy. It is also becoming clear that all CRC patients diagnosed under age 50 and perhaps all CRC patients regardless of age at diagnosis need to be referred to cancer genetics for consideration of germline genetic testing using a panel of cancer susceptibility genes. If this occurs, one could argue that tumor screening for dMMR will no longer be necessary. However, it will likely continue for the following reasons: (1) it will still be necessary to determine which patients need immunotherapy, and (2) even with our best efforts, it is unlikely that 100% of CRC patients will get referred for and/or attend a cancer genetics evaluation; this is an opportunity to actively screen all CRC patients for the most common inherited cancer syndrome (Lynch syndrome) as a matter of course.

REFERENCES

1. American Cancer Society. Cancer facts & figures 2017. Atlanta (GA): American Cancer Society; 2017.
2. Hampel H, Frankel WL, Martin E, et al. Feasibility of screening for Lynch syndrome among patients with colorectal cancer. J Clin Oncol 2008;26:5783–8.
3. Hampel H, Frankel WL, Martin E, et al. Screening for the Lynch syndrome (hereditary nonpolyposis colorectal cancer). N Engl J Med 2005;352:1851–60.
4. Yurgelun MB. Germline Testing for Individuals With Pancreatic Cancer: The Benefits and Challenges to Casting a Wider Net. J Clin Oncol 2017:JCO2017747535.

5. The NCCN Clinical Practice Guidelines in Oncology (NCCN GuidelinesTM). Genetic/familial high-risk assessment: breast and ovarian (version 1.2017). National Comprehensive Cancer Network, Inc; 2017. Available at: https://www.nccn.org/professionals/physician_gls/default.aspx.

6. Giardiello FM, Allen JI, Axilbund JE, et al. Guidelines on genetic evaluation and management of Lynch syndrome: a consensus statement by the US Multi-society Task Force on colorectal cancer. Am J Gastroenterol 2014;109:1159–79.

7. Syngal S, Brand RE, Church JM, et al. ACG clinical guideline: genetic testing and management of hereditary gastrointestinal cancer syndromes. Am J Gastroenterol 2015;110:223–62 [quiz: 63].

8. Le DT, Uram JN, Wang H, et al. PD-1 blockade in tumors with mismatch-repair deficiency. N Engl J Med 2015;372:2509–20.

9. Beamer LC, Grant ML, Espenschied CR, et al. Reflex immunohistochemistry and microsatellite instability testing of colorectal tumors for Lynch syndrome among US cancer programs and follow-up of abnormal results. J Clin Oncol 2012;30: 1058–63.

10. Pearlman R, Frankel WL, Swanson B, et al. Prevalence and spectrum of germline cancer susceptibility gene mutations among patients with early-onset colorectal cancer. JAMA Oncol 2017;3:464–71.

11. Palomaki GE, McClain MR, Melillo S, et al. EGAPP supplementary evidence review: DNA testing strategies aimed at reducing morbidity and mortality from Lynch syndrome. Genet Med 2009;11:42–65.

12. Grosse SD. When is genomic testing cost-effective? Testing for Lynch syndrome in patients with newly-diagnosed colorectal cancer and their relatives. Healthcare (Basel) 2015;3:860–78.

13. Grosse SD, Palomaki GE, Mvundura M, et al. The cost-effectiveness of routine testing for Lynch syndrome in newly diagnosed patients with colorectal cancer in the United States: corrected estimates. Genet Med 2015;17:510–1.

14. Mvundura M, Grosse SD, Hampel H, et al. The cost-effectiveness of genetic testing strategies for Lynch syndrome among newly diagnosed patients with colorectal cancer. Genet Med 2010;12:93–104.

15. Hiraki S, Rinella ES, Schnabel F, et al. Cancer risk assessment using genetic panel testing: considerations for clinical application. J Genet Couns 2014;23: 604–17.

16. Norquist BM, Harrell MI, Brady MF, et al. Inherited mutations in women with ovarian carcinoma. JAMA Oncol 2016;2:482–90.

The Economics of Colon Cancer

Guy R. Orangio, MD

KEYWORDS

- Economic cost of colon cancer • Cancer survivors • Cancer drugs
- Average sales price • Genomic sequencing • Quality
- Value and cost of colon cancer • Quality-adjusted life years (QALYs)

KEY POINTS

- Economists measure cost of medical care in 2 categories: direct medical coast (by resources used) and indirect medical costs (loss of resources and opportunities).
- The economic cost of colorectal cancer care varies by stage of disease at diagnosis, patient age, observation time, medical services included, inpatient hospitalizations, and cancer-related services.
- Oncologists are working to reduce the costs of chemotherapy and supportive drugs, advanced imaging, and acute hospital inpatient care.
- Oncologists must be educated and incorporate economics into their decision-making processes to ensure medical treatments value matches their cost.
- Cancer drug costs are the result of federal and state policymakers, the Medicare average sales price, the impact of expansion of insurance coverage, and the role of genomic sequencing.

INTRODUCTION

The national health expenditure is projected to increase by 5.6% per year from 2016 to 2025, which means that, by 2525, the national health expenditure will be 19% of the gross domestic product. This increase in spending will be influenced by economic growth and aging of the population without significant change in the insured population, it will increase to 91.5% in 2025 from 90.5% in 2015.[1] The numbers presented are "projections," but I think most physicians realize that the cost of health care in the United States is increasing at an unsustainable rate. When attempting to define the economic burden of cancer care, one would think that it would be a simple analysis of data with some rudimentary formula and that the actual "cost" of cancer care would be evident. Unfortunately, there are many challenges to determining cost or assessing

Disclosure Statement: The author has nothing to disclose.
LSU Department of Surgery, 1542 Tulane Avenue, Suite 758, New Orleans, LA 70112, USA
E-mail address: gorang@lsuhsc.edu

Surg Oncol Clin N Am 27 (2018) 327–347
https://doi.org/10.1016/j.soc.2017.11.007
1055-3207/18/© 2017 Elsevier Inc. All rights reserved.

Abbreviations	
ACA	Patient Protection and Affordable Care Act
COME HOME	Community Oncology Medical Home
DMC	Direct medical cost
ED	Emergency department
FDA	US Food and Drug Administration
HH	Home health
HRRs	Hospital referral regions
IPRF	Inpatient rehabilitation facility
IQR	Interquartile range
LOS	Length of stay
PAC	Post acute care
PCCP	Patient Care Connect Program
Q	Quartile
QALYS	Quality-adjusted life-years
QOL	Quality of life
SEER	Surveillance, Epidemiology, and End Results
SSI	Surgical site infection

the economic burden at the population level, and the effects of health care policy and programs on the continuum of care of patients with cancer. The existing data for cost analysis are imperfect and based on claims ("paying bills"), mostly in Medicare beneficiaries. The United States' health care system is fragmented into diverse collection of rural and urban systems, some with "mature" health care networks, but the majority of which are fee-for-service reimbursement models. Cancer care and its treatment result in loss of economic resources, for example, financial loss to cancer survivors and caregivers, owing to morbidity, decreased quality of life (QOL), and premature death. Cost is measured by the monetary value of resources used to treat the disease and the loss of opportunities (patients, families, employers, and society) owing to cancer. The cost is measured longitudinally from the initial diagnosis of cancer to end-of-life care.[2]

ECONOMIC BURDEN OF CANCER

This article discusses in "general terms" the estimates and projections of the national burden of cancer care. When economists measure cost of medical care it is under 2 categories direct medical costs (DMCs; resources used) and indirect medical costs (loss of resources and opportunities). DMCs are services that patients receive include hospitalizations, surgery, physician visits, radiation therapy, chemotherapy, and/or immunotherapy, and these items are measured by insurance payments and patient copayments (deductibles and out-of-pocket costs). Unfortunately, the majority of estimates of the DMCs of cancer are focused on the elderly population aged 65 years and older. There are "incidences costs," which are "estimates" at an individual level and can range from diagnosis to several months or to patient's lifetime. Phase-specific prevalence costs are obtained from cancer incidence and survival data to estimate the costs of cancer care per year.[2]

The indirect costs of cancer are the monetary losses associated with the "morbidity costs" that the patient, the caregiver, and the family incur while receiving medical care, time lost from work and other usual activities combined. The value of lost time can only be approximated by human capital method and calculated by the willingness-to-pay method. The human capital method is defined by using gender- and age-specific average earnings, which are combined with time lost from work or working life lost to owing premature death or unrealized earnings. The willingness-to-pay method incorporates lost productivity and intrinsic value of life by estimating the average amount that an individual or population would pay for an additional year of life. The time data include travel time to and from care, and the wait time while receiving care. This "loss of productivity" is not only viewed with respect to the cancer patient, but also from the perspective of the employer's costs owing to disability and absenteeism, which can be substantial.[2]

ECONOMIC COST OF COLORECTAL CANCER

A 2013 systematic review of the economic costs associated with colorectal cancer care showed that the cost varied by stage of disease at diagnosis, patient age, observation time (12 months after diagnosis vs life time), type of medical services included, the site where care is performed (inpatient hospitalizations), and the type of cancer-related service (eg, chemotherapy). Also included were the cost effectiveness of alternative cancer treatments (DMCs) and the cost of cancer prevention or screening. The cost of time and productivity losses associated with cancer care treatment for the patient and caregiver are substantial, and that affects the societal burden.[3]

FINANCIAL BURDEN ON CANCERS SURVIVORS

Cancer care costs are increasing at 2 to 3 times the rate of other health care cost and this will continue for the next decade.[4] The cost of cancer care in the United States has led to considerable financial hardship for patients and families. A 2012 a survey of 4719 cancer survivors ages 18 to 64 examined the proportions of survivors who report going into debt or filing for bankruptcy as a result of the debt incurred.[5] At least 30% of cancer survivors report financial hardship and bankruptcy rates are 2.5 times higher than those people without a history of cancer.[6] The study results indicated 88% were white, 67% were female, 69% were married, 54% were employed full time, and 85% were privately insured. Sixty-two percent had a bachelor's or advanced degree, and 42% had an annual household income of $81,000.00. Sixty-four percent of patients reporting worrying about having to pay large bills related to their cancer treatment. Thirty-four percent reported that they or a family member had gone in to debt because of cancer, and 3% said, "They or their families filed for bankruptcy as a result of cancer." Forty percent made other financial sacrifices owing to cancer care. When the authors look at the subset of survivors who reported they a family member had gone to debt, 87% worried about paying the large bills related to cancer and 9% reported that they or a family member filed for bankruptcy as a result of their cancer. Sixty-eight percent made other financial sacrifices, and 94% had out-of-pocket spending on medical expenses. The out-of-pocket expense for the 1583 cancer survivors was for medical expenses (90%), transportation (60%), lodging (22%), and childcare and home care (approximately 12%). Of the 1583 cancer survivors who reported that they or a family member had gone in to debt, 1558 reported the amount of debt incurred (**Table 1**).

Table 1	
Debt incurred by cancer survivors or family members	
Percent of Incurred Debt	**Amount ($)**
45	<10,000
30	10,000–24,999
12	24,000–49,000
13	≥50,000

Cancer survivors between the ages of 18 and 54 years were significantly more likely to go in to debt that those 55 to 64 years of age. Filing for bankruptcy because of cancer was significantly more likely with younger age, lower annual household income, those who were unemployed, having Medicaid insurance, and having more than 2 cancers. The mean annual health care expenditure for the working-age cancer survivor population is in the first year $17,170 and then is $9369 after the first year, which is 3 times greater than in the same population without a cancer history.[6]

FINANCIAL BURDEN OF CANCER SURVIVORS: ADOLESCENTS AND YOUNG ADULTS

In 2012, an estimated 614,000 adolescent and young adults (ages 15–39) who were first diagnosed with cancer were alive in the United States.[7] All cancer survivors are at risk of developing chronic health conditions from the treatment of their cancer. Young adults are prone to interruption of normal developmental processes; they also face unique medical, psychosocial, financial, and occupational challenges.[8,9] Young adults who are survivors of cancer need to be screened for secondary cancers or recurrence, infertility, and cardiac conditions over their lifetime. Interruption of normal developmental transitions in young adulthood have had substantial effects on education and employment opportunities. The authors used data from the 2008 to 2011 Medical Expenditure Panel Surveys. The Medical Expenditure Panel Surveys is a nationally representative survey that is conducted annually among the US civilian population.[10] The authors identified 1464 adolescent and young adult cancer survivors and compared them with 86,865 adults without history of cancer. They looked at DMCs and examined the source of payment: out of pocket, private health insurance, Medicare, Medicaid, or other sources. They looked at service type, namely, ambulatory care, inpatient care, prescriptions medication, and other services. Indirect morbidity costs were assessed by employment disability, missed work or school days, and additional days spent in bed. The annual DMC for adolescent and young adult cancer survivors were $7417 versus $4247 for adults without cancer. The annual source of payment for the DMC was broken down into out-of-pocket costs ($4765), private insurance ($3083), Medicare ($1246), Medicaid ($541), and other ($876). The service type costs were broken down to ambulatory care ($2409), inpatient care ($1605), and prescriptions ($1446). The demographics of adolescent and young adult cancer survivors were 77.8% female, 80.8% white, more than 45% high school graduates, 66% with private insurance, 20% on Medicaid or Medicare, 12% uninsured, 21% poor (<125% of the federal poverty level), and 41% low or middle income. Employment status of the cancer survivors were 33.5% unemployed, of which 34% were disable by their illness. In 2008 to 2011, the annual excess economic burden of cancer survivorship was $5420 per survivor with excess medical expenditures accounting for 58.8% of the total burden ($3170 of the $5420). Annual loss of productivity was estimated to be $2250 per adolescent and young adult cancer survivor, which is higher than for older cancer survivors. Most of the lost productivity in younger survivors was due to the interruptions of the developmental transitions experienced by adolescents and your adults.[11]

ECONOMIC COST OF MEDICAL ONCOLOGY

The cost of chemotherapy and supportive drugs, advanced imaging, and acute hospital inpatient care are all considered areas of opportunity for cost reductions in medical oncology. The use of oncology services is one area of concern. There are many rapidly emerging new treatments, some of which lack demonstrated superiority yet provide financial incentives to providers. Chemotherapy regimens can vary among

US community oncology practices and there are regional variations in the use of inpatient services for patients with advanced cancer. Stakeholders have reported reductions in inpatient use through enhanced care management.[12] Some pilot studies have reported that the use of clinical decision support and bundled payment models to incentivize cost-effective treatments are effective when an equally efficacious regimens exists.[13] In a 2015 study on Medicare fee-for-service beneficiaries claims data, the authors examined the magnitude of variation at the medical oncology practice level for key oncology services. They analyzed measures of chemotherapy, advanced imaging, and inpatient payments per beneficiary. The annual payments per beneficiary included both physician and facility payments. They Winsorized[a] values at the 99th percentile of all observations in the sample, and they assigned values above the 99th percentile to mitigate the effect of extreme values; for example, chemotherapy was assigned a value of $91,041, advanced imaging $6753, and acute medical hospitalization $ 50,749. The median (interquartile range [IQR]) payments per beneficiary for chemotherapy was $14,863 (IQR, $12,966-$16,832), advanced imaging $1441 (IQR, $1228-$1667), and inpatient management $5528 (IQR, $4690-$6562). Major differences were found in expenditures for chemotherapy, where the interquartile difference was 8.8 times as great as imaging and twice as great as inpatient management. The following were differences per median payments per beneficiary for chemotherapeutic agents: pegfilgrastim, quartile 1 (Q1) $717 versus quartile 4 (Q4) $364, ratio Q4/Q1 4.4; bevacizumab, Q1 $4,571 versus Q4 $8,104, ratio Q4/Q1 1.8; cetuximab, Q1 $1,671 versus Q4 $ 2,410, ratio Q4/Q1 1.4; and oxaliplatin, Q1 $5136 versus Q4 $6,509, ratio Q4/Q1 1.3. Across all cancers and oncology practices, pegfilgrastim was 21% and bevacizumab 16% of the total difference in chemotherapy spending between quartiles. PET examinations accounted for 54.2% of the differential payments for advanced imaging. The authors demonstrated a substantial variation across medical oncology physician practices in the use of chemotherapy, advanced imaging, and acute medical inpatient admission. They concluded that the evidence on practice-level variation in oncology services warrants an alternative payment model to control costs on these services.[14]

In a 2012 study, medical oncologists in the United States and Canada were surveyed on a hypothetical new chemotherapy drug and were asked how much benefit, in months of life expectancy gained, this drug would need to provide to warrant its use. There were 1365 surveys mailed with an overall response rate of 59%. In the section of the questionnaire assessing the general attitudes toward cost of cancer care, oncologists were asked, "What do you think is a reasonable definition of good value for money or cost-effectiveness per life-year gained?" Responses categories were: $0 to $50,000, $50,001 to $100,000, $100,001 to $150,000, $150,001 to $200,000 and more than $200,000. The clinical scenario involved a patient with metastatic cancer who was expected to survive for 12 months with standard chemotherapy at a cost of $25,000 per year. The survey asked, "What minimum improvement in median survival would cause you to prescribe a new medication instead of standard treatment?" (Assume the patient has no out-of-pocket expense). The cost of the new drug varied at either $75,000 or $150,000. A second scenario focused on treatments that improve QOL but that do not extend the duration of life. The study showed that Canadian oncologists endorsed higher cost-effective thresholds than US oncologists (P = .04). Only 30% of US oncologists and 35% of Canadian oncologists endorsed

---

[a] Winsorized is the transformation of statistics by limiting extreme values in the statistical data to reduce the effect of spurious outliers.

cost-effectiveness thresholds of greater than $100,000 per life year. Overall, the US and Canadian oncologists did not differ when the cost of the drug was $150,000; they demanded a longer survival. The results of the study show that oncologists do not have consistent opinions about how many months an expensive new therapy should extend a person's life before the cost of the therapy is justified. They concluded that oncologists are relatively insensitive to the costs of the drugs when making these decisions, and that this finding was not surprising, because physicians receive little training in how to factor cost-effectiveness information into their decision making. The investigators concluded that physicians must be educated and supported in incorporating economic consequences in to their decision-making process, to ensure that medical treatments bring good value for their patients.[15]

HIGH COST OF CANCER DRUGS

Over the past 2 decades, the price of anticancer drugs set by manufactures, after US Food and Drug Administration (FDA) approval, has been increasing by 10% per year.[16] It is difficult to determine whether these drugs offer sufficient benefits to justify their costs. Clinical trials examine whether new anticancer medications improve survival, but tell us little about the cost of the new treatments. The clinical trials are guided by protocols, but different patterns of use is governed by physicians' experience in the "real world," so use can vary by drug. In a 2016 study data from the Surveillance, Epidemiology, and End Results (SEER) Medicare database was used to access the "value of new cancer treatments" for patients with metastatic breast, lung, or kidney tumors, or chronic myelogenous leukemia. The study examined changes in life expectancy and lifetime medical costs for 1996 to 2013. Outcomes for patients with metastatic tumors were measured in terms of median survival, the value of care, and average life expectancy. The authors used a "phase-of-care" approach from point of diagnosis until death to determine lifetime medical costs (including drugs, outpatients visits, and hospital admissions). The average increase in life expectancy for patients with metastatic breast cancer, treated with physician-administered chemotherapy increased by 13.2 months with a lifetime increase of medical costs of $72,200. Among those patients who did not received those drugs, life expectancy increased by a more modest 2.0 months with increased costs of only $8900. The authors wondered whether improvements in life expectancy could be attributable to improvements in supportive care or lead-time bias. Life expectancy among patients with lung cancer and kidney cancer treated increased by 3.9 months with increased costs of $23,200 and 7.9 months and increased costs of $44,700, respectively. The authors concluded that the increases in the cost of treating patient with metastatic breast, lung, or kidney tumors were accompanied by meaningful improvements in survival. Life expectancy remains low and there is a lot of potential for future research and development on new drugs to produced substantial benefits.[17] Another extremely important factor increasing cancer drug cost is the revolution in the understanding of the molecular biology of cancer, which is a direct result of the human genome project.[18]

Medicare's Average Sales Price

Before 2005, drug manufacturers' common practice was to charge medical oncologists a deeply discounted price for the purchase of cancer drugs. Because Medicare allowed providers to bill those drugs at a rate of 95% of average wholesale price, the difference between the buying and selling price with the administrative fees accounted for up to 50% of the income in oncology practices. Then in 2005, Medicare changed the way it paid for cancer drugs to average sales price plus 6%. Because manufacturers are still free to set prices for new drugs and discounts that ultimately determine the average sales price, there remains a healthy margin for physicians under the average sales price plus 6% rule.[18]

Policies That Mandate Cancer Drug Coverage

The Social Security Act, sections 1861 (t) (2) (B) (ii) (I) and (II), stipulates that Medicare and Medicaid must cover anticancer drugs and biologics for on- and off-label uses as long as they are listed in at least one of a number of compendia. These compendia are authoritative sources for determining "medically accepted "indications of drugs and biologic agents. According to FDA-approved indications (on label) or non–FDA-approved indications (off label). Commercial insurance plans are not bound to follow Medicare's policies; however, manufacturer lobbyists in many states have stepped in to override possible insurance restrictions on cancer drugs.[18]

Impact of Coverage Expansion

The Patient Protection an Affordable Care Act (ACA) has increase insurance coverage for millions of lower income Americans. Medicaid accounts for much of this increase, and much of this coverage is for children. Combined Medicare and Medicaid coverage now insures 100 million people. Realizing that cancer incidence is somewhat a bimodal disease with a higher incidence in children and older adults, the federal and state government pays for approximately 70% of all new patients with cancer in the United States each year. The ACA's exchanges and employer mandates have further expanded coverage to millions of working-age adults who are supported by government subsidies.[18]

Role of Genomic Sequencing

Technology is fueling cancer drug therapy through reductions in the cost of genomic sequencing. This technology allows the manipulation by drugs or biological agents in DNA mutations and changes in cellular process. The author concludes that cancer drug pricing decisions are driven by factors that have very little to do with the intrinsic value of the products themselves. Developing policies that address the uncertainly that drug makers face in a landscape or rapid technologic change may provide a better solution for society than price controls.[18]

EARLY COLON CANCER MEASURES, QUALITY, VALUE, AND COST

A 2008 study focusing on colorectal cancer because of its high prevalence in the United States looked at service use in high-spending areas and whether or not recommended care is linked to improved patient outcomes.[19] It looked at the SEER program of the National Cancer Institute for 11 population-based cancer registries (about 14% of the US population), sampling 55,549 patients diagnosed at age 64 or older with colorectal cancer. It measured area-level spending of inpatient care at the end of life (based on the last 6 months of life) and calculated an end-of-life inpatient expenditure index. The study examined 6 measures of appropriateness of care for patients diagnosed with colorectal cancer (**Box 1**). Using Medicare administrative data, the authors examined those patients who received chemotherapy within 6 months of diagnosis. They examined the use treatment that was recommended (stage III; n = 11,261), not recommended (stage I; n = 10,998), or discretional because the benefits and risks are less clear (stage II [n = 16,371] and stage IV [n = 8661]). The authors found mixed results in the association between area-level inpatient end-of-life spending and recommended care. There was consistently higher use of costly

---

Box 1
Six measures for assessing appropriateness of care in colorectal patients

Measures

1. Stage at diagnosis as a measure of quality of screening services, classifying patients according to diagnosis with late (stage IV) versus early (stage I/II/III) disease.

2. Adjuvant chemotherapy (in addition to surgery) for patients with stage III colon cancer.

3. Adjuvant chemotherapy and radiation therapy for patients with stage II/III rectal cancer.

4. Receipt of surveillance colonoscopy within 1 year after surgery for patient and for surgery patients undergoing curative surgery.

5. Complete diagnostic colonoscopy before or at surgery.

6. Surveillance testing for the carcinoembryonic antigen.

Data from Adjuvant therapy for patients with colon and rectum cancer. Consens Statement 1990;8(4):1–25. Available at: https://consensus.nih.gov/1990/1990adjuvanttherapycolonrectal cancer079html.htm.

---

chemotherapy and few differences in patient outcomes across areas. There was also on association between end-of-life spending and 3 of the 6 quality measures in high-spending areas. In the high versus low areas, there was an increased use of chemotherapy among older patients with more comorbid illnesses. They suggested that high-spending areas may be treating patients unlikely to benefit owing to significant comorbidities and limited life expectancy. The authors found that high end-of-life inpatient expenditure index areas were more likely to provide recommended care, but that was offset by increased use of care that was ineffective or potentially harmful. The authors recommend that policy should focus on cost containment, but that an across-the-board reduction in services may eliminate valuable care in addition to reducing wasteful care. Policies that were designed to rein in discretionary and nonrecommended care while encouraging the use of recommended care would yield greater value for medical spending.[19]

Value

A 2015 study examined how recent treatment advances in colorectal cancer and multiple myeloma have altered both the cost of health care and the value to patients. The net cost of health care is measured in quality-adjusted cost of care. This allows for incorporating value into measurements of growth by (1) constructing conventional growth curves in health care costs and (2) measuring that growth in value to patients, in terms of monetized gains in quality-adjusted life-years (QALYs), a metric that incorporates increases in both life expectancy and QOL. The difference between the change in costs and the change in benefits defines the net change in the quality-adjusted cost of care.[20] The authors focused on patients receiving postoperative chemotherapy, one of the most important drivers of both cost growth and improvement in patient health outcome. They constructed a weighted average market price for treatment for an individual patient. In early 2000, 4 new treatment options (capecitabine, oxaliplatin, bevacizumab, and cetuximab) were approved by the FDA. By 2005, the average cost of treatment cycle exceeded $35,000.[20]

Although the costs increased, these new treatments also improved patient health outcomes. In 1991 and using fluorouracil and leucovorin, patients could expect to survive on average 12.5 months. In 2004, patients on oxaliplatin and bevacizumab could expect to live 23.2 months. The authors defined the cost as the increase in health care costs to the net of the value of improved health outcomes. The change was computed as the difference between the cost of the new therapies and the cost of the baseline therapy. The value of life-years has been calculated to be between $100,000 and $300,000 per year, and the authors used the lower end of this range for their calculations. The difference between the growth in cost and the growth in value was the change in the equality-adjusted cost of care. Health care costs increased by $34,493 as a result of the new technology; however, patients' health improved by 0.33115 QALYs, which is a value of $33,115 per person. Therefore, the quality-adjusted cost of care increased by only $1277 during the time period. The authors concluded that this study provided a simple, transparent framework, based on existing economic tools, to help policymakers incorporate value into consideration of health care cost by using a quality an adjusted care metric.[20]

Value of Cancer Care in the United States

In the United States, cancer care gains are assessed in survival time after cancer diagnosis. A 2013 study, comparing US health care spending with 10 European countries looked at survival differences for patients with cancer compared with the relative cost of cancer care. The authors found that US patients experience greater survival gains than those in European countries, even after considering the higher US health care costs. This investment generated $598 billion of additional value for US patients who were diagnosed with cancer from 1983 to 1999.[21] The US spending on cancer care, in 2011 US dollars, increased from $47,000 (1983–1999) to $70,000 per case, a 49% increase. Over the same time, European countries saw an increase of only by 16%. The net social value of survival in the United States for an individual cancer patient was on average $61,000 (range, $51,000-$94,000) over the 17-year analysis period, or approximately $443 billion annually. The authors felt the differences in US costs reflect an appropriate unitization of new technology.[21]

A 2015 study compared cancer care from 1982 to 2010 in the United States with care in 20 Western European counties. The evaluation was performed on population-level cancer mortality rates, cost of cancer care, number of cancer deaths averted, life-years saved, and the value of cancer QALYs. The estimated value of US cancer care, per tumor, relative to Western Europe cancer care was calculated as the ratio US cancer costs minus Western European cancer costs to the number of QALYs saved. US colorectal cancer mortality rates were lower that those of Western European countries throughout the entire study period and led to 264,632 averted deaths. The authors concluded that the greater number of averted colorectal cancer deaths in the United States was due to screening, when compared with Western Europe.[22] There are multiple studies in the United States, demonstrating that the increase in colorectal cancer screening preceded the steepest decrease in colorectal cancer mortality. Between 1975 and 2000, there was a 53% decrease in colorectal cancer mortality in the United States because of screening programs. The combination of higher screening rates, greater use of curative-intent surgery, and adjuvant chemotherapy in the United States contributed to a decrease in colorectal cancer deaths.[23–25]

COLORECTAL CANCER SCREENING HEALTH LITERACY

Section 5002 of the ACA states that it is important that individuals have the capacity to obtain, process, communicate, and understand basic health information and services needed to make appropriated health decisions. Health outcomes are linked to health literacy, including the ability to interpret labels and health care messages, take medications, receive preventive care, and avoid hospitalizations and excessive use of emergency care.[26,27] There have been, over the past several years, major federal policy initiatives that establish remedies for limited health literacy including the ACA, the National Action Plan to Improve Health Literacy of the Department of Health and Human Services, and the Plain Writing Act of 2010, which requires all federal documents to be written in a "clear, concise, well-organized" manner. To navigate successfully though health care systems, patients need to possess and demonstrate multiple skills and use major components of health literacy. Limited health literacy can lead to the cycle of "crisis care."[28] Improving providers' communication skill is an important aspect to remedying limited health literacy. In a 2004 study, the authors compared 2 groups of providers and the rates patient participation in colon cancer screening. The patients paired with the first group of providers had a higher rate of colon cancer screening than patients paired with the second group of providers (41.3% vs 32.4%). Group 1 providers received feedback on their patients' health literacy status and underwent training in establishing effected communication with patients who had limited literacy skills. Group 2 providers did not receive this training. The group 1 providers (with communication training) had an effected colon cancer screening rate of 55.7% screening versus 30% for the group 2 providers.[28] In a second 2012 study on health literacy and bowel preparation, it was demonstrated that comprehension and health literacy influenced the outcome of the screening colonoscopy. In this study, the authors recruited 764 patients of mixed social and demographic backgrounds with a median age of 63 years and an adequate health literacy score of 79%. The participant's comprehension of an "open book" test, on a bowel preparation for colonoscopy was tested. There were 5 questions and the mean number of correct answers was 3.2 (standard deviation, 1.2). The authors concluded that poor comprehension of colonoscopy preparation had negative implications for the safety and economic impact of on these procedures.[29]

Heath Care Access and Colorectal Cancer Screening

Over the last 20 years, Medicare policies have changed. The 1997 Balanced Budget Act began covering colorectal screening Medicare Part B beneficiaries with an annual deductible; however, colonoscopy was initially covered for people only with a high risk of developing colorectal cancer. In 2001, the Consolidated Appropriations Act added coverage colonoscopy for all Part B Medicare beneficiaries and later the Deficit Reduction Act of 2005 exempted all screening colonoscopies from Part B annual deductible by 2007. Finally, in 2010 the ACA made preventive services more affordable and accessible. In 2011, ACA Medicare mandated that all cost sharing be waived for routine initial colorectal cancer screening and that beneficiaries would not have to pay a deductible. In a population-based study from 2008 to 2013 of patients with an initial diagnosis of cancer, the data from the SEER Program, sponsored by the National Cancer Institute, was analyzed. The authors used the American Joint Committee on Cancers Cancer Staging Manual, and defined stages III and IV disease as late stage cancers. The results showed that the incidence of early stage colorectal cancer decreased for people 65 or older but remained constant for those ages 50 to 64 years. The authors estimated that ACA Medicare increased the number of early stage colorectal cancer diagnoses by 8% per year. Individuals age 65 to 75 years had an increase in early stage colorectal cancer diagnoses by 6.7% and in those 75 years or older had an increase of 10.5%. There was an interestingly greater impact on the number of women (12.8%) compared with men (3.8%) diagnosed with early stage colorectal cancer.[30]

SURGICAL COST OF COLON CANCER

There is no debate that the primary treatment for colon cancer is surgery. Colon resection is the single most important and effective modality for establishing a long-term cure. The principles of surgical resection include en bloc resection of the primary tumor with its draining lymph node distribution, defined by is primary blood supply to the involved segment. The concept of complete mesocolic excision with central vascular ligation is new nomenclature for what has been the hallmark of resection for colon cancer.[31–33] The Clinical Outcomes of Surgical Therapy (COST) study, comparing laparoscopically assisted with open colectomy for colon cancer, was a randomized prospective multicenter trial that evaluated the utility of laparoscopic resection for patients with colon cancer. A total of 872 patients with right and sigmoid colon carcinomas were randomly assigned to either open or laparoscopic resection. Follow-up at 3 years did not show any difference in survival or recurrence.[34] In a study in 2007, the COST Study Group Trial evaluated long-term survival and recurrence rates at 5 and 7 years; there were no differences between the open and laparoscopic groups.[35] Since these early studies, the cost effectiveness of minimally invasive versus open colectomy has been established.

COST EFFECTIVENESS OF LAPAROSCOPIC VERSUS ROBOTIC VERSUS OPEN RESECTION

Evaluation of the cost-effectiveness of any operative procedure needs to take into account the costs incurred by the patient and society as well as the patients' QOL. Surgical procedures are associated with significant equipment costs, as well as the potential to increase or decrease QOL. There is also an associated increase in costs secondary to complications. Laparoscopic resection does have an associated decrease in hospital length of stay (LOS), but it is also associated with an increase in operating room costs. In a 2012 study, data from large randomized trials from 1994 to 2010 comparing open versus laparoscopic resections, the authors developed a model to analyze cost and QALYs for each approach. Laparoscopy has higher initial costs related to operating room equipment and operation length; however, this increase was overcome by a decrease in hospital LOS, rate of ileus, wound infection, time off of work, and indirect cost of caregiver time. When the authors look at sensitivity analyses, they found that laparoscopic surgery was cost effective under a variety of conditions, including cost of equipment, operating room time, hospital LOS, recovery time, conversion rate, rate of ileus, and wound infection. Laparoscopic approaches were less costly compared the open approaches with no difference in QOL. The overall saving of laparoscopic resection was $4283 and sensitivity analyses indicate that it is cost effective at less than $50,000 per QALYs under most conditions.[36]

The use of a robotic platform for colectomy is controversial because of higher costs and a paucity of data regarding outcomes on a national level. In a study to evaluate this was published in 2016, using data from the National Inpatient Sample consisted of 509,026 patients who underwent elective colectomy from 2009 to 2012. Variables included age, sex, race, and procedure status (only elective colectomies). They compared open, robotic, and laparoscopic right and left colectomies; robotic (n = 7686 [right = 2755; left = 4931]), laparoscopic (n = 235,080 [right = 117,005; left = 118,075]) and open (n = 266,263 [right = 123,009; left = 143,254]). The mean patient age was 62.5 years, 80.6% were white, 54.4% were women, and more than 36% of cases were for colon cancer. There was a statistically significant decrease in the percent of open cases over the 3 study years from 55.5% to 49.0% (P<.0001), with a corresponding increase in laparoscopy from 44.0% to 48.2% (P = .0001) and robotic surgery procedures from 0.6% to 2.8% (P = .0001).[37]

Outcomes included in-hospital mortality, and cardiovascular, pulmonary, infectious, iatrogenic injury, urinary, and gastrointestinal complications of surgery. The costs were determined by applying group- and facility-level costs to charge ratios, applied to the Diagnosis Related Group. There was no difference between laparoscopy versus robotic analyses of cardiovascular complications, mortality, and urinary, gastrointestinal, or pulmonary complications. However, there was a greater probability of iatrogenic complications with the robotic platform; including puncture and bleeding complications (R = 1.73; 95% confidence interval, 1.20–2.47). The median estimated cost of robotic surgery was higher at $15,649 (IQR, $11,840-$20,071) versus for laparoscopic surgery at $12,071 (IQR, $9338-$16,203; P<.0001). There was no variation in hospital outcomes among robotic, laparoscopic, and open surgeries. The median LOS was significantly less for laparoscopic (4 days) and robotic (4 days) colectomies as compared with open colectomy (6 days; P<.0001). The authors concluded that the majority of colectomies in the United States are still being done open. There is, however, an increasing volume and rate of laparoscopic in higher volume centers. Robotic colectomy still seems to be in the learning stage, with a higher rate of iatrogenic complications. The authors recommended that robotic colectomy be monitored closely within a registry over the next several years.[37]

Hospital Duration of Stay and Readmission Rates

The use of minimally invasive surgical platforms, and over the last 10 years, enhanced recovery after surgery programs for colectomy has resulted in cost savings for hospitals. However, there was a concern that a decreased LOS and early discharge (to home) would be offset by a higher rate of readmissions. A recent metaanalysis of randomized trials of enhanced recovery after surgery programs for colectomy revealed a significant improvement in outcomes. There was a decrease in LOS by 2.5 days, and a reduction in 30-morbidity.[38] In a 2011 study on the Medicare population, the authors looked at the relationship between early discharges (to home) after colectomy and the rate of readmissions. The patients were from the national Medicare Provider Analysis and Review database for 2003 to 2008. There were 477,461 Medicare patients who were diagnosed with colon cancer and who underwent laparoscopic or open colectomy. Risk factors including age, sex, race, socioeconomic status, admission (elective, urgent, or emergent), and the Elixhauser comorbidity index (a method of categorizing comorbidities of patients based on the *International Classification of Diseases*). LOS was defined as the date of discharge minus the date of surgery. Hospitals were divided into 3 groups based on median LOS for colectomy surgery for cancer: early discharge hospitals, defined by a median LOS of 5 or fewer days; usual hospitals, defined by a median LOS of 5 to 9 days; and long hospitals, defined by a median LOS of greater than 9 days. Readmission was defied as any readmission to any hospital within 30 days of discharge. The readmission rates were compared between the 3 hospitals groups. Risk-adjusted readmission to any hospital was calculated for each hospital by dividing the observed readmission rate by the expected readmission rate (based on patients comorbidity) and multiplying by the average readmission rate. The risk-adjusted readmission rates were assigned to each patient based on hospital and averaged across all patients assigned to each hospital median LOS group. Expected readmission rates were calculated using multiple logistic regression models of patient risk factors for readmission: 29 comorbid conditions, 8 postoperative complications, and laparoscopic versus open surgery. The analyses were repeated with early discharges defined as 4 or fewer days to determine whether results were sensitive to this definition.[39] The results showed that the readmissions rates decreased from 16% to 14% overall from 2003 to 2008. There was no significant increase in the readmission rate in the early discharge hospital versus the usual LOS hospitals (adjusted odds ratio, 1.04; 95% confidence interval, 1.2–1.09), whereas the long LOS hospitals had a significantly higher risk-adjusted readmission rate. Omitting complications from the multivariable model did not alter the results. When the early discharge median was defined as a LOS of 4 or fewer days, there was a statistically significant association between early discharge and readmission. A patient-level analysis was performed to determine risk factors for readmission after colectomy. Independent risk factors included older age, male sex, black race, comorbidities, complications, lower socioeconomic status, urgent or emergent surgery, an open approach (vs laparoscopic), and a longer LOS for the index hospitalization. The ACA of 2010 had a readmission rate reduction as a priority for health care reform. In 2004, the Medicare unplanned readmission rate of 19.6% cost $17 billion to the Medicare fee-for-service program. This study indicated a strong association between patient risk factors and readmission risk, including comorbidity, emergency surgery, and lower socioeconomic status, and that potentially preventable complications were not the major driver of readmission risk. The conclusion were hospitals with a pattern of early discharge defined as a median LOS of 5 or fewer days after surgery do not have a higher risk-adjusted readmission rate than other hospitals. However, hospitals with aggressive early discharge rates have a higher rate of readmissions.[39]

Cost of Readmission

The Centers for Medicare and Medicaid Services in 2013 targeted hospitals with higher than expected risk-adjusted 30-day readmission rates for patients after colorectal surgery, and has chosen this as a metric for value-based hospital payments. A study in 2011 examined a private insurance health plan database for procedure-related risk factors for patients undergoing colorectal surgery. The data included administrative claims from 2002 to 2008 in 9 BlueCross BlueShield health plans, representing 3.8 million insured lives. The patients selected were aged 18 to 64, excluding those 65 years of age and older. Indications for the operation were grouped into colon cancer, diverticulitis or inflammatory bowel disease, and other. The study identified postoperative patients with either surgical site infections (SSIs; superficial, deep, or organ space infections) and/or ostomies. Readmission was defined as a hospitalization with in 30 and 90 days after discharge after the index surgical procedure. Reasons for readmission were divided into groups: cardiovascular, venous thromboembolic, gastrointestinal including dehydration, infectious complications, hemorrhage, respiratory complications, and genitourinary. Costs associated with the readmission were calculated from the paid claims for all hospital, emergency department (ED), home health (HH), and outpatient pharmacy services (amount paid by insurance) starting from the day of surgery (Current Procedural Terminology) and continuing for that hospitalization (diagnostic related group). The main outcomes of the study were the rate of readmission, duration of readmission, total costs, and the costs associated with the readmission. A total of 10,882 patients were identified who underwent colorectal operations between 2002 and 2008. The mean age was 53.9 years with 51.2% men. Indications for surgery were 43.9% colon cancer (4772), 30.4% diverticulitis (3310), and 4.5% inflammatory bowel disease (493). The mean LOS was 9.5 days for open and 6 days for laparoscopic resections. The readmission rate for the laparoscopic group was 8.4% and for the open group was 18.5%. The percent of patients with an SSI on the index hospitalization was 11.3% (1233) and as an outpatient or at time of readmission was 7.5% (815). The overall 30-day SSIs rate for all groups was 18.8%. The overall patient readmission rate for 30 days was 11.4% (1239/10,882), for 31 to 90 days 11.9% (1027/10,882) and for 90 days 32.3%. The mean number of readmission per patient was 1.16 (range, 1–7), with 2 or more readmissions occurring in 1.5% of patients (n = 155) at 30 days and 5.2% of patients (n = 570) at 90 days. In patients with an SSI on the index admission, 19.6% (242/1233) were readmitted within the 30 days and 34.7% (428) were readmitted within the 90 days. There were 13.6% of patients (n = 1483) with or who underwent construction of ostomy during the index admission. Of those, 18% of patients (n = 267) were readmitted within 30 days and 34.7% of patients (n = 428) were readmitted within 90 days. The median cost of all patients was $8885 (range, $4173-$19,915). The cost was higher in patients with an SSI was $12,835 (range, $6143-$31,778), and in patients with ostomies $8523 (range, $3812-$17,306). Patients with ostomies and no SSI cost $7902 (range, $3909-$16,995). The reoperation rate of readmitted patients was 14%, with 21 for ostomy closure (planned closures) and 280 for wound dehiscence, repair of perforation, removal of foreign body, and control of hemorrhage.

On multivariate analysis, the predictors of readmission after colorectal surgery were index hospitalization LOS of greater than 7 days, a Patient-Refined Diagnostic Related Group severity of illness score of 3 or 4, a new ostomy construction, or a discharge to nursing facility. The authors concluded that readmission rate in patients with an SSI and/or ostomy is greatly increased; patients with an ostomy were 3 times more likely to be readmitted, whereas SSI patients were 2 times as likely. They concluded that improved coordination between hospital discharge and outpatient management of patients undergoing colorectal resections may prevent a subset of readmissions and have potential for major cost savings.[40]

Post Acute Care Spending After Surgery

Post acute care (PAC) is one of the fastest growth spending areas of US health care. More than 40% of Americans ages 65 and older age discharged from a hospital use PAC, either HH, skilled nursing facilities, or inpatient or outpatient rehabilitation. The Hospital Value-Based Purchasing Program is holding hospitals accountable for care that occurs after discharge. A hospital will be penalized for spending more than its peer institutions for an episode of care. The ACA of 2010 included 2 Bundled Payments for Care Improvement initiatives: a cardiac and orthopedic bundled payment model. In both bundled payment models, hospitals can accept payments for longitudinal, condition-specific episodes of care that include PAC.[41] A 2017 study was done of fee-for-service Medicare beneficiaries ages 65 years or older undergoing total hip replacement, coronary artery bypass grafting, or colectomy. The authors started with 283,194 patients in 3926 hospitals undergoing colectomy and, after applying exclusion criteria, collected data on 189,229 patients and 1876 hospitals (**Box 2**). They defined PAC for 4 types of services: HH, skilled nursing facility, inpatient rehabilitation facility (IPRF) and outpatient rehabilitation within 90 days after discharge from the initial procedure.

Each PAC setting has different patient social supports and different payment models:

1. Patients are discharged home with outpatient rehabilitation and must be able to attend regular therapy sessions out side the home with reimbursement per service tied to relative value units; or
2. Patients are discharged with HH care who have only limited ability to leave their homes and require intermittent skilled nursing and physical or occupational therapy; or
3. Patients are discharged to a skilled nursing facility who are reimbursed per diem; or
4. Patients are discharged to IPRF care and are reimbursed per stay.

Box 2
Exclusion criteria
Exclusion for patients
Hospice care
Long-term hospital
Inpatient rehabilitation facility
Skilled nursing facility (within 90 days of procedure)
Not eligible for Medicare parts A and B
Hospitals that performed fewer than 10 of the procedures per year

The overall goal was to determine the causes for differences across PAC spending quintiles, defined as average PAC spending per patient at a given hospital. The authors assessed the variation in spending on PAC is affected by several factors: actual cost (actual Medicare payments), different regional prices and variations in wages across regions, and adjusted for case mix. Overall, at least 50% of postcolectomy patients used PAC services. The highest spending quintile was teaching hospitals and for for-profit hospitals that were mostly located in the Northeast. The difference lowest spending quartile versus the highest spending quartile in the use a PAC services was in the 40% and 60% range with an associated mean spending of $2694 and $7491, respectively. When the authors considered the intensity of PAC and the variation in price-standardized total payments for PAC, spending on IPRF care had the greatest increase in spending across quartiles. The variation in price standardization and risk-adjusted payments for PAC was due to the choice of care settings rather than the intensity of the care. When the payments were also adjusted for case mix, the difference between the lowest and the highest spending quintiles decreased because patients in the lowest quintile were not as sick as the patients in the hospitals in the highest quintile. When adjusting for the site of PAC, there was a further reduction in cost. High-cost hospitals and their patients also choose to discharge patients to a skilled nursing facility and IPRF setting more often, which increased the cost. Cost saving may be obtained by decreasing the LOS of stay in these skilled nursing facilities. Patients play an important role in the choice of PAC settings, and their choice is influenced based on patient preference and available social support.[42]

END-OF-LIFE SPENDING

There were approximately 900,000 Medicare beneficiaries with cancer in the last year of life in 2010 with that number expected to increase to 1.2 million by 2020. In 2010, the total costs of cancer care in the last year of life was $37 billion, and by 2020 it will be $50 billion. The costs are based on spending for high rates of ED visits and stays in the intensive care unit during the last months of life.[4] High use of cancer treatment at the end of life is a burden to health care systems and also may represent poor outcomes. A 2012 study used patient behavior to infer the value of oncology therapies in the treatment of metastatic colorectal cancer (second most common cancer-related cause of death in the United States). The authors' study of the patients' decisions on how much to spend on treatment reveals the value they place on alternative treatment choices, as measured in dollars rather than in QALYs. This dollar measure of benefit is compared directly with the cost of therapy to measure the ratio of benefits to costs of the treatment. This was similar to a cost-effectiveness study that measures benefits using QALYs. The authors looked at the principle of consumer economics: the amount that someone is willing to pay for a good is the best measure of its social value. The trade off between price and demand is called the "demand cure." The study sample was based on the medical and pharmacy claims for US patients with metastatic colorectal, breast, head and neck, and lung cancers enrolled in health plans of 45 Fortune 500 companies from 1997 to 2006. The final database information was on 4800 patients with 9206 patient-years. Value of therapy in this model was measured as the ratio between the benefit, the value to the consumer, and its cost. If this ratio is greater than some "threshold," it indicates that the drug is cost effective: the benefit outweighs its cost, which is distinct from the value that the patient ascribes to therapy. They looked at the mean value of all drugs used in the same year and the copayment averages. Looking at patients with metastatic colorectal cancer with 1718 patient-years, the annual total expenditure per drug was $8928 with an annual number of 9.7 claims per drug. A key finding was that higher out-of-pocket expenses led to modest but statistically significant decreases in the average number of claims. The estimated impact of change in price on demand for the drug was −0.062. This is the "price elasticity of demand," the measure of the responsiveness, or elasticity, of quantity demanded of a good or service to a change in its price. For example, a 10% increase in price was associated with a decrease of 0.6 in the number of claims. The average annual total cost of therapy and the estimated value of that therapy to the patients are defined as how much patients were willing to pay for therapy. For patients with colorectal cancer, the average cost of therapy per year was $10,775 with an estimated annual willingness to pay for that therapy of $251,567, a cost benefit ratio of 23. There is a distinction between value and "ability to pay." The value a person places on a life-year will exceed his or her annual income. The authors estimated the expected benefit of therapy divided by accepted cost was valued at $100,000 per QALY, with an average survival gain of about 1.34 times the average QALY for patients with metastatic colorectal cancer (about 10.7 months of survival gains). This study found that patients with metastatic colorectal cancer placed a greater value on survival gains, something that was not recognized by health care regulators and payers. This finding has important implications for the reimbursement of health care technologies that treat terminal illnesses. In conclusion, the authors suggest that empirical data on patients' choices can provide important information to regulators and payers about how to value the survival gains from oncology treatment and that ignoring patients' preferences for life extension might lead to a major misstatement of value in health care.[43] However, there are many patients with advanced cancer who prefer less aggressive treatment and more spiritual support and palliative care to avoid intensive inpatient settings at the end of life. The Centers for Medicare and Medicaid Services has recognized 3 innovative models of cancer care with their Health Care Innovation awards. These awards recognized care innovations that reduced costs and use, yet improved quality of care for Medicare beneficiaries with cancer. Only one looked at the end-of-life care, but all 3 provided improved access to care services for patients with cancer. Model one is the Community Oncology Medical Home (COME HOME) from Innovative Oncology Business Solutions, created 7 sites across the United States. This model addressed the challenges of practice variation, care fragmentation, and high overall costs of care. The model developed triage pathways to help first responders and nurses identify and manage patient symptoms. They provided enhanced access to care through a round-the-clock triage phone line, same-day appointments, extended night and weekend hours, and on-call providers. The program used diagnosis and treatment pathways (based on national evidence-based standards) to guide clinical decision making and supported patient self-management to improve quality of care and health outcomes. It was support by an electronic medial record system that enabled real-time access to patient information. Model 2 is the Patient Care Connect Program (PCCP) from the University of Alabama at Birmingham. This navigation intervention was implemented at 12 sites in 5 southern states. The PCCP used nonclinical navigators to educate and empower patients with cancer and survivors, connect patients and caregivers with resources, and improve adherence to care plans. Lay navigators acted as liaisons between patents and health care providers to clarify treatment plans and to voice patients' concerns. The PCCP has a program called Respecting Choices that focuses on advance care planning and goal setting with the patient and their family at the end of life. Model 3 is the University of Virginia's palliative care for patients with advanced stage cancer through CARE Track. A nurse coordinator using the Patient-Reported Outcomes Measurement Information System identifies patients in most need of pain and symptom management, and refers them for more intensive palliative care services. The goal of the study was to examine how each model affects end-of-life outcomes for patients with cancer. The study population included patients enrolled in all 3 models from June 2012 to December 2105 and who died before December 31, 2015, with a comparative group. The participants were linked to the models by fee-for-service Medicare claims in the Centers for Medicare and Medicaid Services Chronic Conditions Data Warehouse. Practices were identified that were similar in organization to the each of the models for comparison. For COME HOME, they selected similar outpatient oncology practices; for the PCCP, they selected similar outpatient comprehensive cancer centers; and for the CARE Track, they identified cancer centers with a similar volume of oncology care. All comparison groups were in the same geographic region as the models. Then, they matched patient demographics, comorbidities, and cost use and indicators for cancer treatment: surgery, chemotherapy, and radiation therapy for metastatic and high-risk cancers to adjust for differences in severity. Then they measured cost outcomes as the average total Medicare cost of care in the last 30, 90, and 180 days of life per patient. Cost outcomes were continuous and presented in dollars per patient. They assessed use outcomes for hospital and ED by number visits or admissions in the last 30 days of life. Quality of care outcomes included hospice and chemotherapy by the number of patients using each service in the last 2 weeks of life. In each of the models, one-third of patients had metastatic cancer. The COME HOME model decreased the average cost in participants versus comparators in the last 30 days ($959), 90 days ($3346), and 180 days ($5790). There was a similar pattern in PCCP, with an estimated difference between the participants versus comparators at a 6% decrease in costs at 30 days and an 18% decrease in costs at 90 days. There was not a statistically significant decrease in cost for the CARE Track, secondary to small sample. The use of palliative care in the last 30 days of life resulted in the COME HOME having fewer hospitalizations, namely, in 57 of 1000 people and a nonsignificant decrease in the number of ED visits. PCCP also had fewer hospitalizations and ED visits, and CARE Track had a nonsignificant decrease in the number of hospitalizations and ED visits. Quality of care in the last 2 weeks of life was not significantly different in any of the models with regard to hospice admission and chemotherapy in the last 2 weeks of life; however, there was a decreased number of visits overall. The authors concluded that the COME HOME, patient navigation, and palliative care models show promise in reducing the cost of end-of-life care for patients with cancer.[44]

Medicare spending on end-of-life care amounts to 25% of the total annual Medicare spending for 5% of Medicare enrollees, with 70% of all terminal-year expense concentrated in the last 6 moths of life. Approximately 1 in 5 deaths among the elderly is from cancer and the financial impact of cost from hospice care has been increasing, from 26% of patients in 2002% to 47% of those who died in 2012.[45] Geographic variation in end-of-life care spending is driven by physician behavior, differences in health care supply, patient demographics, the severity of the underlying illness, and patient preference. The authors hypothesized that, in regions characterized by high-end-of-life care expenditures, duration of hospice service would be inversely associated with end-of-life care expenditures in contrast with regions characterized by low end-of-life care expenditures. Using the SEER Medicare dataset, they identified patients who died as a result of cancer and calculated their end-of-life care expenditures using the last 6 months of claims for each decedent. They looked at factors such as age, duration of hospice service, and local health care spending patterns in the hospital referral regions (HRR) where the patients resided. They then scored the HRRs into quintiles based on mean end-of-life care expenditures across these quintiles (quintile 1 lowest mean spending vs quintile 5 highest mean spending). Then they looked at the proportion of the variation in end-of-life care expenditures between the highest and lowest quintile regions that could be explained by hospice use (yes vs no) and duration of service in hospice. They categorized the length of service in days into 6 groups (none, 1–3, 4–7, 8–28, 29–56, and >59 days). They identified beneficiaries who had breast, prostate, lung, colorectal, pancreatic, liver, kidney, or hematologic cancers or melanoma diagnosed from 2004 to 2011 between the ages of 66.5 and 94.9 years who died from cancer within 3 years of diagnosis. The control variables included age, race, sex, income, education, year of death, marital status, SEER registry region, urban status of residence, disability status, comorbidities, and tumor characteristics (site, stage IV, multiple cancer, death [6–12, 12–24, and 24–36 months]).

They identified 103,745 people who died of cancer (mean age, 77.8 years), in 129 HRRs during the study period. The unadjusted mean end-of-life care expenditure per decedent in quintile 1 was $39,600 and ranged up to quintile 5 at $49,680. There was a mean duration of hospice service of 10.9 days and a range of duration of hospice service of 13.0 in quintile 1 up to 7.9 days in quintile 5 regions. Quintile 1 patients were more likely to be female, white, and from low-income neighborhoods in nonmetropolitan areas with no additional comorbidities ($P<.001$). More than 30% of all patients in all quintiles were diagnosed with state IV cancers. The study found that hospice use and the duration of hospice enrollment explained only 8% of the variation in end-of-life expenditures between the highest and lowest quintile regions, and this finding suggested that the duration of hospice enrollment had no impact on spending variation. The analysis revealed that, in regions with higher levels of spending, end-of-life care expenditures were associated with duration of hospice service, which was in sharp contrast with regions with lower levels of spending on end-of-life expenditures. The association between hospice expenditures and duration of hospice service is similar across HRRs because hospice payment is based on per diem rates. The driving force for the regional variation in spending is physician behavior. Physicians in different geographic regions practice differently; for example, in high-expenditure regions they are more likely than those in low-expenditure regions to recommend discretionary services to their patients that lack strong evidence.[46] Physicians seek approval from colleagues of equal or higher status to avoid being criticized and may "follow the pack," especially when decisions fall in to the gray areas.[47,48] The authors concluded that the implementation of local incentives in high-expenditure regions to promote hospice use might be effective in decreasing individual expenses and reducing aggressive end-of-life care. Such targeted cost-saving measures may provide substantial economic benefits on a national scale, given that intense end-of-life care expenditures constitute a significant proportion of annual Medicare expenditures.[46]

SUMMARY

The purpose of this article was to identify the economic complexities of the United States health care system. There are many challenges in determining the economic burden of cancer care in the United States, because the existing data are imperfect and are based mostly on the Medicare beneficiaries' fee-for-service payment model, which is being dismantled through Medicare Payment Reform. Since the ACA of 2010, the Medicare Access CHIP Reauthorization Act of 2015 and the Medicare Quality Payment Program, there has been a shift to payment reimbursement linked to quality and value of care. The economic burden of cancer care has so many variables—regionalization of care, physician behavior, practice patterns, patient preferences, high cost of anticancer drugs, site of service, index hospital care, postdischarge acute care services, readmissions, and end-of-life care. We must also recognize the economic burden of limited health literacy and how it affects the quality of care that we deliver. Physicians must remain aware of the economic payment models that are being developed and how they will be shaping reimbursement today and beyond.

REFERENCES

1. Keehan SP, Stone DA, Poisal JA, et al. National health expenditure projections, 2016-25: price increases, aging push sector to 20 percent of economy. Health Aff 2017;36(3):553–63.
2. Yabroff KR, Borowski L, Lipscomb J. Economic studies in colorectal cancer: challenges in measuring and comparing costs. Cancer Epidemiol Biomarkers Prev 2011;20(10):2006–14.
3. Yabroff KR, Borowski L, Lipscomb J. Economic studies in colorectal cancer: challenges in measuring and comparing costs. J Natl Cancer Inst Monogr 2013;46: 62–78.
4. Mariotto AB, Yabroff KR, Shao Y, et al. Projections of the cost of cancer care in the United States: 2010-2020. J Natl Cancer Inst 2011;103(2):117–28.
5. Banegas MP, Guy GP Jr, de Moor JS, et al. For working-age cancer survivors medical debt and bankruptcy created financial hardships. Health Aff 2016; 35(1):54–61.
6. Ramsey S, Blough D, Kirchhoff A, et al. Washington State cancer patients found to be at greater risk for bankruptcy than people without a cancer diagnosis. Health Aff 2013;32(6):1143–52.
7. DeSantis SR, Stein VK, Mariotto K, et al. Cancer treatment and survivorship statistics, 2012. CA Cancer J Clin 2012;62(4):220–41.
8. Bleyer A. Young adult oncology: the patients and their survival challenges. CA Cancer J Clin 2007;57(4):242–55.
9. Bellizzi A, Bar R, Hayes-Lattin B, et al. Positive and negative psychosocial impact of being diagnosed with cancer as an adolescent or your adult. Cancer 2012; 118(20):5155–62.
10. Cohen JW, Monheit AC, Beauregard KM, et al. The medical expenditure panel survey: a national health information resource. Inquiry 1996;33(4):373–89.
11. Guy GP Jr, Yabroff KR, Exwueme DU, et al. Estimating the health and economic burden of cancer among those diagnosed as adolescents and young adults. Health Aff 2014;33(6):1024–31.

12. Hoverman JR, Klein I, Harrison DW, et al. Opening the black box: the impact of on oncology management program consisting of level 1 pathways and an outbound nurse call system. J Oncol Pract 2014;10(1):63–7.
13. Newcomer LN, Gould B, Page RD, et al. Changing physicians incentives for affordable, quality cancer care: results of an episode payment model. J Oncol Pract 2014;10(5):322–6.
14. Clough JD, Patel K, Riley GF, et al. Wide variation in payments for Medicare beneficiary oncology services suggests room for practice-level improvement. Health Aff 2012;34(4):601–8.
15. Ubel PA, Berry SR, Nadler E, et al. In a survey, marked inconsistency in how oncologists judged value of high-cost cancer drugs in relation to gains in survival. Health Aff 2012;31(4):709–17.
16. Howard DH, Bach PB, Berndt ER, et al. Pricing in the market for anticancer drugs. J Econ Perspect 2015;29(1):139–62.
17. Howard DH, Chernew ME, Abdelgawad T, et al. New anticancer drugs associated with large increases in costs and life expectancy. Health Aff 2016;35(9):1581–7.
18. Ramsey SD. How state and federal policies as well as advancers in genome science contributes to the high cost of cancer drugs. Health Aff 2015;34(4):571–5.
19. Landrum MB, Meara ER, Chandra A, et al. Is spending more always wasteful? The appropriateness of care and outcomes among colorectal cancer patients. Health Aff 2008;27(1):159–68.
20. Lakdawalla D, Shafrin J, Lucarelli C, et al. Quality-adjusted cost of care; a meaningful way to measure growth in innovation cost versus the value of health gains. Health Aff (Millwood) 2015;34(4):555–61.
21. Philipson T, Eber M, Lakdawalla DN, et al. An analysis of whether higher health care spending in the United States versus Europe is "worth it" in the case of cancer. Health Aff 2012;31(4):667–75.
22. Soneji S, Yang JW. New analysis reexamines the value of cancer care in the United States compared to Western Europe. Health Aff 2015;34(3):390–9.
23. Hoff G, Dominitz HA. Comparing US and European approaches to colorectal cancer screening: which is best? Gut 2010;59(3):407–14.
24. Edwards BK, Ward E, Kohler BA, et al. Annual report to the nation on the status of cancer 1975-2006. Cancer 2010;116(3):544–73.
25. Bosetti C, Levi F, Rosato V, et al. Recent trends in colorectal cancer mortality in Europe. Int J Cancer 2011;129(1):180–9.
26. Berkman ND, Sheridan SL, Donauhe KE, et al. Low health literacy and health outcomes: an updated systemic review. Ann Intern Med 2011;155(2):97–107.
27. Kohn HK, Berwick DM, Clancy CM, et al. New federal policy initiatives to boost health literacy can help the nation move beyond the cycle of costly "crisis care". Health Aff 2012;31(2):434–43.
28. Ferreira MR, Dolan NC, Fitzgibbon ML, et al. Health care provider-directed intervention to increase colorectal cancer screening among veterans: results of a randomized controlled trial. J Clin Oncol 2005;23(7):1548–54.
29. Smith SG, von Wagner C, McGregor LM, et al. The influence of health literacy on comprehension of a colonoscopy preparation information leaflet. Dis Colon Rectum 2012;55:1074–80.
30. Lissenden B, Yao NA. Affordable care act changes to Medicare led to increased diagnoses of early-stage colorectal cancer among seniors. Health Aff 2017;36(1):101–7.

31. Chang GJ, Kaiser AM, Mills S, et al. Standards practice task force of the American Society of Colon and Rectal Surgeons. Practice parameters for the management of colon cancer. Dis Colon Rectum 2012;55:831–43.

32. Nelson H, Petrelli N, Carlin A, et al. National Cancer Institute Expert Panel. Guidelines 2000 for colon and rectal cancer surgery. J Natl Cancer Inst 2001;93: 583–96.

33. Sterns MW Jr, Schottenfeld D. Techniques for the surgical management of colon cancer. Cancer 1971;28:165–9.

34. Clinical Outcomes of Surgical Therapy Study Group (COST). A comparison of laparoscopically assisted and open colectomy for colon cancer. N Engl J Med 2004;350:2050–9.

35. Fleshman J, Sargent DJ, Green E, et al. Laparoscopic colectomy for cancer is not inferior to open surgery based on 5-year data from the cost study group trial. Ann Surg 2007;245:655–64.

36. Jensen CC, Prasad LM, Abcarian H. Cost-effectiveness of laparoscopic vs open resection for colon and rectal cancer. Dis Colon Rectum 2012;55:1017–23.

37. Yeo HL, Isaacs A, Abelson JS, et al. Comparison of open, laparoscopic, and robotic colectomies using a large national database: outcomes and trends related to surgery center volume. Dis Colon Rectum 2016;59:535–642.

38. Adamant M, Kehlet H, Tomlinson GA, et al. Enhanced recovery pathways optimized health outcomes and resourced utilization: a meta-analysis of randomized controlled trials in colorectal surgery. Surgery 2011;149:830–40.

39. Hendren S, Morris AM, Zhang W, et al. Early discharge and hospital readmission after colectomy for cancer. Dis Colon Rectum 2011;54:1362–7.

40. Wick EC, Shore AD, Hirose K, et al. Readmission rates and cost following colorectal surgery. Dis Colon Rectum 2011;54:1475–9.

41. Centers for Medicare and Medicaid Services. CMS.gov. Bundled payments for care improvement (BPCI) initiative general information. Baltimore (MD): Centers for Medicare and Medicaid Services; 2016. Available at: http://innovation.cms.gov/initiatives/bundled-payments/. Accessed November 8, 2016.

42. Chen LM, Norton EC, Banerjee B, et al. Spending on care after surgery driven by choice of care settings instead of intensity of services. Health Aff 2017;36(1): 83–90.

43. Seabury SA, Goldman DP, Maclean JR, et al. Patients value metastatic cancer therapy more highly than is typically shown through tradition estimates. Health Aff 2012;31(4):691–9.

44. Colligan EM, Ewald E, Ruiz S, et al. Innovative oncology care models improve end-of-life quality, reduce utilization and spending. Health Aff 2017;36(3):433–40.

45. Hogan C. Spending in the last year of life and the impact of hospice on Medicare outlays. Washington (DC): Medicare Payment Advisory Commission; 2015. Available at: http://www.medpac.gov/docs/defauli-source/contractor-reports/spending-in-the-last-year-of-life-and-the-impact-of-hospice-on-medicare-ouylays-updated-august-2015-.pdf?sfvrsn=0. Accessed January 9, 2017.

46. Wang S, Hsu SH, Huang S, et al. Longer periods of hospice service associated with lower end-of life spending in regions with high expenditures. Health Aff 2017; 36(2):328–36.

47. Sirovich BE, Gottlieb DJ, Welch HG, et al. Variation in the tendency of primary care physicians to intervene. Arch Intern Med 2005;165(19):2252–6.

48. Sirovich BE, Gallagher PM, Wennberg DE, et al. Discretionary decision making by primary care physicians and cost of US health care. Health Aff 2008;27(3): 813–23.

Clinical Trials and Progress in Metastatic Colon Cancer

Kabir Mody, MD[a], Tanios Bekaii-Saab, MD[b],*

KEYWORDS

- Colorectal cancer • Clinical trials • KRAS • BRAF • Her2 • Immunotherapy

KEY POINTS

- Presence of mutations in KRAS, NRAS, or BRAF and potentially amplifications in Her2 should be used to guide the use of anti–endothelial growth factor receptor therapies for patients with metastatic colorectal cancer.
- The elucidation of several molecular alterations in metastatic colorectal cancer, including KRAS, NRAS, BRAF, Her2, cMET, mismatch repair, and others, are guiding drug development, clinical trials, and individualized therapy for patients with metastatic colorectal cancer.
- Beyond the rise of immunotherapy for patients with mismatch repair deficiency–related colorectal cancer, several other novel immunotherapy strategies are being evaluated.

INTRODUCTION

Colorectal cancer (CRC) is a leading cause of cancer-related deaths worldwide but mortality associated with this disease has declined in recent decades due to improved screening, better surgical techniques enabling resection of both local and metastatic disease in more patients, improved preoperative and postoperative care, and more effective systemic therapies across all stages of the disease.[1–3] The availability of fluoropyrimidines (5-fluorouracil and capecitabine), oxaliplatin, and irinotecan as the backbones of therapy for metastatic disease has resulted in median overall survival (OS) of up to 24 months.[4] With the addition of agents inhibiting angiogenesis via targeting vascular endothelial growth factor (VEGF) (bevacizumab, ramucirumab, and ziv-aflibercept) and agents inhibiting the epidermal growth factor receptor (EGFR)

Disclosure: K. Mody has contributed research to FibroGen, Inc, Ipsen, Senwha Biosciences, Ariad Pharmaceuticals, Tracon Pharmaceuticals, AstraZeneca/MedImmune, and Genentech. He is also a consultant for Celgene, Merrimack Pharmaceuticals, and Genentech. T. Bekaii-Saab has contributed research to Boston Biomedical, Bayer, Celgene, and Merrimack. He is also a consultant for Bayer, Boehringer Ingelheim, Merrimack, Ipsen; Glenmark, Amgen, Genentech, BMS, Exelixis, Merck, Silajen, and Armo.
^a Gastrointestinal Cancer Program, Mayo Clinic Cancer Center, Mayo Clinic Florida, 4500 San Pablo Road, Jacksonville, FL 32224, USA; ^b Gastrointestinal Cancer Program, Mayo Clinic Cancer Center, Mayo Clinic Arizona, 5777 East Mayo Boulevard, Phoenix, AZ 85054, USA
* Corresponding author.
E-mail address: Bekaii-Saab.Tanios@mayo.edu

signaling pathway (cetuximab and panitumumab), median survival has risen to 30 months in the RAS wild-type patient population.[4] More recently, 2 agents, regorafenib (a broad-spectrum multikinase inhibitor) and trifluridine/tipiracil (a fluoropyrimidine compound), have added to the armamentarium in the salvage setting.

CRC was one of the first tumors to undergo comprehensive genomic characterization that demonstrated several genes and pathways implicated in the disease's development and progression.[5–8] It has transformed CRC into a disease of genomic/transcriptomic subtypes. Additionally the field has recognized that tumors undergo genomic/molecular evolution while under treatment. Critical pathways include TP53, BRAF, KRAS, Her2, PIK3CA, APC, transforming growth factor (TFG)-β, CTNNB and WNT signaling, epithelial-to-mesenchymal transition, MYC amplification, mismatch repair (MMR), and others.[9]

Based on this work, several molecular classifications have arisen, although there are differences among them and none has emerged as a standard in clinical practice.[8,10–17] One such classification system, the consensus molecular subtypes (CMSs), was developed from a comprehensive effort of the CRC Subtyping Consortium. Recognizing that transcriptomics is closely linked to tumor phenotype and clinical behavior, they sought to characterize, in a common set of samples, the key biological features of core subtypes while integrating all other available data sources (mutation, copy number, methylation, microRNA, and proteomics) and assessing correlations with patient outcome.[18] The subtypes developed were the following: CMS1 (microsatellite instability immune) characterized by a hypermutated, microsatellite unstable and strong immune activation state; CMS2 (canonical) characterized by epithelial nature with marked WNT and MYC signaling activation; CMS3 (metabolic) characterized by epithelial nature and evident metabolic dysregulation; and CMS4 (mesenchymal) characterized by prominent TGF-β activation, stromal invasion, and angiogenesis. On integration with clinical data, CMS1 tumors were noted to be more frequently diagnosed in women with right-sided lesions, presenting more often with higher histopathologic grade; CMS2 tumors were mainly left-sided; CMS4 tumors tended to be diagnosed at more advanced stages (III and IV). Analysis of combined data sets, and additionally in a subset of patients from the PETACC-3 clinical trial, revealed that CMS4 tumors resulted in decidedly worse OS and worse relapse-free survival. Conversely, superior survival rates after relapse were seen in CMS2 patients, with a larger proportion of long-term survivors in this subset. The CMS1 population had a poor survival rate after relapse.[14,18,19]

Also of emerging importance, and likely rooted in differences in embryologic origin and associated molecular variances, is the role of primary tumor location—right colon versus left colon—as predictive and prognostic subtypes in metastatic CRC.[20] In at least 2 large analyses, tumors arising in the right colon versus left colon were clinically different, with left-sided primary tumors having superior OS and progression-free survival (PFS) compared with right-sided tumors.[20,21] This difference in location was independently predictive in the face of multiple molecular parameters analyzed, including CMS subtypes. These developments are in need of incorporation into prospective trials to validate and advance individualized treatment of patients. This, taken together with the presence of several molecular alterations, including KRAS, BRAF, Her2, cMET, MMR, and others, are guiding drug development, clinical trials, and individualized therapy for patients with CRC.

MUTATIONS IN THE RAS PATHWAY AND THEIR IMPLICATIONS ON CHOICE OF THERAPY

The Kirsten Ras (KRAS) oncogene encodes for a guanosine triphosphateguanosine diphosphate binding protein downstream of the EGFR in the RAS/RAF/MAPK signaling pathway. KRAS mutations occur in up to 45% of patients with CRC and are driver mutations, critically involved in initiation, proliferation, and progression of CRC.[22–27] A majority of KRAS mutations occur at codons 12, 13, and 61 of the KRAS gene, with the most common a glycine-to-aspartic acid substitution in codon 12. An additional 10% of patients have tumor mutations in other RAS genes, including most importantly NRAS.[22,23] The presence of a KRAS mutation correlates with worse OS, increased invasive stage, liver and lung metastases, and risk of relapse after disease resection compared with KRAS wild-type disease.[28–33] There is also a high concordance rate (96%) between primary CRC tumors and their liver metastases in regard to the presence or absence of KRAS mutations.[34]

The presence of RAS mutations in patients with metastatic CRC is critical given its predictive value regarding the use of EGFR inhibitors.[35] A meta-analysis of 45 clinical studies concluded that the absence of *KRAS* mutations is predictive of improved PFS and OS in patients with advanced CRC treated with anti-EGFR antibodies compared with those harboring KRAS-mutated disease.[36] In patients with tumors harboring RAS mutations, the addition of anti-EGFR therapy to combination chemotherapy adversely affects outcome.[22,37,38]

For patients with RAS wild-type tumors, both bevacizumab and anti-EGFR agents (cetuximab or panitumumab) represent options for addition to chemotherapy. At least 2 large studies have evaluated, in patients with KRAS wild-type disease, for superior efficacy with the addition of either an anti-EGFR agent (cetuximab in both cases) or antiangiogenic therapy with bevacizumab. The FIRE-3 study was a randomized, open-label, phase 3 trial comparing FOLFIRI chemotherapy with either bevacizumab or cetuximab in patients with KRAS (exon 2, codons 12/13) wild-type metastatic CRC[37]; 592 patients with KRAS exon 2 wild-type tumors were randomized to FOLFIRI plus cetuximab or FOLFIRI plus bevacizumab. The objective response rate (ORR) (primary endpoint) was 62.0% in the cetuximab arm compared with 58.0% in the bevacizumab arm (OR 1.18; 95% CI, 0.85–1.64; $P = .18$). Median PFS was 10.0 months in the cetuximab arm and 10.3 months in the bevacizumab arm (hazard ratio [HR] 1.06; 95% CI, 0.88–1.26; $P = .55$); however, the secondary endpoint of median OS was 28.7 months in the cetuximab arm compared with 25.0 months in the bevacizumab arm (HR 0.77; 95% CI, 0.62–0.96; $P = .017$). Patients in the FIRE-3 trial were retrospectively more widely tested for BRAF and RAS mutations and 188 patients with RAS-mutant tumors and 48 with BRAF-mutant tumors were identified. RAS mutations were associated with a trend toward lower ORR (37% vs 50.5%; $P = .11$) and shorter PFS (7.4 vs 9.7 months; HR 1.25; $P = .14$) in patients receiving FOLFIRI plus cetuximab versus bevacizumab, but OS was comparable (19.1 vs 20.1 months; HR 1.05; $P = .73$), respectively.[39] In the CALGB 80405 trial, 1137 patients with *KRAS* wild-type (codons 12 and 13) metastatic CRC received FOLFIRI or mFOLFOX6 chemotherapy at the investigator's discretion and were randomized to the addition of either cetuximab or bevacizumab.[40] Median OSs (primary endpoints) for chemotherapy with bevacizumab versus chemotherapy with cetuximab were 29.04 months and 29.93 months, respectively (HR 0.92; $P = .34$). Median PFS for chemotherapy with bevacizumab versus chemotherapy with cetuximab was 10.84 versus 10.45 months. In a combined analysis of data from 3 trials, including 1096 patients with *RAS* wild-type metastatic CRC, OS (HR 0.80 [95% CI, 0.68–0.93]) and ORR (OR 0.57) favored chemotherapy plus anti-EGFR agents versus bevacizumab plus chemotherapy. PFS (HR 0.98) and resection rates (OR 0.93) were similar between treatments.

Unfortunately, not all patients with *KRAS* exon 2 wild-type disease respond to anti-EGFR monoclonal antibodies. Extended RAS testing to identify non–exon 2 mutations in these patients has been shown to help identify additional patients who may, with anti-EGFR therapy, suffer harm and ineffectiveness. Retrospective analysis of data from the PRIME study initiated the concept of extended *RAS* analysis.[22] Of the study population, 48% patients had tumors with completely wild-type *RAS* (no *KRAS* or *NRAS* mutations in exons 2, 3, or 4 of either gene). In those with extended RAS wild-type disease, panitumumab-FOLFOX treatment was associated with a significant 2.3 months improvement in PFS (10.1 vs 7.9 months, $P = .004$) and 5.6 months improvement in OS (25.8 vs 20.2 months; $P = .009$) compared with FOLFOX alone, respectively. Patients with wild-type *KRAS* tumors at exon 2, but with mutations in other *RAS* exons (*KRAS* exon 3 or 4; *NRAS* exon 2, 3, or 4; or *BRAF* exon 15), showed shorter PFS (7.3 months vs 8 months; $P = .04$) and OS (17.1 months vs 17.8 months; $P = .01$) in the panitumumab-FOLFOX group than in the FOLFOX group, similar to those seen in patients with any *RAS* mutations. Additional evaluations of data from the FIRE-3 and PEAK studies have also shown improved PFS and OS outcomes in those with extended RAS wild-type disease.[38,39] Given these and other available data, it is clear that extended RAS testing should be performed in all patients to identify those with mutations, given the lack of benefit and added cost and toxicities in these patients.

Outcomes with anti-EGFR therapy may also be independently affected by primary tumor location within the colon. For example, among patients with all wild-type disease enrolled in the CALGB 80405 study, those with left-sided primary tumors receiving first-line chemotherapy with the anti-EGFR agent cetuximab had significantly better OS (40.3 vs 18.4 months ($P = .003$; HR 1.68)) compared with those having right-sided tumors.[41] Similarly, data from the FIRE-3 study show PFS and OS of 10.8 months and 38.7 months, respectively, in patients with left-sided disease getting cetuximab. Conversely, in patients with right-sided diseases, PFS and OS were 6.9 months and 16.1 months, respectively, in a population of patients who were RAS wild-type. Analysis of several other studies evaluating bevacizumab and anti-EGFR therapies with chemotherapy in the first-line treatment of patients with metastatic CRC have demonstrated benefit with the addition of anti-EGFR agents (cetuximab or panitumumab) in patients with left-sided primary tumors but no benefit for anti-EGFR therapeutics in right-sided cancers.[42–48] This finding further refines the personalization of anti-EGFR therapies and has clear implications in that tumor sidedness should now be taken into account with all patients when discussing treatment options. The National Comprehensive Cancer Network (NCCN) guidelines for the management of patients with metastatic CRC now recommend against the use of anti-EGFR therapies in patients with RAS wild-type right-sided disease. For left-sided RAS wild-type tumors, both anti-EGFR and anti-VEGF strategies are considered acceptable. Beyond its impact on decisions regarding the use of anti-EGFR therapies, tumor sidedness likely is related to other molecular features of a patient's colon cancer, including, for example, MMR, RAS, Her2, amphiregulin, and epiregulin. Incorporation of tumor sidedness information into clinical trials and further exploration of how these factors have an impact on current and future treatments are ongoing.

Given the high incidence and critical importance of RAS mutations in CRC, therapeutics targeting mutated RAS have been a sought after capability in this disease. Numerous therapeutic strategies targeting components of the KRAS signaling pathway have yielded limited clinical success. The limited clinical success of targeting RAF–MEK–ERK components could be resultant from a nonessential role for mutated KRAS in CRC maintenance, the abundance of downstream pathways from activated KRAS, the existence of alternative KRAS-independent proliferation/survival signaling pathways such as YAP, or the intratumoral genomic heterogeneity of the mutant

KRAS allele.[49,50] KRAS mutation has been shown heterogenous in primary CRC tumors and selected for during EGFR inhibitor therapy.[51,52]

One approach to inhibiting KRAS is via targeting of pathways and effectors downstream of the mutant RAS. This too has been met with limited clinical success.[53] One approach logically thought of is to target MEK alone. Several selective inhibitors of MEK have entered clinical trial evaluation; however, clinical activity with single MEK inhibitors is rarely observed. The first-generation MEK inhibitor, CI-1040, was evaluated in a phase II trial of 4 tumor types, including 20 patients with CRC. The drug was well tolerated but failed to show sufficient antitumor activity to warrant further development. No complete or partial responses were observed. Stable disease (SD) lasting a median of 4.4 months (range: 4–18 months) was seen in 8 patients (2 CRCs).[54] In addition, the second-generation MEK1/2 inhibitor, selumetinib (AZD6244), has not demonstrated activity in an unselected patient population with metastatic CRC. Selumetinib showed similar efficacy to capecitabine in terms of the number of patients with a disease progression event PFS.[55] With approximately 34 patients per arm, disease progression was noted in 28 patients (approximately 80%) in both the AZD6244 and capecitabine treatment groups. Median PFSs were 2.7 months and 2.9 months in the AZD6244 and capecitabine groups, respectively. Ten patients in the AZD6244 treatment arm had a best response of SD. Despite these disappointing results, treatment strategies in RAS-mutant CRC continue and include the combined use of multiple agents targeting several genes involved in the MAPK pathway. Ideally this would cause significant suppression of activated RAS activity. An example of this is a study that evaluated the gene signatures in KRAS mutated versus KRAS wild-type colon cancers and demonstrated that up-regulated genes showed significant enrichment in pathways related to cell cycle and mitosis with FOXM1, the master transcription regulator of mitosis, present in the signature.[56] CDK4/6, an upstream regulator of FOXM1, was thought to potentially be a codriver to the MAPK pathway, promoting the growth of KRAS-mutant CRC.[57–60] Combination treatment in vitro and in vivo of KRAS mutated colon cancer cells and normal with colon epithelial lines with the CDK4/6 inhibitor palbociclib and MEK inhibitor PD0325901 was tested to determine their efficacy and toxicity. Inhibiting CDK4/6 and MEK synergistically depleted FOXM1 and KRAS-associated gene signature, suggesting that CDK4/6 and MEK coregulate the KRAS gene signature. The combined inhibition of CDK4/6 and MEK elicited a robust therapeutic response in KRAS-dependent CRC but not in normal colon epithelial cells, both in vitro and in vivo, and this correlated with downregulation of the KRAS-associated gene signature.[56] Based on these promising data, clinical trial investigations are under way and more investigation regarding alternative strategies in ongoing.

TARGETING BRAF-MUTATED TUMORS

BRAF mutations, largely BRAF V600E, are present in approximately 5% of patients with metastatic CRC and result in constitutive activation of signaling through the MAPK pathway. This mutation is often associated with a more aggressive phenotype, with patients responding poorly to standard combination chemotherapy, with poor survival typically not surpassing a median of 1 year.[61–65] In the TRIBE study, an open-label, multicenter, phase 3 randomized study of patients with unresectable metastatic CRC, FOLFOXIRI plus bevacizumab significantly improved PFS of patients compared with FOLFIRI plus bevacizumab.[66] In the updated analysis, the results for OS and treatment efficacy in RAS and BRAF molecular subgroups are reported.[67] At a median follow-up of 48.1 months, median OS was 13.4 months in the BRAF mutation–positive subgroup (HR 2.79; 95% CI, 1.75–4.46; likelihood ratio test P<.0001). This result established FOLFOXIRI plus bevacizumab as the preferred standard of care in the management of eligible patients with BRAF-mutated CRC.

In BRAF-mutated metastatic melanoma, BRAF inhibition has led to significant improvement in clinical outcomes.[68–71] The efficacy of single-agent strategies with BRAF inhibitors, however, has not been replicated in patients with BRAF-mutant metastatic CRC, with response rates in the single digits.[71,72] This resistance to BRAF inhibition in colon cancer is likely secondary to a feedback loop causing persistent MAPK signaling activation.[73–75] Although transient inhibition of the downstream pERK by BRAF inhibitor vemurafenib was observed in CRC, rapid ERK reactivation occurred through EGFR-mediated activation of RAS and CRAF.[75] BRAF-mutant CRC was also noted to express greater levels of pEGFR than did BRAF-mutant melanomas, suggesting that CRC is more optimally positioned for EGFR-mediated resistance.[75] It has thus been postulated that multitarget inhibition of multiple actors in this pathway is necessary.

In SWOG 1406, 99 patients were randomized to receive irinotecan and cetuximab either with (VIC) or without (IC) the BRAFV600 targeting agent vemurafenib. More than 50% of these patients were exposed to 1 prior treatment regimen for their disease and an additional 34% to 39% to 2 prior regimens. Treatment was generally well tolerated, with 6% and 16% of patients in the IC and VIC arms, respectively, discontinuing therapy due to adverse events. Median PFS was 2 months in the IC arm and 4.3 months in the VIC arm (P = .001; HR 0.48; 95% CI, 0.31–0.75). Partial response, SD, and progression rates were statistically significantly different between arms—4%, 17%, and 66%, respectively, in the IC arm and 16%, 50%, and 18%, respectively, in the VIC arm (P = .001), for a disease control rate (DCR) of 22% and 67%; 48% of patients treated in the IC arm crossed over to the VIC arm after progression of their disease, and these patients experienced a DCR of 72%. Median OS showed a trend toward significance with 5.9 months in the IC arm versus 9.6 months in the VIC arm (P = .19; HR 0.73; 95% CI, 0.45–1.17), with a high rate of crossover of patients from the IC arm into the VIC group. The ongoing BEACON CRC trial (NCT02928224) is examining, in patients with BRAF V600E mutated metastatic CRC, the combination of an MEK inhibitor (binimetinib), a selective BRAF kinase inhibitor (encorafenib), and the EGFR inhibitor cetuximab compared with the combination of encorafenib and cetuximab or control (investigator's choice of irinotecan and cetuximab or FOLFIRI and cetuximab).

Data from a large cohort of patients with metastatic CRC show that non–V600 BRAF mutations occur in 2.2% of patients and represented 22% of all BRAF mutations identified. Compared with patients harboring both V600E BRAF mutations and BRAF wild-type disease, these patients had significantly longer median OS.[76] Identifying the true functional consequences of these alternative mutations in CRC will be important to recognize treatment strategies that may be applicable in this unique subset of patients. Given the serious prognostic and therapeutic implications of BRAF mutation presence in colorectal tumors, testing for such mutations should be considered standard of care for all patients with metastatic CRC.

TARGETING THE AMPLIFIED HER2 PATHWAY

ERBB2 (Her2) is amplified and its protein is overexpressed in various malignancies, including breast and gastric cancers, where this phenomenon has been exploited clinically with the use of ant-Her2 agents with relative good success.[77–80] The Cancer Genome Atlas project identified Her2 mutations and gene amplification in 7% of patients with CRC. Her2 amplification criteria were recently elucidated (HERACLES Diagnostic Criteria). In a large cohort (n = 1086) of patients with KRAS wild-type CRC, 5% of patients demonstrated Her2 positive/amplified based on this CRC-specific scoring criteria.

Novel therapeutic options for patients with Her2-amplified CRC were sought out by a large group of investigators in Italy.[81] They identified a subpopulation of mice bearing Her2-amplified, cetuximab-resistant xenografts and treated these mice with various Her2-targeted therapies either alone or in combination. Monotherapy with any of the drugs was ineffective, but combination therapy with an antibody (trastuzumab) and a tyrosine kinase inhibitor (lapatinib) led to sustained tumor responses. This work supported the HERACLES-A trial, which investigated the combination of trastuzumab and lapatinib in patients (n = 27) with KRAS wild-type (exon 2 codons 12 and 13), metastatic CRC (74% colon and 26% rectal) resistant to EGFR therapies, and after failure of standard therapies.[81] A majority of patients (74%) had received greater than or equal to 4 prior lines of therapy. Her2 3positive expression by immunohistochemistry (IHC) was noted in 74% of the patients, with the remainder Her2 2positive. Of the 27 patients, the ORR was 30% (n = 8; 4% complete response and 26% partial response), and 44% had SD. A majority of patients demonstrating an objective response (88%) had tumors with 3positive Her2 scoring on IHC. Overall, 59% of patients had disease response and/or disease control lasting for 4 months or longer. Thus, disease was controlled in 74%, with median follow-up of 94 weeks. The treatment was well tolerated with the most common adverse effects diarrhea, rash, dry skin, fatigue, and paronychia, although the only grade 3 to 4 adverse effect occurring in greater than 10% of patients was fatigue. Further investigations of similar targeted therapy approaches for Her2-amplified disease are being investigated. These include the ongoing MY-PATHWAY study, which is evaluating pertuzumab and trastuzumab in patients with Her2-amplified tumors, including metastatic CRC.[82] Also, the HERACLES-B study is evaluating the combination of pertuzumab and trastuzumab, which both target Her2, as second-line or third-line therapy in chemorefractory metastatic CRC. Additionally, the HERACLES-RESCUE is a phase 2 trial assessing the efficacy of trastuzumab emtansine in Her2-amplified metastatic CRC progressing on anti-Her2 therapy with lapatinib and trastuzumab. T-DM1 is an antibody-drug conjugate whereby trastuzumab (the T portion) is connected via a stable thioether linker to emtansine (the DM1 portion), a potent microtubule chemotherapy agent. Once trastuzumab binds to Her2-expressing cells, the linker is broken down, releasing DM1 intracellularly. Finally, another study of tucatanib (Cascadian Therapeutics, Seattle, WA), a small molecule selective Her2 inhibitor with trastuzumab, the MOUNTAINEER trial, is under way (NCT03043313).

It has also recently been demonstrated that activation of Her2 signaling, as happens with Her2 amplification, may result in resistance to anti-EGFR therapies, which are already prevalent agents in use clinically, as discussed previously.[83] This finding needs to be validated further prospectively. Overall, testing of Her2 alterations should be strongly considered for incorporation into clinical practice to allow for proper identification of patients with Her 2-amplified disease.

OTHER TARGETS

The fibroblast growth factor receptors (FGFRs) are a group of 4 tyrosine kinase receptors (FGFR1, 2, 3, and 4) that bind to any of 18 secreted glycoprotein ligands, fibroblast growth factors (FGFs).[84] Binding results in activation of signaling pathways, including the MAPK, PI3K/Akt, and STAT pathways.[85] FGFR overexpression has been identified in CRC samples and is postulated to play a key role in this disease.[53]

In tumor samples where FGFR signaling has been identified as playing an important role, it has been in the tumor microenvironment, with a correlation between FGFR overexpression and tumor invasion, advanced-stage disease, and chemotherapy resistance.[86–89] Preclinical studies have demonstrated reversal of chemotherapy resistance by combining FGFR inhibitors with chemotherapy in CRC cell lines. This may represent a potential therapeutic strategy to overcome resistance in CRC.[53] There are now several agents in clinical trials in a variety of malignancies, and at least 1 Food and Drug Administration (FDA)-approved agent with anti-FGFR activity (ponatinib). Additionally, Regorafenib, an oral multikinase inhibitor with relative activity against FGFRs 1 and 2, is already approved for treatment of refractory metastatic CRC and is an agent being built on in this regard.

Hepatocyte growth factor receptor, otherwise known as c-MET, is overexpressed in up to 67% of CRC samples. Its overexpression is a negative prognostic marker rand contributes to oncogenesis, invasiveness, recurrence, and chemoresistance.[90–93] Blockade of c-MET inhibits tumor growth in CRC cell lines, thus these agents targeting MET/HGF (eg, crizotinib, tivantinib, cabozantinib, AMG102, and AV299) are under investigation for the treatment of CRC, although many of the efforts to target c-MET in this disease have thus far been unsuccessful.[94,95]

THE ROLE OF IMMUNOTHERAPY

Immunotherapy agents, specifically therapies targeting immune checkpoint proteins, have recently revolutionized cancer treatment; however, heretofore, only a subset of patients with any given tumor type have responses. Determinants of this subset are still somewhat obscure although several molecular markers have been evaluated. What is evident is that tumor mutational load has emerged as a biomarker of immunotherapy success with tumors bearing higher mutational loads more likely to respond. Biomarkers with some evidence of capability in prediction of responses to immune checkpoint blockade include genes with impact on this mutational load, including microsatellite instability and mutations in POLE and POLD.

Mutations in POLE and POLD map to proofreading domains of DNA polymerases ε and δ, with the effect of impairing correction of mispaired bases, markedly affecting the process of DNA replication.[96,97] The true frequency of POLE/POLD mutations in patients with CRC is unclear and estimates at frequency have ranged from 1.3% to 12.3%.[96,98,99] There are clinical reports of success with immune checkpoint blockade therapies in patients with POLE-mutant endometrial cancer and also POLE-mutant colorectal cancer.[100,101] Microsatellite instability (MSI) is a marker of impaired MMR protein function within a tumor. MSI is a polymerase chain reaction–based assay in which 5 microsatellites are evaluated for instability; if greater than or equal to 2/5 are unstable, the sample is deemed to be MSI-high (MSI-H). Otherwise, tumors are termed microsatellite stable (MSS). Another assay involves assessment of the MMR proteins (MLH1, MSH2, MSH6, and PMS2) by IHC. An absence of staining is equivalent to MSI-H status and referred to as MMR deficient (dMMR). MSI-H tumors, on pathologic analysis, are characterized by a strong lymphocytic infiltrate.[102] This lymphocytic response has been thought to be secondary to an immunogenic, high mutational, and thus neoantigen, burden. This has now been demonstrated to be the case in genomic analysis.[103–107]

Microsatellite Instability High Disease

The concept that MSI-H tumors have a higher mutational burden and thus bear a higher neoantigen load formed the rationale for an initial study of anti–Programmed

Cell Death protein–1 therapy in patients with dMMR CRCs, which demonstrated impressive efficacy in mostly refractory patients.[108] In the follow-up study to this, 86 consecutive patients with dMMR malignancies of 12 types were enrolled to receive anti–PD-1 therapy (pembrolizumab).[109] Therapy was well tolerated with a vast majority of patients experiencing adverse effects of low grade. Objective responses were seen in 53% of patients, with 21% having complete responses. These response rates were similar between CRC and other cancer types. The overall DCR was 77%. Different from traditional chemotherapy, the median time to any response of disease was 21 weeks, and the median time to complete response was 42 weeks. After a median follow-up of 12.5 months, neither median PFS nor median OS had been reached. The investigators sought to determine the percentage of patients to whom these results might be applicable; 12,019 cancers representing 32 tumor types were evaluated for dMMR using next-generation sequencing. They noted that greater than 5% of adenocarcinomas of 11 different types, including CRC (6%), demonstrated dMMR status, accounting for an estimated 60,000 patients in the United States alone.[109] A second study evaluated another agent targeting PD-1, nivolumab, in patients with metastatic dMMR CRCs who had progressed on greater than or equal to 1 prior line of therapy. With 84% of patients having received greater than or equal to 2 prior lines of therapy, the ORR was 27% and the DCR was 62%. Median time to response was approximately 2.7 months, with PFS rate at 12 months of 45.6%. Median OS had not yet been reached. No differences in outcomes were noted when evaluated regarding PD-L1 tumor positivity versus negativity or to tumoral KRAS or BRAF mutation status. Again, treatment was well tolerated with just 20% of patients having grade 3 to grade 4 treatment-related adverse events. Based on these data, the FDA earlier this year approved the anti–PD-1 antibodies pembrolizumab for use in any tumor with MSI-H status and nivolumab only for those with metastatic CRC. Additionally, the most recent NCCN guidelines include both pembrolizumab and nivolumab as options for metastatic and unresectable MSI-H CRC.

Combination immune checkpoint inhibition with PD-1 inhibitor nivolumab and CTLA-4 inhibitor ipilimumab has also been clinically evaluated. In CheckMate 142, nivolumab was combined with ipilimumab × 4 doses followed by nivolumab monotherapy[110]; 30 patients were initially enrolled, with 27 patients evaluable at the interim analysis. The ORR was 41%, with 37% achieving SD, for a DCR of 78%, with 82% of responses ongoing at 6 months. Median PFS and OS had not been reached yet. Because responses can be slower to evolve with immunotherapy and data continue to mature, no clear clinical conclusions can be made at this time. This combination therapy comes at the cost of significantly worse grade 3 to grade 4 adverse events.[110,111] Multiple other studies are planned or ongoing to further evaluate the role of PD-1/L1 inhibition in MSI-H CRC in combination with various immomodulating strategies.

Microsatellite Instability Low Disease or Stable Disease

When pembrolizumab was evaluated in patients with MSI-H disease, a cohort of patients specifically with MSS CRC was also enrolled.[108] Importantly, in this cohort no responses were observed, with a median PFS of 2.2 months and OS of 5 months. As with other malignancies the combination of anti–PD-1 and anti–CTLA-4 therapies has also been investigated in MSS CRC. Preliminarily, the Checkmate 142 study demonstrated no efficacy in MSS tumors with combination therapy in 2 dosing cohorts.[110] Median PFS was 2.3 months at best in the 2 dosing cohorts. Thus, the data so far suggest no activity of anti–PD-1 therapy given singly or in combination with anti–CTLA-4 therapy.

In the MSS cohort of patients, representing more than 95% of patients with metastatic CRC, immune-enhancing approaches are being explored. One such approach stems from preclinical data that suggested, in melanoma, colorectal, and breast cancer models, that MEK inhibition up-regulates interferon-γ–mediated HLA molecule and PD-L1 expression, and synergizes with PD-1 inhibition.[112,113] A phase I study was thus undertaken investigating the combination of MEK inhibition with cobimetinib and PD-L1 inhibition with atezolizumab, with an expansion cohort in KRAS-mutant CRC.[114,115] Interim results demonstrated, in 23 patients with metastatic CRC, 20 with KRAS-mutant disease, a 17% overall response rate, and a 6-month OS of 72%. Three of the 4 responders had known MSS disease. Serial tumor biopsy samples demonstrated effects commensurate with the preclinical rationale for the study. A phase III randomized study evaluating the role of the cobimetinib and atezolizumab combination in patients with refractory metastatic MSS CRC compared with atezolizumab alone or regorafenib is now completed accrual and is pending analysis of final results. Other strategies include MEK inhibition combined with the anti–PD-1/anti–CTLA-4 (NCT02060188), and triple combination with anti-VEGF and anti–PD-1 agents (NCT02876224).

The future of immunotherapy in CRC seems bright because, in addition to the strategies discussed previously, multiple other approaches are being investigated. These include further work combining multiple immune checkpoint blockade agents targeting such proteins as indoleamine 2,3-dioxygenase or LAG-3. Drugs that target proteins acting as direct immune stimulators, such as KIR and 4-1BB (CD137), are also being studied in multiple combinations. Immune checkpoint therapeutics are also being combined with other agents targeting epigenetic mechanisms, such as DNA methyltransferase inhibitors and angiogenesis via VEGF and its receptors. Immunotherapy agents are also being combined with radiation, believed to increase antigenicity of tumors, in various forms.

SUMMARY

Over the past several years, genomic sequencing of colon cancer has resulted in a deeper understanding of the genomic landscape of metastatic CRC. This has enabled the field to develop and tailor therapies for patients. Despite these improvements, much work remains and future studies will add to the understanding of the functional and impact of various gene alterations, how the landscape changes with treatment, and how genomic alterations may have an impact on nongenomically targeted therapies, such as chemotherapy and immunotherapy. Additionally, new technologies will improve the ability to evaluate patients' tumors in several ways and personalize therapies. For example, the promise of liquid biopsies, using circulating cell-free DNA (cfDNA) released by tumor cells, for genomic profiling provides a comprehensive evaluation of a patient's advanced disease. This allows for real-time tracking of clonal evolution and mechanisms of resistance while on therapy, in a way that is more relevant than the use of tissue from prior biopsies. Both focused analysis for several genes and multigene assays are already being used.[52,116] cfDNA is already in use in clinical trials, and trials evaluating genomically guided personalized therapies determined by cfDNA analysis, such as the COLOMATE study, are in development. Additionally, progress has been made regarding the use of immunotherapy in patients with colon cancer, particularly in the MSI-H subpopulation, and further progress in the larger MSS population seems close behind. Despite the knowledge that further failures may lie ahead, there is certainly reason for great optimism on behalf of patients suffering from metastatic CRC.

REFERENCES

1. Siegel RL, Miller KD, Fedewa SA, et al. Colorectal cancer statistics, 2017. CA Cancer J Clin 2017;67(3):177–93.
2. Welch HG, Robertson DJ. Colorectal cancer on the decline–why screening can't explain it all. N Engl J Med 2016;374(17):1605–7.
3. Torre LA, Bray F, Siegel RL, et al. Global cancer statistics, 2012. CA Cancer J Clin 2015;65(2):87–108.
4. Cremolini C, Schirripa M, Antoniotti C, et al. First-line chemotherapy for mCRC-a review and evidence-based algorithm. Nat Rev Clin Oncol 2015;12(10):607–19.
5. Fearon ER. Molecular genetics of colorectal cancer. Annu Rev Pathol 2011;6: 479–507.
6. Fearon ER, Vogelstein B. A genetic model for colorectal tumorigenesis. Cell 1990;61(5):759–67.
7. Vogelstein B, Fearon ER, Hamilton SR, et al. Genetic alterations during colorectal-tumor development. N Engl J Med 1988;319(9):525–32.
8. Vogelstein B, Papadopoulos N, Velculescu VE, et al. Cancer genome landscapes. Science 2013;339(6127):1546–58.
9. Cancer Genome Atlas Network. Comprehensive molecular characterization of human colon and rectal cancer. Nature 2012;487(7407):330–7.
10. Sjoblom T, Jones S, Wood LD, et al. The consensus coding sequences of human breast and colorectal cancers. Science 2006;314(5797):268–74.
11. Leary RJ, Lin JC, Cummins J, et al. Integrated analysis of homozygous deletions, focal amplifications, and sequence alterations in breast and colorectal cancers. Proc Natl Acad Sci U S A 2008;105(42):16224–9.
12. Martin ES, Tonon G, Sinha R, et al. Common and distinct genomic events in sporadic colorectal cancer and diverse cancer types. Cancer Res 2007;67(22): 10736–43.
13. De Sousa EMF, Wang X, Jansen M, et al. Poor-prognosis colon cancer is defined by a molecularly distinct subtype and develops from serrated precursor lesions. Nat Med 2013;19(5):614–8.
14. Dienstmann R, Vermeulen L, Guinney J, et al. Consensus molecular subtypes and the evolution of precision medicine in colorectal cancer. Nat Rev Cancer 2017;17(4):268.
15. Sadanandam A, Lyssiotis CA, Homicsko K, et al. A colorectal cancer classification system that associates cellular phenotype and responses to therapy. Nat Med 2013;19(5):619–25.
16. Marisa L, de Reynies A, Duval A, et al. Gene expression classification of colon cancer into molecular subtypes: characterization, validation, and prognostic value. PLoS Med 2013;10(5):e1001453.
17. Roepman P, Schlicker A, Tabernero J, et al. Colorectal cancer intrinsic subtypes predict chemotherapy benefit, deficient mismatch repair and epithelial-to-mesenchymal transition. Int J Cancer 2014;134(3):552–62.
18. Guinney J, Dienstmann R, Wang X, et al. The consensus molecular subtypes of colorectal cancer. Nat Med 2015;21(11):1350–6.
19. Van Cutsem E, Labianca R, Bodoky G, et al. Randomized phase III trial comparing biweekly infusional fluorouracil/leucovorin alone or with irinotecan in the adjuvant treatment of stage III colon cancer: PETACC-3. J Clin Oncol 2009;27(19):3117–25.
20. Venook A, Niedzwiecki D, Innocenti F, et al. Impact of primary (1°) tumor location on overall survival (OS) and progression-free survival (PFS) in patients (pts) with

metastatic colorectal cancer (mCRC): Analysis of CALGB/SWOG 80405 (Alliance). J Clin Oncol 2016;34 [abstract: 3504].

21. Schrag D, Weng S, Brooks GA, et al. The relationship between primary tumor sidedness and prognosis in colorectal cancer. J Clin Oncol 2016;34(34 Suppl) [abstract: 3505].

22. Douillard JY, Oliner KS, Siena S, et al. Panitumumab-FOLFOX4 treatment and RAS mutations in colorectal cancer. N Engl J Med 2013;369(11):1023–34.

23. Douillard JY, Rong A, Sidhu R. RAS mutations in colorectal cancer. N Engl J Med 2013;369(22):2159–60.

24. Van Cutsem E, Kohne CH, Lang I, et al. Cetuximab plus irinotecan, fluorouracil, and leucovorin as first-line treatment for metastatic colorectal cancer: updated analysis of overall survival according to tumor KRAS and BRAF mutation status. J Clin Oncol 2011;29(15):2011–9.

25. Peeters M, Price TJ, Cervantes A, et al. Randomized phase III study of panitumumab with fluorouracil, leucovorin, and irinotecan (FOLFIRI) compared with FOLFIRI alone as second-line treatment in patients with metastatic colorectal cancer. J Clin Oncol 2010;28(31):4706–13.

26. Maughan TS, Adams RA, Smith CG, et al. Addition of cetuximab to oxaliplatin-based first-line combination chemotherapy for treatment of advanced colorectal cancer: results of the randomised phase 3 MRC COIN trial. Lancet 2011; 377(9783):2103–14.

27. Tveit KM, Guren T, Glimelius B, et al. Phase III trial of cetuximab with continuous or intermittent fluorouracil, leucovorin, and oxaliplatin (Nordic FLOX) versus FLOX alone in first-line treatment of metastatic colorectal cancer: the NORDIC-VII study. J Clin Oncol 2012;30(15):1755–62.

28. Vauthey JN, Zimmitti G, Kopetz SE, et al. RAS mutation status predicts survival and patterns of recurrence in patients undergoing hepatectomy for colorectal liver metastases. Ann Surg 2013;258(4):619–26 [discussion: 626–7].

29. Yaeger R, Cowell E, Chou JF, et al. RAS mutations affect pattern of metastatic spread and increase propensity for brain metastasis in colorectal cancer. Cancer 2015;121(8):1195–203.

30. Karagkounis G, Torbenson MS, Daniel HD, et al. Incidence and prognostic impact of KRAS and BRAF mutation in patients undergoing liver surgery for colorectal metastases. Cancer 2013;119(23):4137–44.

31. Li HT, Lu YY, An YX, et al. KRAS, BRAF and PIK3CA mutations in human colorectal cancer: relationship with metastatic colorectal cancer. Oncol Rep 2011; 25(6):1691–7.

32. Mannan A, Hahn-Stromberg V. K-ras mutations are correlated to lymph node metastasis and tumor stage, but not to the growth pattern of colon carcinoma. APMIS 2012;120(6):459–68.

33. Modest DP, Stintzing S, Laubender RP, et al. Clinical characterization of patients with metastatic colorectal cancer depending on the KRAS status. Anticancer Drugs 2011;22(9):913–8.

34. Knijn N, Mekenkamp LJ, Klomp M, et al. KRAS mutation analysis: a comparison between primary tumours and matched liver metastases in 305 colorectal cancer patients. Br J Cancer 2011;104(6):1020–6.

35. Peeters M, Douillard JY, Van Cutsem E, et al. Mutant KRAS codon 12 and 13 alleles in patients with metastatic colorectal cancer: assessment as prognostic and predictive biomarkers of response to panitumumab. J Clin Oncol 2013; 31(6):759–65.

36. Dahabreh IJ, Terasawa T, Castaldi PJ, et al. Systematic review: Anti-epidermal growth factor receptor treatment effect modification by KRAS mutations in advanced colorectal cancer. Ann Intern Med 2011;154(1):37–49.

37. Heinemann V, von Weikersthal LF, Decker T, et al. FOLFIRI plus cetuximab versus FOLFIRI plus bevacizumab as first-line treatment for patients with metastatic colorectal cancer (FIRE-3): a randomised, open-label, phase 3 trial. Lancet Oncol 2014;15(10):1065–75.

38. Schwartzberg LS, Rivera F, Karthaus M, et al. PEAK: a randomized, multicenter phase II study of panitumumab plus modified fluorouracil, leucovorin, and oxaliplatin (mFOLFOX6) or bevacizumab plus mFOLFOX6 in patients with previously untreated, unresectable, wild-type KRAS exon 2 metastatic colorectal cancer. J Clin Oncol 2014;32(21):2240–7.

39. Stintzing S, Miller-Phillips L, Modest DP, et al. Impact of BRAF and RAS mutations on first-line efficacy of FOLFIRI plus cetuximab versus FOLFIRI plus bevacizumab: analysis of the FIRE-3 (AIO KRK-0306) study. Eur J Cancer 2017;79: 50–60.

40. Venook A, Niedzwiecki D, Lenz HJ, et al. CALGB/SWOG 80405: phase III trial of irinotecan/5-FU/leucovorin (FOLFIRI) or oxaliplatin/5-FU/leucovorin (mFOLFOX6) with bevacizumab (BV) or cetuximab (CET) for patients (pts) with KRAS wild-type (wt) untreated metastatic adenocarcinoma of the colon or rectum (MCRC). J Clin Oncol 2014;32 [abstract: LBA3].

41. Venook A, Ou F-S, Lenz HJ, et al. Primary tumor location as an independent prognostic marker from molecular features for overall survival in patients with metastatic colorectal cancer: analysis of CALGB/SWOG 80405 (Alliance). J Clin Oncol 2017;35(Suppl) [abstract: 3503].

42. Loupakis F, Yang D, Yau L, et al. Primary tumor location as a prognostic factor in metastatic colorectal cancer. J Natl Cancer Inst 2015;107(3) [pii:dju427].

43. Lenz HJ, lee F, Yau L, et al. MAVERICC, a phase 2 study of mFOLFOX6-bevacizumab (BV) vs FOLFIRI-BV with biomarker stratification as first-line (1L) chemotherapy (CT) in patients (pts) with metastatic colorectal cancer (mCRC). J Clin Oncol 2016;34(Suppl 4S) [abstract: 493].

44. Wong HL, Lee B, Field K, et al. Impact of primary tumor site on bevacizumab efficacy in metastatic colorectal cancer. Clin Colorectal Cancer 2016;15(2): e9–15.

45. Brule S, Jonker DJ, Karapetis CS, et al. Location of colon cancer (right-sided [RC] versus left-sided [LC]) as a predictor of benefit from cetuximab (CET): NCIC CTG CO.17. J Clin Oncol 2013;31(Suppl) [abstract: 3528].

46. Brule SY, Jonker DJ, Karapetis CS, et al. Location of colon cancer (right-sided versus left-sided) as a prognostic factor and a predictor of benefit from cetuximab in NCIC CO.17. Eur J Cancer 2015;51(11):1405–14.

47. Heinemann V, Modest DP, von Weikersthal LF, et al. Gender and tumor location as predictors for efficacy: influence on endpoints in first-line treatment with FOLFIRI in combination with cetuximab or bevacizumab in the AIO KRK 0306 (FIRE3) trial. J Clin Oncol 2014;32(Suppl) [abstract: 3600].

48. Boeckx N, Toler A, Op de Beeck K, et al. Primary tumor sidedness impacts on prognosis and treatment outcome: results from three randomized studies of panitumumab plus chemotherapy versus chemotherapy. Ann Oncol 2016; 27(6):15–42.

49. Pylayeva-Gupta Y, Grabocka E, Bar-Sagi D. RAS oncogenes: weaving a tumorigenic web. Nat Rev Cancer 2011;11(11):761–74.

50. Kapoor A, Yao W, Ying H, et al. Yap1 activation enables bypass of oncogenic Kras addiction in pancreatic cancer. Cell 2014;158(1):185–97.
51. Diaz LA Jr, Williams RT, Wu J, et al. The molecular evolution of acquired resistance to targeted EGFR blockade in colorectal cancers. Nature 2012; 486(7404):537–40.
52. Misale S, Yaeger R, Hobor S, et al. Emergence of KRAS mutations and acquired resistance to anti-EGFR therapy in colorectal cancer. Nature 2012;486(7404): 532–6.
53. Ahn DH, Ciombor KK, Mikhail S, et al. Genomic diversity of colorectal cancer: changing landscape and emerging targets. World J Gastroenterol 2016; 22(25):5668–77.
54. Rinehart J, Adjei AA, Lorusso PM, et al. Multicenter phase II study of the oral MEK inhibitor, CI-1040, in patients with advanced non-small-cell lung, breast, colon, and pancreatic cancer. J Clin Oncol 2004;22(22):4456–62.
55. Bennouna J, Lang I, Valladares-Ayerbes M, et al. A Phase II, open-label, randomised study to assess the efficacy and safety of the MEK1/2 inhibitor AZD6244 (ARRY-142886) versus capecitabine monotherapy in patients with colorectal cancer who have failed one or two prior chemotherapeutic regimens. Invest New Drugs 2011;29(5):1021–8.
56. Pek M, Yatim S, Chen Y, et al. Oncogenic KRAS-associated gene signature defines co-targeting of CDK4/6 and MEK as a viable therapeutic strategy in colorectal cancer. Oncogene 2017;36(35):4975–86.
57. Malumbres M, Barbacid M. Cell cycle, CDKs and cancer: a changing paradigm. Nat Rev Cancer 2009;9(3):153–66.
58. Choi YJ, Anders L. Signaling through cyclin D-dependent kinases. Oncogene 2014;33(15):1890–903.
59. Anders L, Ke N, Hydbring P, et al. A systematic screen for CDK4/6 substrates links FOXM1 phosphorylation to senescence suppression in cancer cells. Cancer Cell 2011;20(5):620–34.
60. Harbour JW, Dean DC. The Rb/E2F pathway: expanding roles and emerging paradigms. Genes Dev 2000;14(19):2393–409.
61. Yokota T, Ura T, Shibata N, et al. BRAF mutation is a powerful prognostic factor in advanced and recurrent colorectal cancer. Br J Cancer 2011;104(5):856–62.
62. Tran B, Kopetz S, Tie J, et al. Impact of BRAF mutation and microsatellite instability on the pattern of metastatic spread and prognosis in metastatic colorectal cancer. Cancer 2011;117(20):4623–32.
63. Price TJ, Hardingham JE, Lee CK, et al. Impact of KRAS and BRAF gene mutation status on outcomes from the phase III AGITG MAX trial of capecitabine alone or in combination with bevacizumab and mitomycin in advanced colorectal cancer. J Clin Oncol 2011;29(19):2675–82.
64. Morris V, Overman MJ, Jiang ZQ, et al. Progression-free survival remains poor over sequential lines of systemic therapy in patients with BRAF-mutated colorectal cancer. Clin Colorectal Cancer 2014;13(3):164–71.
65. Samowitz WS, Sweeney C, Herrick J, et al. Poor survival associated with the BRAF V600E mutation in microsatellite-stable colon cancers. Cancer Res 2005;65(14):6063–9.
66. Loupakis F, Cremolini C, Masi G, et al. Initial therapy with FOLFOXIRI and bevacizumab for metastatic colorectal cancer. N Engl J Med 2014;371(17):1609–18.
67. Cremolini C, Loupakis F, Antoniotti C, et al. FOLFOXIRI plus bevacizumab versus FOLFIRI plus bevacizumab as first-line treatment of patients with metastatic colorectal cancer: updated overall survival and molecular subgroup

analyses of the open-label, phase 3 TRIBE study. Lancet Oncol 2015;16(13): 1306–15.

68. Flaherty KT, Puzanov I, Kim KB, et al. Inhibition of mutated, activated BRAF in metastatic melanoma. N Engl J Med 2010;363(9):809–19.

69. Sosman JA, Kim KB, Schuchter L, et al. Survival in BRAF V600-mutant advanced melanoma treated with vemurafenib. N Engl J Med 2012;366(8): 707–14.

70. Falchook GS, Long GV, Kurzrock R, et al. Dabrafenib in patients with melanoma, untreated brain metastases, and other solid tumours: a phase 1 dose-escalation trial. Lancet 2012;379(9829):1893–901.

71. Hauschild A, Grob JJ, Demidov LV, et al. Dabrafenib in BRAF-mutated metastatic melanoma: a multicentre, open-label, phase 3 randomised controlled trial. Lancet 2012;380(9839):358–65.

72. Kopetz S, Desai J, Chan E, et al. Phase II pilot study of vemurafenib in patients with metastatic BRAF-mutated colorectal cancer. J Clin Oncol 2015;33(34): 4032–8.

73. Hong DS, Morris VK, El Osta B, et al. Phase IB study of vemurafenib in combination with irinotecan and cetuximab in patients with metastatic colorectal cancer with BRAFV600E mutation. Cancer Discov 2016;6(12):1352–65.

74. Corcoran RB, Dias-Santagata D, Bergethon K, et al. BRAF gene amplification can promote acquired resistance to MEK inhibitors in cancer cells harboring the BRAF V600E mutation. Sci Signal 2010;3(149):ra84.

75. Corcoran RB, Ebi H, Turke AB, et al. EGFR-mediated re-activation of MAPK signaling contributes to insensitivity of BRAF mutant colorectal cancers to RAF inhibition with vemurafenib. Cancer Discov 2012;2(3):227–35.

76. Jones JC, Renfro LA, Al-Shamsi HO, et al. Non-V600 BRAF mutations define a clinically distinct molecular subtype of metastatic colorectal cancer. J Clin Oncol 2017;35(23):2624–30.

77. Gutierrez C, Schiff R. HER2: biology, detection, and clinical implications. Arch Pathol Lab Med 2011;135(1):55–62.

78. Arteaga CL, Engelman JA. ERBB receptors: from oncogene discovery to basic science to mechanism-based cancer therapeutics. Cancer Cell 2014;25(3): 282–303.

79. Slamon DJ, Leyland-Jones B, Shak S, et al. Use of chemotherapy plus a monoclonal antibody against HER2 for metastatic breast cancer that overexpresses HER2. N Engl J Med 2001;344(11):783–92.

80. Bang YJ, Van Cutsem E, Feyereislova A, et al. Trastuzumab in combination with chemotherapy versus chemotherapy alone for treatment of HER2-positive advanced gastric or gastro-oesophageal junction cancer (ToGA): a phase 3, open-label, randomised controlled trial. Lancet 2010;376(9742):687–97.

81. Sartore-Bianchi A, Trusolino L, Martino C, et al. Dual-targeted therapy with trastuzumab and lapatinib in treatment-refractory, KRAS codon 12/13 wild-type, HER2-positive metastatic colorectal cancer (HERACLES): a proof-of-concept, multicentre, open-label, phase 2 trial. Lancet Oncol 2016;17(6):738–46.

82. Hurwitz HH, Raghav K, Burris H 3rd, et al. Pertuzumab + trastuzumab for HER2-amplified/overexpressed metastatic colorectal cancer (mCRC): interim data from MyPathway. J Clin Oncol 2017;35(Suppl 4S) [abstract: 676].

83. Raghav K, Overman MJ, Yu R, et al. HER2 amplification as a negative predictive biomarker for anti-epidermal growth factor receptor antibody therapy in metastatic colorectal cancer. J Clin Oncol 2016;34(Suppl) [abstract: 3517].

84. Belov AA, Mohammadi M. Molecular mechanisms of fibroblast growth factor signaling in physiology and pathology. Cold Spring Harb Perspect Biol 2013; 5(6) [pii:a015958].

85. Kouhara H, Hadari YR, Spivak-Kroizman T, et al. A lipid-anchored Grb2-binding protein that links FGF-receptor activation to the Ras/MAPK signaling pathway. Cell 1997;89(5):693–702.

86. Stevenson L, Allen WL, Turkington R, et al. Identification of galanin and its receptor GalR1 as novel determinants of resistance to chemotherapy and potential biomarkers in colorectal cancer. Clin Cancer Res 2012;18(19):5412–26.

87. Bange J, Prechtl D, Cheburkin Y, et al. Cancer progression and tumor cell motility are associated with the FGFR4 Arg(388) allele. Cancer Res 2002; 62(3):840–7.

88. Liu R, Li J, Xie K, et al. FGFR4 promotes stroma-induced epithelial-to-mesenchymal transition in colorectal cancer. Cancer Res 2013;73(19):5926–35.

89. Henriksson ML, Edin S, Dahlin AM, et al. Colorectal cancer cells activate adjacent fibroblasts resulting in FGF1/FGFR3 signaling and increased invasion. Am J Pathol 2011;178(3):1387–94.

90. Al-Maghrabi J, Emam E, Gomaa W, et al. c-MET immunostaining in colorectal carcinoma is associated with local disease recurrence. BMC Cancer 2015;15: 676.

91. Di Renzo MF, Olivero M, Serini G, et al. Overexpression of the c-MET/HGF receptor in human thyroid carcinomas derived from the follicular epithelium. J Endocrinol Invest 1995;18(2):134–9.

92. Osada S, Matsui S, Komori S, et al. Effect of hepatocyte growth factor on progression of liver metastasis in colorectal cancer. Hepatogastroenterology 2010;57(97):76–80.

93. Gayyed MF, Abd El-Maqsoud NM, El-Hameed El-Heeny AA, et al. c-MET expression in colorectal adenomas and primary carcinomas with its corresponding metastases. J Gastrointest Oncol 2015;6(6):618–27.

94. Sun Y, Sun L, An Y, et al. Cabozantinib, a novel c-met inhibitor, inhibits colorectal cancer development in a xenograft model. Med Sci Monit 2015;21:2316–21.

95. Song EK, Tai WM, Messersmith WA, et al. Potent antitumor activity of cabozantinib, a c-MET and VEGFR2 inhibitor, in a colorectal cancer patient-derived tumor explant model. Int J Cancer 2015;136(8):1967–75.

96. Stadler ZK, Battaglin F, Middha S, et al. Reliable detection of mismatch repair deficiency in colorectal cancers using mutational load in next-generation sequencing panels. J Clin Oncol 2016;34(18):2141–7.

97. Palles C, Cazier JB, Howarth KM, et al. Germline mutations affecting the proofreading domains of POLE and POLD1 predispose to colorectal adenomas and carcinomas. Nat Genet 2013;45(2):136–44.

98. Spier I, Holzapfel S, Altmuller J, et al. Frequency and phenotypic spectrum of germline mutations in POLE and seven other polymerase genes in 266 patients with colorectal adenomas and carcinomas. Int J Cancer 2015;137(2):320–31.

99. Stenzinger A, Pfarr N, Endris V, et al. Mutations in POLE and survival of colorectal cancer patients–link to disease stage and treatment. Cancer Med 2014; 3(6):1527–38.

100. Mehnert JM, Panda A, Zhong H, et al. Immune activation and response to pembrolizumab in POLE-mutant endometrial cancer. J Clin Invest 2016;126(6): 2334–40.

101. Gong J, Wang C, Lee PP, et al. Response to PD-1 blockade in microsatellite stable metastatic colorectal cancer harboring a POLE mutation. J Natl Compr Canc Netw 2017;15(2):142–7.
102. Boland CR, Goel A. Microsatellite instability in colorectal cancer. Gastroenterology 2010;138(6):2073–87.e3.
103. Giannakis M, Mu XJ, Shukla SA, et al. Genomic correlates of immune-cell infiltrates in colorectal carcinoma. Cell Rep 2016;17(4):1206.
104. Lengauer C, Kinzler KW, Vogelstein B. Genetic instabilities in human cancers. Nature 1998;396(6712):643–9.
105. Kim H, Jen J, Vogelstein B, et al. Clinical and pathological characteristics of sporadic colorectal carcinomas with DNA replication errors in microsatellite sequences. Am J Pathol 1994;145(1):148–56.
106. Smyrk TC, Watson P, Kaul K, et al. Tumor-infiltrating lymphocytes are a marker for microsatellite instability in colorectal carcinoma. Cancer 2001;91(12): 2417–22.
107. Dolcetti R, Viel A, Doglioni C, et al. High prevalence of activated intraepithelial cytotoxic T lymphocytes and increased neoplastic cell apoptosis in colorectal carcinomas with microsatellite instability. Am J Pathol 1999;154(6):1805–13.
108. Le DT, Uram JN, Wang H, et al. PD-1 blockade in tumors with mismatch-repair deficiency. N Engl J Med 2015;372(26):2509–20.
109. Le DT, Durham JN, Smith KN, et al. Mismatch-repair deficiency predicts response of solid tumors to PD-1 blockade. Science 2017;357(6349):409–13.
110. Overman MJ, Kopetz S, Mcdermott RS, et al. Nivolumab ± ipilimumab in treatment (tx) of patients (pts) with metastatic colorectal cancer (mCRC) with and without high microsatellite instability (MSI-H): CheckMate-142 interim results. J Clin Oncol 2016;34:3501.
111. Overman MJ, Lonardi S, Leone F, et al. Nivolumab in patients with DNA mismatch repair deficient/microsatellite instability high metastatic colorectal cancer: update from checkmate 142. J Clin Oncol 2017;35(4, Suppl):519.
112. Liu L, Mayes PA, Eastman S, et al. The BRAF and MEK inhibitors dabrafenib and trametinib: effects on immune function and in combination with immunomodulatory antibodies targeting PD-1, PD-L1, and CTLA-4. Clin Cancer Res 2015; 21(7):1639–51.
113. Loi S, Dushyanthen S, Beavis PA, et al. RAS/MAPK activation is associated with reduced tumor-infiltrating lymphocytes in triple-negative breast cancer: therapeutic cooperation between MEK and PD-1/PD-L1 immune checkpoint inhibitors. Clin Cancer Res 2016;22(6):1499–509.
114. Bendell J, Powderly JD, lieu CH, et al. Safety and efficacy of MPDL3280A (anti-PDL1) in combination with bevacizumab (bev) and/or FOLFOX in patients (pts) with metastatic colorectal cancer (mCRC). J Clin Oncol 2015;33(Suppl S3):704.
115. Diaz LA Jr, Bardelli A. Liquid biopsies: genotyping circulating tumor DNA. J Clin Oncol 2014;32(6):579–86.
116. Siravegna G, Mussolin B, Buscarino M, et al. Clonal evolution and resistance to EGFR blockade in the blood of colorectal cancer patients. Nat Med 2015;21(7): 827.

Maximizing the Effectiveness of Colonoscopy in the Prevention of Colorectal Cancer

John F. Sullivan, MD[a], John A. Dumot, DO[b],*

KEYWORDS

- Colonoscopy • Colorectal cancer • Interval cancer • Adenoma detection rate
- Polypectomy • Assistive devices • Advanced techniques

KEY POINTS

- Colonoscopy is the gold standard for colon cancer prevention and maximizing its efficacy leads to a decrease in interval colorectal cancer rates.
- The adenoma detection rate is the most widely accepted surrogate marker for an effective provider of screening colonoscopy, in addition to specific quality metrics identified within individual procedures.
- Methods to improve adenoma detection rate include adopting endoscopic techniques, using updated and high-definition endoscopy equipment, and using assistive devices in the appropriate clinical setting.
- Proper polypectomy technique decreases the chances for residual polyp and thus decreases interval colorectal cancer rates.
- Advanced polypectomy techniques, including endoscopic mucosal resection and endoscopic submucosal dissection, have a developing role in the nonsurgical management of large polyps.

EFFECTIVENESS OF COLONOSCOPY FOR COLORECTAL CANCER PREVENTION

Colorectal cancer is the third most commonly diagnosed cancer and the third most common cause of death related to cancer in the United States.[1] Colonoscopy with polypectomy of adenomatous polyps results in a 76% to 90% reduction in the incidence of colon cancer in appropriately screened individuals.[2] Although colonoscopy

Disclosure: J.F. Sullivan and J.A. Dumot have nothing to disclose.
[a] Department of Gastroenterology and Liver Disease, University Hospitals Cleveland Medical Center, 11100 Euclid Avenue, Cleveland, OH 44106, USA; [b] Digestive Health Institute, University Hospitals Cleveland Medical Center, 11100 Euclid Avenue, Cleveland, OH 44106, USA
* Corresponding author.
E-mail address: john.dumot@uhhospitals.org

is considered the gold standard test in the prevention of colorectal cancer, variations in physician performance and other technical issues limit its effectiveness. In this article, we summarize pertinent data to incorporate into practice to maximize the efficacy of screening colonoscopy and achieve the greatest benefit in terms of colorectal cancer prevention.

INTERVAL COLORECTAL CANCER

Interval colorectal cancers are cancers that are diagnosed after a screening or surveillance examination in which no cancer is detected, and before the date of the next recommended examination.[3] Large, population-based studies have demonstrated that approximately 6% of colorectal cancers are interval cancers.[4] Interval cancers are more likely to be diagnosed in patients over the age of 60, in those who have a family history of colorectal cancer, in those who have an index colonoscopy with a previously detected adenoma, and to occur on the right side of the colon.[4,5]

The cause of interval cancers is thought to be 3-fold: undetected adenomatous polyps, incomplete resection of adenomatous polyps, and the interval growth of aggressive adenomatous lesions.[6] Therefore, a key to decreasing the rate of interval colorectal cancer is to maximize the effectiveness of colonoscopy with an increased rate at detecting and completely removing precancerous polyps. In addition to a sound procedural technique, proper surveillance interval recommendations will take the quality of the bowel preparation, size and number of adenomatous polyps into consideration to reduce the risk of an interval colorectal cancer.

Physicians finding or removing large polyps should consider marking the proximal and distal segment containing the lesion with carbon ink when the lesion cannot be easily identified by a normal anatomic landmark such as the cecal base or ileocecal valve. Special attention to avoid injecting into or under the base of the lesion is necessary to avoid causing scar formation by targeting a fold or two away from the lesion. Also, physicians must avoid partial polypectomy, which makes further endoscopic therapy difficult.

INCREASING THE ADENOMA DETECTION RATE

The proportion of screening colonoscopy examinations performed by a physician that detect 1 or more adenomas is the adenoma detection rate (ADR). The ADR is a very simple calculation and serves as a basic quality measure in physician performance because it has been inversely correlated with the rate of interval colorectal cancer.[7] An ADR of 25% is considered to be an acceptable rate for the standard physician.[8] Based on the inverse relationship between ADR and interval colorectal cancer, it would ensue that increasing the ADR would lead to a decrease in interval colorectal cancers, with recent studies mentioned elsewhere in this article demonstrating an even higher ADR with careful procedural techniques. In fact, ADR has been validated as an independent predictor of the risk of interval cancer.[9] Therefore, determining techniques and methods to maximize the ADR has been at the forefront of the literature seeking to maximize the effectiveness of screening colonoscopy.

Withdrawal time is the amount of time a physician spends examining the colonic mucosa after intubation and identification and photo documentation of the cecum landmarks of appendicular orifice and ileocecal valve, until the endoscope is withdrawn from the anus. A longer withdrawal time has been shown to correlate with significantly higher ADRs. Physicians with a withdrawal time of more than 6 minutes detect a neoplastic lesion in 23.8% of colonoscopies compared with 11.8% for those with a withdrawal time of less than 6 minutes.[10] The authors also found a higher detection rate for advanced neoplastic lesions in the group with a withdrawal time of more than 6 minutes (6.4% vs 2.6%). These data have led to the widespread acceptance of at least a 6-minute withdrawal time being a surrogate marker for an adequate screening colonoscopy.

The technological advancements leading to high-definition colonoscopy and processors has also led to a small but statistically significant increase in ADR. Compared with standard video endoscopy, there was an incremental yield of 3.5% more adenomatous polyps with high-definition white light colonoscopy. The greatest benefit was in the detection of small adenomatous polyps; there was no statistically significant increase in the detection of larger or high-risk adenomas.[11] Given its widespread availability and use, high-definition endoscopy is now the standard of care.

Based on a Cochrane Review, there is no convincing evidence that narrow band imaging (NBI) significantly increases the rate of adenoma detection over high-definition white light colonoscopy.[12] Although NBI may not lead to a higher ADR, there is a developing role for the use of NBI in the real-time visual diagnosis of adenomatous polyps. NBI led to a significantly higher sensitivity and specificity for diagnosing adenomas (96% and 93%, respectively) compared with high-definition white light colonoscopy (38% and 61%, respectively).[13] These data suggest that in the future it may be feasible to pursue polypectomy and polyp discard with the diagnosis of adenomatous polyps being made visually rather than having to rely on histopathology.[14] This trend would lead to a significant cost reduction and decrease the risks associated with polypectomy of benign distal hyperplastic polyps.

Chromoendoscopy is the use of dye spraying of the colonic mucosa to enhance the contrast difference between normal colonic mucosa and polyps. A Cochrane review looking at the efficacy of chromoendoscopy showed that it did lead to a 30% increase in adenomatous polyp detection compared with standard colonoscopy in the general screening population without inflammatory bowel disease.[15] However, in the inflammatory bowel disease population, there is no compelling evidence that chromoendoscopy is superior to colonoscopy with targeted and random biopsies, because there was no statistically significant difference in the detection of dysplastic lesions between these 2 groups.[16] A systematic review of 10 randomized trials found a higher dysplasia detection rate with a major drawback of longer procedural times without evidence of preventing cancer mortality.[17] These longer withdrawal times owing to the need for dye spraying in chromoendoscopy may also be a confounding variable in the increased detection of adenomatous polyps and are likely to be too cumbersome a process to be used in the setting of general colorectal cancer screening.

Water exchange colonoscopy is the infusion of water into the colon with suctioning of the water primarily during scope insertion.[18] Water immersion colonoscopy is the infusion of water into the colon with suctioning of the water primarily during scope withdrawal. A Cochrane review showed that water infusion colonoscopy with either water immersion or water exchange leads to detection of an adenoma in 3 more patients for every 100 screening colonoscopies when compared with standard colonoscopy.[19] Further differentiating between the 2 types of water infusion, multiple studies suggest water exchange leads to higher ADRs, particularly in the right side of the colon.[20–22]

Given the predominance of interval colorectal cancers being right sided, there have been many studies in the literature looking at techniques to increase ADR specifically in this segment of the colon. The 2 well-studied techniques are cecal retroflexion and a second forward view examination of the right colon. The literature suggests that these 2 techniques do provide a modest increase in right colon ADR compared with standard colonoscopy.[23] Although cecal retroflexion seems to be slightly more effective at increasing the ADR compared with a second forward view examination of the right colon, retroflexion can be difficult to accomplish even for experienced physicians, and relying on either technique should be adequate to improve the sensitivity of colonoscopy over the general technique of insertion and single forward view examination of the right colon.[23–26]

The quality of the bowel preparation has been shown to affect the ADR. A majority of studies have shown that a poor bowel preparation leads to missed lesions and a lower ADR. However, there is not necessarily a direct relationship between the quality of the bowel preparation and the ADR; multiple studies have demonstrated that there is no increase in the ADR between an adequate or intermediate quality preparation and an excellent bowel preparation.[27,28] There are even a few studies that suggest that a pristine bowel preparation may lead to overconfidence on the part of the physician and lower ADRs.[29]

The use of carbon dioxide insufflation does not lead to an increase in the ADR when compared with air insufflation.[30,31] Carbon dioxide insufflation has been shown to reduce both procedural and postprocedural pain, and to possibly decrease cecal intubation time.[32,33] In addition, the use of anesthesia administered propofol also leads to an increase in patient comfort in comparison with moderate conscious sedation, but again there is no difference in the ADR between these 2 types of sedation.[34]

The use of antispasmodic medications to improve luminal distention and thus increase the ADR is not widespread and is currently limited to clinical trials. Hyoscine butyl bromide, peppermint oil, and glucagon have all either shown no efficacy at increasing the ADR or have such limited data that they cannot be routinely recommended for use in screening colonoscopy.[35]

There are some promising data from randomized controlled trials that indicate that patient position change to the left lateral side on withdrawal increases ADR, especially in the right colon and if the baseline ADR of the physician is low.[36,37] However, a recent systematic review called these results into question because there is also high-quality evidence from other studies that suggests that position change does not affect the ADR.[38] Consequently, routine position change during withdrawal cannot be recommended until further studies confirm its efficacy. Position change may be used selectively when visualization of a particular colonic segment is difficult.

Physician awareness of the ADR being monitored has also been shown to lead to a statistically significant increase in both withdrawal time and the ADR. The withdrawal time went from a less than recommended 4.5 minutes in the group that was unaware that they were being monitored to a 7-minute withdrawal time in the monitored group for a screening colonoscopy not requiring polypectomy. In addition, the ADR increased from 21% in the unaware group to 36% in the monitored group.[39] These data suggest that there is a benefit to the routine monitoring and updating of physicians regarding their ADRs.

ASSISTIVE DEVICES

The use of assistive devices applied to the end of the endoscope have been studied to determine if they have the ability to improve visualization of the colonic mucosa thereby improving on standard colonoscopy. These assistive devices mechanically stretch colonic folds, allowing for optimal visualization for polyps on withdrawal.[40] Newer endoscopes with wider fields of view are also being used. Many of the studies regarding these potential assistive devices or newer endoscopes have used the adenoma miss rate (AMR) in tandem colonoscopy as their benchmark rather than the ADR.

The transparent plastic cap is the most basic assistive device that has been studied. Although cap-assisted colonoscopy has been shown to marginally improve the cecal intubation rate, there was no increase in the ADR when compared with standard colonoscopy.[41,42] A Cochrane review of cap-assisted colonoscopy concluded that studies were mixed and, at best, there was only marginal improvement in the polyp detection rate.[43] We have found the cap-assisted colonoscopy technique extremely valuable when visualization behind folds is difficult, as well as in performing wide area mucosal resection as outlined elsewhere in this article.

The Endocuff is a device placed on the end of the endoscope that has 2 rows of soft arms that help to spread open the colonic mucosa upon withdrawal. A metaanalysis of 9 studies regarding this device demonstrated that colonoscopy with the cuff had a higher rate of adenoma detection (odds ratio, 1.49) compared with standard colonoscopy. This study also found that the use of the cuff resulted in a higher rate of superficial mucosal injury but not frank perforation.[44] However, a subsequent randomized, controlled trial in the fecal occult blood–positive patient population demonstrated that there was no increase in adenoma detection using this device.[45] The study also showed that in 6% of patients the cuff had to be removed owing to the inability to pass it through the sigmoid colon.

The Endoring is another device with multiple flexible rings made from silicone-rubber that again is attached to the end of the endoscope. This device was shown to significantly decrease the AMR from 48.3% to 10.3% when compared with standard colonoscopy in a tandem colonoscopy study. The mean overall procedure time was increased in the group using the device, but this was attributed to the need for more polypectomies compared with the standard colonoscopy group.[46]

There are several wide-angle viewing endoscopes but the most-studied is the full-spectrum endoscopy (FUSE). FUSE is a newer endoscope with multiple imagers at the tip that provide a panoramic 330° views as opposed to the traditional forward viewing (TFV) endoscopes that provide a 170° view. The initial company-funded study for FUSE looked at the AMR in tandem colonoscopy compared with TFV endoscopy and showed that the AMR was significantly lower at 7% in the FUSE group compared with 41% in the TFV group. There was no increase in procedure time or complication rate.[47] Another more recent study found that the ADR was unchanged between FUSE and TFV endoscopy, but the AMR was again significantly higher in the TFV group. However, none of the missed adenomas were greater than 5 mm, and none were advanced lesions.[48]

There are 2 other novel systems not currently available for use in the United States that need further study before being considered for general use. The G-Eye is an inflatable balloon that flattens and spreads mucosa and folds.[49] The Third Eye Panoramic is a clip-on accessory camera that increases field of view.

Although the data regarding these assistive devices and colonoscopes with wider fields of view are promising, the data are not definitive enough to recommend their use for routine screening colonoscopy.[49] In addition, the use of these devices, many of which are single use, comes with an additional cost that currently make them prohibitive for use in routine screening. Further studies are necessary to determine if the cost to benefit ratio makes any of these devices feasible for use in routine screening colonoscopy. Until then, these devices should be used on a case-by-case basis, based on physician preference and patient risk stratification.

POLYPECTOMY

Incomplete polypectomy of adenomatous polyps leading to residual adenomatous polyps is one of the etiologies of interval colon cancer.[50] Complete resection of adenomatous polyps depends on proper endoscopic technique and the selection of the appropriate tool for polypectomy based on the size and characteristics of the polyp.

For diminutive adenomatous polyps (<5-7 mm), there are multiple studies that demonstrate that complete polypectomy is more regularly achieved using cold snare polypectomy (93%–97%) in comparison with cold forceps biopsy polypectomy (75%–83%).[51,52] These results were validated in a metaanalysis that demonstrated that incomplete diminutive polyp resection was decreased by 60% when cold snare polypectomy or jumbo cold forceps biopsy polypectomy was used in comparison with standard cold forceps biopsy polypectomy.[53]

For larger adenomatous polyps (<6 mm), hot snare polypectomy results in a higher complete resection rate (70.5%) compared with cold snare polypectomy (47.3%).[54] Hot snare carries the benefit of having collateral cautery of the mucosa surrounding the polyp, helping to obliterate any perimeter adenomatous tissue that may be missed by the actual snare.

Based on these studies, it can generally be recommended that, to achieve the most complete polypectomy, a cold snare should be used for diminutive polyps and a hot snare should be used for larger polyps. However, the location and characteristics of the polyp in addition to physician skill and preference should also play a role in the decision of what polypectomy tool is best suited to a particular polyp. Judicial use of electrocautery is necessary to limit postpolypectomy burn syndrome and delayed bleeding.

ADVANCED POLYPECTOMY

Two advanced polypectomy techniques, endoscopic mucosal resection (EMR) and endoscopic submucosal dissection (ESD) are beginning to supplant the need for surgical resection in the case of many large polyps. EMR is used for large, superficial precancerous and cancerous polyps and uses suctioning and/or submucosal injection to separate the muscularis propria from the lesion before cutting out the lesion, usually with a snare.[55] For EMR, a physician should be skilled with the injection of lifting substances such as saline or Hespan mixed with methylene blue, because these substances can help to delineate the edges of precancerous polyps and allow for a more complete and en bloc resection, especially in the case of flat polyps. With EMR, sometimes very large polyps must be removed in a piecemeal fashion and there is the possibility that a lesion will not lift, thereby signaling that its depth of invasion is deeper than expected and is not suitable for EMR.[55,56]

ESD was born out of EMR and is a 3-step process: injection of fluid into the submucosa to elevate the lesion away from the muscle layer, circumferential cutting of the surrounding mucosa of the lesion often times using specially designed knives, and subsequent dissection of the connective tissue of the submucosa beneath the lesion.[57] There is some evidence that ESD may be more effective than EMR, leading to higher en bloc resection and curative rates, but ESD is associated with a higher perforation rate. It is also more commonly used in Eastern countries such as Japan and used in only a limited number of advanced endoscopy centers in the United States.[58] ESD is also associated with several other disadvantages, including longer procedure times, high procedure-related complication rates, and technical difficulty in the resection of large polyps.[59] Unlike EMR, which is a technique that most well-trained physicians can use for the removal of large polyps, ESD is a more specialized skill that requires more specific and individualized training.[60,61] Generally, ESD for large, laterally spreading colorectal polyps has a high value in the distal colon and rectum, where surgical resection is associated with higher risks and costs. In the proximal colon, ESD has not been shown to be more effective than wide area piecemeal mucosal resection or laparoscopic colectomy for the recurrent or defiant laterally spreading tumor.

REFERENCES

1. Siegel RL, Miller KD, Jemal A. Cancer statistics, 2015. CA Cancer J Clin 2015; 65(1):5–29.
2. Winawer SJ, Zauber AG, Ho MN, et al. Prevention of colorectal cancer by colonoscopic polypectomy: the National Polyp Study Workgroup. N Engl J Med 1993; 329(27):1977–81.
3. Sanduleanu S, le Clercq CM, Dekker E, et al. Definition and taxonomy of interval colorectal cancers: a proposal for standardising nomenclature. Gut 2015;64(8): 1257–67.
4. Samadder NJ, Curtin K, Tuohy TM, et al. Characteristics of missed or interval colorectal cancer and patient survival: a population-based study. Gastroenterology 2014;146(4):950–60.
5. Richter JM, Campbell EJ, Chung DC. Interval colorectal cancer after colonoscopy. Clin Colorectal Cancer 2015;14(1):46–51.
6. Benedict M, Neto AG, Zhang X. Interval colorectal carcinoma: an unsolved debate. World J Gastroenterol 2015;21(45):12735–41.
7. Corley DA, Jensen CD, Marks AR, et al. Adenoma detection rate and risk of colorectal cancer and death. N Engl J Med 2014;370(14):1298–306.
8. Kaminski MF, Thomas-Gibson S, Bugajski M, et al. Performance measures for lower gastrointestinal endoscopy: a European Society of Gastrointestinal Endoscopy (ESGE) quality improvement initiative. United European J Gastroenterol 2017;5(3):309–34.
9. Kaminski MF, Regula J, Kraszewska E, et al. Quality indicators for colonoscopy and the risk of interval cancer. N Engl J Med 2010;362(19):1795–803.
10. Barclay RL, Vicari JJ, Doughty AS, et al. Colonoscopic withdrawal times and adenoma detection during screening colonoscopy. N Engl J Med 2006;355(24): 2533–41.
11. Subramanian V, Mannath J, Hawkey CJ, et al. High definition colonoscopy vs standard video endoscopy for the detection of colonic polyps: a meta-analysis. Endoscopy 2011;43(6):499–505.
12. Nagorni A, Bjelakovic G, Petrovic B. Narrow band imaging versus conventional white light colonoscopy for the detection of colorectal polyps. Cochrane Database Syst Rev 2012;(1):CD008361.
13. Rastogi A, Keighley J, Singh V, et al. High accuracy of narrow band imaging without magnification for the real-time characterization of polyp histology and its comparison with high-definition white light colonoscopy: a prospective study. Am J Gastroenterol 2009;104(10):2422–30.
14. Utsumi T, Iwatate M, Sano W, et al. Polyp detection, characterization, and management using narrow-band imaging with/without magnification. Clin Endosc 2015;48(6):491–7.
15. Brown SR, Baraza W, Din S, et al. Chromoscopy versus conventional endoscopy for the detection of polyps in the colon and rectum. Cochrane Database Syst Rev 2016;(4):CD006439.
16. Mooiweer E, van der Meulen-de Jong AE, Ponsioen CY, et al. Chromoendoscopy for surveillance in inflammatory bowel disease does not increase neoplasia

detection compared with conventional colonoscopy with random biopsies: results from a large retrospective study. Am J Gastroenterol 2015;110(7):1014–21.

17. Iannone A, Ruospo M, Wong G, et al. Chromoendoscopy for surveillance in ulcerative colitis and Crohn's disease: a systematic review of randomized trials. Clin Gastroenterol Hepatol 2017;15(11):1684–97.e11.

18. Rex DK. Water exchange vs water immersion during colonoscope insertion. Am J Gastroenterol 2014;109(9):1401–3.

19. Hafner S, Zolk K, Radaelli F, et al. Water infusion versus air insufflation for colonoscopy. Cochrane Database Syst Rev 2015;(5):CD009863.

20. Cadoni S, Falt P, Rondonotti E, et al. Water exchange for screening colonoscopy increases adenoma detection rate: a multicenter, double-blinded, randomized controlled trial. Endoscopy 2017;49(5):456–67.

21. Hsieh YH, Koo M, Leung FW. A patient-blinded randomized, controlled trial comparing air insufflation, water immersion, and water exchange during minimally sedated colonoscopy. Am J Gastroenterol 2014;109(9):1390–400.

22. Leung FW, Amato A, Ell C, et al. Water-aided colonoscopy: a systematic review. Gastrointest Endosc 2012;76(3):657–66.

23. Kushnir VM, Oh YS, Hollander T, et al. Impact of retroflexion vs second forward view examination of the right colon on adenoma detection: a comparison study. Am J Gastroenterol 2015;110(3):415–22.

24. Chandran S, Parker F, Vaughan R, et al. Right-sided adenoma detection with retroflexion versus forward-view colonoscopy. Gastrointest Endosc 2015;81(3): 608–13.

25. Lee HS, Jeon SW, Park HY, et al. Improved detection of right colon adenomas with additional retroflexion following two forward-view examinations: a prospective study. Endoscopy 2017;49(4):334–41.

26. Triantafyllou K, Tziatzios G, Sioulas AD, et al. Diagnostic yield of scope retroflexion in the right colon: a prospective cohort study. Dig Liver Dis 2016;48(2): 176–81.

27. Clark BT, Rustagi T, Laine L. What level of bowel prep quality requires early repeat colonoscopy: systematic review and meta-analysis of the impact of preparation quality on adenoma detection rate. Am J Gastroenterol 2014;109(11):1714–23.

28. Anderson JC, Butterly LF, Robinson CM, et al. Impact of fair bowel preparation quality on adenoma and serrated polyp detection: data from the New Hampshire colonoscopy registry by using a standardized preparation-quality rating. Gastrointest Endosc 2014;80(3):463–70.

29. Calderwood AH, Thompson KD, Schroy PC, et al. Good is better than excellent: bowel preparation quality and adenoma detection rates. Gastrointest Endosc 2015;81(3):691–9.

30. Bretthauer M, Kaminski MF, Loberg M, et al. Population-based colonoscopy screening for colorectal cancer: a randomized clinical trial. JAMA Intern Med 2016;176(7):894–902.

31. Perbtani YB, Riverso M, Shuster JJ, et al. Does carbon dioxide insufflation impact adenoma detection rate: a single-center retrospective analysis. Endosc Int Open 2016;4(12):1275–9.

32. Memon A, Memon B, Yunus RM, et al. Carbon dioxide versus air insufflation for elective colonoscopy: a meta-analysis and systematic review of randomized controlled trials. Surg Laparosc Endosc Percutan Tech 2016;26(2):102–16.

33. Sajid MS, Caswell J, Bhatti MI, et al. Carbon dioxide insufflation vs conventional air insufflation for colonoscopy: a systematic review and meta-analysis of published randomized controlled trials. Colorectal Dis 2015;17(2):111–23.

34. Metwally M, Agresti N, Hale WB, et al. Conscious or unconscious: the impact of sedation choice on colon adenoma detection. World J Gastroenterol 2011;17(34): 3912–5.

35. Sanagapalli S, Agnihotri K, Leong R, et al. Antispasmodic drugs in colonoscopy: a review of their pharmacology, safety and efficacy in improving polyp detection and related outcomes. Therap Adv Gastroenterol 2017;10(1):101–13.

36. Ball AJ, Johal SS, Riley SA. Position change during colonoscope withdrawal increases polyp and adenoma detection in the right but not in the left side of the colon: results of a randomized controlled trial. Gastrointest Endosc 2015;82(3): 488–94.

37. Lee SW, Chang JH, Ji JS, et al. Effect of dynamic position changes on adenoma detection during colonoscope withdrawal: a randomized controlled multicenter trial. Am J Gastroenterol 2016;111(1):63–9.

38. Zhao SB, Wan H, Fu HY, et al. Quantitative assessment of the effect of position changes during colonoscopy withdrawal. J Dig Dis 2016;17(6):357–65.

39. Vavricka SR, Sulz MC, Degen L, et al. Monitoring colonoscopy withdrawal time significantly improves the adenoma detection rate and the performance of endoscopists. Endoscopy 2016;48(3):256–62.

40. Gkolfakis P, Tziatzios G, Dimitriadis GD, et al. New endoscopes and add-on devices to improve colonoscopy performance. World J Gastroenterol 2017;23(21): 3784–96.

41. Pohl H, Bensen SP, Toor A, et al. Cap-assisted colonoscopy and detection of adenomatous polyps (CAP) study: a randomized trial. Endoscopy 2015;47(10): 891–7.

42. Tee HP, Corte C, Al-Ghamdi H, et al. Prospective randomized controlled trial evaluating cap-assisted colonoscopy vs standard colonoscopy. World J Gastroenterol 2010;16(31):3905–10.

43. Morgan J, Thomas K, Lee-Robichaud H, et al. Transparent cap colonoscopy versus standard colonoscopy to improve caecal intubation. Cochrane Database Syst Rev 2012;(12):CD008211.

44. Chin M, Karnes W, Jamal MM, et al. Use of the Endocuff during routine colonoscopy examination improves adenoma detection: a meta-analysis. World J Gastroenterol 2016;22(43):9642–9.

45. Bhattacharyya R, Chedgy F, Kandiah K, et al. Endocuff-assisted vs. standard colonoscopy in the fecal occult blood test-based UK Bowel Cancer Screening Programme (E-cap study): a randomized trial. Endoscopy 2017;49(11):1043–50.

46. Dik VK, Gralnek IM, Segol O, et al. Multicenter, randomized, tandem evaluation of EndoRings colonoscopy-results of the CLEVER study. Endoscopy 2015;47(12): 1151–8.

47. Gralnek IM, Siersema PD, Halpern Z, et al. Standard forward-viewing colonoscopy versus full-spectrum endoscopy: an international, multicentre, randomised, tandem colonoscopy trial. Lancet Oncol 2014;15(3):353–60.

48. Facciorusso A, Del Prete V, Buccino V, et al. Full-spectrum versus standard colonoscopy for improving polyp detection rate: a systematic review and meta-analysis. J Gastroenterol Hepatol 2017. [Epub ahead of print].

49. Konda V, Chauhan SS, Abu Dayyeh BK, et al. Endoscopes and devices to improve colon polyp detection. Gastrointest Endosc 2015;81(5):1122–9.

50. Anderloni A, Jovani M, Hassan C, et al. Advances, problems, and complications of polypectomy. Clin Exp Gastroenterol 2014;7:285–96.

51. Kim JS, Lee BI, Choi H, et al. Cold snare polypectomy versus cold forceps polypectomy for diminutive and small colorectal polyps: a randomized controlled trial. Gastrointest Endosc 2015;81(3):741–7.

52. Lee CK, Shim JJ, Jang JY. Cold snare polypectomy vs cold forceps polypectomy using double-biopsy technique for removal of diminutive colorectal polyps: a prospective randomized study. Am J Gastroenterol 2013;108(10):1593–600.

53. Raad D, Tripathi P, Cooper G, et al. Role of the cold biopsy technique in diminutive and small colonic polyp removal: a systematic review and meta-analysis. Gastrointest Endosc 2016;83(3):508–15.

54. Yamamoto T, Suzuki S, Kusano C, et al. Histological outcomes between hot and cold snare polypectomy for small colorectal polyps. Saudi J Gastroenterol 2017; 23(4):246–52.

55. Mannath J, Ragunath K. Endoscopic mucosal resection: who and how? Therap Adv Gastroenterol 2011;4(5):275–82.

56. Arezzo A, Passera R, Marchese N, et al. Systematic review and meta-analysis of endoscopic submucosal dissection vs endoscopic mucosal resection for colorectal lesions. United European Gastroenterol J 2016;4(1):18–29.

57. Kakushima N, Fujishiro M. Endoscopic submucosal dissection for gastrointestinal neoplasms. World J Gastroenterol 2008;14(19):2962–7.

58. Saito Y, Fukuzawa M, Matsuda T, et al. Clinical outcome of endoscopic submucosal dissection versus endoscopic mucosal resection of large colorectal tumors as determined by curative resection. Surg Endosc 2010;24(2):343–52.

59. Wang J, Zhang XH, Ge J, et al. Endoscopic submucosal dissection vs endoscopic mucosal resection for colorectal tumors: a meta-analysis. World J Gastroenterol 2014;20(25):8282–7.

60. Cao Y, Liao C, Tan A, et al. Meta-analysis of endoscopic submucosal dissection versus endoscopic mucosal resection for tumors of the gastrointestinal tract. Endoscopy 2009;41(9):751–7.

61. Hochberger J, Kohler P, Kruse E, et al. Endoscopic submucosal dissection. Internist 2013;54(3):287–301.

Surgical Treatment of Metastatic Colorectal Cancer

Jeffery Chakedis, MD[a,1], Carl R. Schmidt, MD[b,*]

KEYWORDS

- Stage IV • Colorectal cancer • Metastases • Surgical management • Surgery

KEY POINTS

- Surgical treatment of metastatic colorectal cancer offers a chance for cure or prolonged survival.
- Advanced surgical techniques, adjuncts to resection, and modern chemotherapy all contribute to best outcomes for patients with hepatic metastases.
- Patients with peritoneal metastatic disease may benefit from surgical cytoreduction and intraperitoneal chemotherapy (HIPEC). Best outcomes are achieved in those for whom complete cytoreduction is surgically feasible.
- Pulmonary metastases are rarely isolated yet surgical resection is associated with prolonged survival in selected patients.

MANAGEMENT OF METASTATIC COLORECTAL CANCER

Metastatic disease occurs in half of people with colorectal cancer (CRC). Metastasis spread through hematogenous or lymphangitic routes and may occur in lymph nodes, liver, lung, peritoneum, brain, and bone. Synchronous presentation at the time of diagnosis of the primary tumor occurs in 21% of patients and is associated with worse survival compared with those who present with metachronous disease.[1] For patients who present with advanced-stage disease and receive no treatment, the median life expectancy is 9 months and 5-year survival is 3%.[2] Improvements in therapy over the past 15 to 20 years have led to improved outcomes because even those who can receive chemotherapy only

---

Disclosures: The authors have nothing to disclose.
[a] Division of Surgical Oncology, Department of Surgery, Complex General Surgical Oncology, The Ohio State University Wexner Medical Center, Arthur G. James Cancer Hospital and Solove Research Institute, 395 West 12th Avenue, Suite 670, Columbus, OH 43210-1267, USA; [b] Division of Surgical Oncology, Department of Surgery, The Ohio State University Wexner Medical Center, Arthur G. James Cancer Hospital and Solove Research Institute, 395 West 12th Avenue, Suite 670, Columbus, OH 43210-1267, USA
[1] Present address: N924 Doan Hall, 410 West 10th Avenue, Columbus, OH 43210.
* Corresponding author. The Ohio State University Wexner Medical Center, Arthur G. James Cancer Hospital and Solove Research Institute, 320 West 10th Avenue, M256 Starling Loving Hall, Columbus, OH 43210-1267.
E-mail address: Carl.Schmidt@osumc.edu

Surg Oncol Clin N Am 27 (2018) 377–399
https://doi.org/10.1016/j.soc.2017.11.010
1055-3207/18/© 2017 Elsevier Inc. All rights reserved.

surgonc.theclinics.com

Abbreviations

CALI	Chemotherapy-associated liver injury
CC	Completeness of cytoreduction
CEA	Carcinoembryonic antigen
CRC	Colorectal cancer
CRLM	Colorectal liver metastasis
CRS	Cytoreductive surgery
CT	Computed tomography
DFS	Disease-free survival
EGFR	Epidermal growth factor receptor
FUDR	5-fluoro 2-deoxyuridine
HIPEC	Hyperthermic intraperitoneal chemotherapy
HR	Hazard ratio
MWA	Microwave ablation
OS	Overall survival
PC	Peritoneal carcinomatosis
PCI	Peritoneal carcinomatosis index
RFA	Radiofrequency ablation

have a median survival of 30 months.[3] Furthermore, multimodal therapies in some cases may even provide cure in the setting of metastatic disease. Understanding the natural history of metastatic CRC in the context of patient- and tumor-specific factors is critical to making treatment decisions when there are a variety of options.

Although most patients with metastatic CRC are incurable, the combination of modern chemotherapy with improved surgical and radiation therapy techniques has led to prolonged cancer control and extended survival for many. Staging work-up for metastatic disease includes computed tomography (CT) of the chest, abdomen, and pelvis with consideration of PET/CT for selected patients with indeterminate findings. Routine laboratory work-up, carcinoembryonic antigen (CEA) level, and determination of RAS and BRAF status of the primary tumor should be performed. Biopsy of metastasis may be needed, or preferred, in the setting of first recurrence or again with indeterminate imaging findings. A multidisciplinary evaluation is of critical importance for most patients with metastatic CRC because choice and order of therapies differ depending on presentation, number of sites and location of metastases, and potential for surgical resection.

Genetic Mutation and Sites of Metastasis

Stage IV CRC encompasses a wide range of possibilities with strikingly different patterns of disease presentation and progression. Prognosis declines as number of metastatic sites of increases and staging has been changed to reflect this heterogeneity.[4] The American Joint Committee on Cancer seventh edition in 2010 changed stage IV disease to subcategories of IVA (metastasis to one site) and IVB (metastasis to more than one site). Although this distinction denotes a difference in overall survival (OS), there is yet more diversity because site of metastasis and the possibility of surgical resection also help determine prognosis.[5,6] The chance of developing metastasis increases with worse primary tumor T and N stage.[7] In general, potentially curative treatments are the goal for patients with one site of surgically resectable metastatic disease especially in the metachronous setting. For those with more than one site of metastatic disease, the general goal is cancer control.

Underlying molecular mechanisms explaining the exact route of metastatic spread of CRC have not yet been determined.[8] There is a high concordance of genetic mutations between primary and metastatic tumors, and sequencing of the primary tumor for RAS, BRAF, and PIK3CA has actionable consequences for metastatic disease in terms of therapy options, such as use of anti–epidermal growth factor receptor (EGFR) therapies.[9] Some studies support the concept that site-specific patterns of metastatic disease may be predicted by underlying mutation pattern (**Fig. 1**).[10–14] Currently, we use clinical and pathologic characteristics of the primary tumor to estimate the prognosis and expected disease course. It is exciting that molecular signatures may be used in the future to offer the most effective therapies based on tumor genetic subtype and may even allow better estimation of timing and location of first recurrence, which could help tailor adjuvant therapy choices.

Perioperative Chemotherapy for Liver Metastases

For patients with liver metastases amenable to surgical resection, the addition of chemotherapy to the overall treatment plan is controversial. Large cohort studies suggest outcomes are good with surgical resection alone in selected patients, and the addition of chemotherapy may not add much benefit.[15,16] To more formally analyze the question, a landmark randomized controlled trial comparing a perioperative chemotherapy approach with hepatectomy alone was done (EORTC 40983) in 2008 with long-term survival published in 2013.[17,18] The study found no statistically significant difference in OS with 50% of patients alive at 5 years in both the surgery alone arm and the perioperative chemotherapy and surgery arm. The group undergoing chemotherapy and surgery had a higher incidence of postoperative complications (25% vs 16%). It should be mentioned that the total number of metastases in the study were limited to four maximum and most patients had solitary metastasis. Thus, the trial results may not be applicable to all patients especially those with a higher burden of disease. Use of biologic inhibitor therapy has also been studied using the EGFR antibody cetuximab for patients with KRAS wild-type tumors and similarly this strategy did

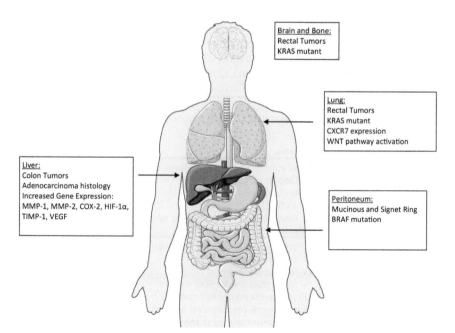

Fig. 1. Mutation analysis of primary CRC tumor and relation to site-specific metastases. (*From* Servier Medical Art. Available at: http://smart.servier.com/ under a Creative Commons Attribution 3.0 Unported License. Accessed October 6, 2017; and *Data from* Refs.[10–14,116])

not improve survival.[19] For the patient with liver metastases amenable to surgical resection, some factors that may influence the choice of liver operation first approach versus perioperative chemotherapy are shown in **Table 1**.

Some potential drawbacks to use of perioperative chemotherapy include the possibility of progression (5%–7%) and chemotherapy-associated liver injury (CALI).[20] The distinct pathologic entities of liver toxicity related to chemotherapy are oxaliplatin-associated sinusoidal obstruction syndrome (blue liver) and irinotecan-associated with steatohepatitis (yellow liver).[21] CALI depends on the number of cycles of therapy received, with more than nine cycles increasing risk of postoperative liver failure. Some of the associated liver damage is often reversible the longer the interval between chemotherapy and resection.[22,23] The concurrent use of bevacizumab is found to be protective of the liver and decreases rates of CALI in many studies.[24]

Treatment Order with Synchronous Metastases

When metastatic disease is diagnosed at the same time as a primary CRC (synchronous disease), there may be multiple therapy options available especially if all metastatic disease is amenable to surgical resection. The prognosis is generally considered worse than those with metachronous presentation of metastatic disease, with only around 6% eligible for potentially curative therapy compared with 17%.[25] A traditional approach has been to surgically remove the primary colon or rectal tumor first, followed by systemic chemotherapy and later consideration of resection of the metastatic disease. This may not be the optimal approach for every patient and several patient-specific factors must be taken into consideration when deciding the order of treatments. We present a treatment algorithm that takes into consideration the patient's symptoms and patient-specific tumor factors adapted from an international consensus (**Fig. 2**).[26]

The symptomatic primary tumor, such as obstructive symptoms or bleeding, in the setting of resectable metastatic disease is usually treated with resection of the primary first followed by systemic chemotherapy and then local or regional treatment of metastatic disease when appropriate. Bleeding that is slow and subacute may be safely managed with temporizing transfusion to allow a chemotherapy-first approach because bleeding often stops after treatment begins. Colon tumors that are nearly obstructing or

---

Table 1
Factors used to guide use of perioperative chemotherapy with hepatic resection for metastatic CRC

Treatment Approach	Factors
Liver operation first	Low volume of liver metastases • Largest <5 cm • Unilobar disease • <5 total liver tumors • Favorable location allowing minor hepatectomy Metachronous presentation
Perioperative chemotherapy	Higher volume of liver metastases • Largest >5 cm • Bilobar disease • More than 4 total liver tumors Extrahepatic metastatic disease Synchronous presentation or short disease-free interval <12 mo Tumor response may change surgical strategy • Decrease size of hepatic resection • Achieve R0 resection May not receive postoperative chemotherapy

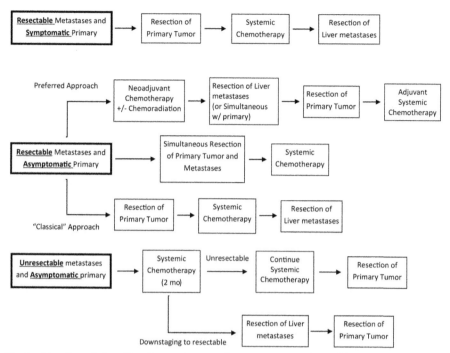

Fig. 2. A treatment algorithm for synchronous liver metastases adapted from an international consensus (Expert Group on OncoSurgery management of Liver Metastases [EGOSLIM]) group. (*Data from* Adam R, de Gramont A, Figueras J, et al. Managing synchronous liver metastases from colorectal cancer: a multidisciplinary international consensus. Cancer Treat Rev 2015;41(9):729–41; and Adam R, De Gramont A, Figueras J, et al. The oncosurgery approach to managing liver metastases from colorectal cancer: a multidisciplinary international consensus. Oncologist 2012;17(10):1225–39.)

have perforated should be managed surgically with diverting ostomy or in some cases primary tumor resection with either ostomy or primary anastomosis depending on the clinical scenario. The use of colonic stents is not recommended in this setting because results are poor and there is no advantage over emergency surgery.[27] Rectal tumors causing obstruction that require advanced surgical techniques for oncologic resection (total mesorectal excision and low rectal anastomosis) should be managed with diverting ostomy followed by systemic chemotherapy or chemoradiation. Radiation therapy to primary rectal tumors is an important component of therapy for rectal cancer in the setting of resectable metastatic disease. Its use in the setting of unresectable, incurable metastatic disease should be more selective and generally for palliative purposes.

Managing patients with asymptomatic primary tumors and resectable metastatic disease is controversial with no data showing a clear advantage to one strategy over another. A common approach is use of four to six cycles of systemic chemotherapy followed by surgical resection of primary tumor and metastatic disease during the same or staged operations.[28] Simultaneous resection of the primary tumor and metastatic liver disease is done with low rates of complication and mortality especially when less than a major hepatic resection is needed.[29,30] Major hepatectomy in combination with segmental colectomy is also safe in experienced hands and is done especially in healthier patients. Simultaneous resection shortens the length of overall hospital stay, length of gap between treatments, and is especially advantageous if operations are done with a minimally invasive approach.[31]

Unfortunately, most patients presenting with synchronous metastatic disease are not amenable to complete surgical resection of all tumors. Asymptomatic primary tumors in the setting of unresectable metastatic disease have been shown to not require resection because more than 90% of patients experience no complications from the primary tumor during initial chemotherapy.[32] Some studies have suggested a possible oncologic benefit of primary tumor resection in this setting. One study examining data from SEER-matched patients using propensity scoring found improved OS and disease-specific survival (hazard ratio [HR], 0.40 and 0.39, respectively; $P<.001$).[33] Although there is a bit of selection bias that may confound these data, other studies have found similar results.[34–36] Another consideration for removal of the primary tumor is the risk of bowel perforation with use of bevacizumab.[37,38]

SURGICAL MANAGEMENT OF HEPATIC METASTASES

Of all patients diagnosed with colorectal liver metastases (CRLM), only 10% to 20% initially are candidates for surgical resection of liver tumors.[39] Encouragingly, modern chemotherapy regimens have response rates up to 70% to 80%, which allows some initially not resectable patients to have a chance at metastasectomy.[40] The combination of chemotherapy and surgical resection of liver metastases allows for 5-year survival around 50%.[18] A more sobering statistic is that at least 70% of patients recur within 5 years of partial hepatectomy in the liver (30%–50%), extrahepatic sites (60%), or both.[41] As such, the 10-year survival rate after partial hepatectomy is estimated at 10% to 15%, and one-third of patients who survive 5 years still ultimately die from recurrent cancer.

Indications for Resection and Outcomes

The definition of resectability for patients with CRLM has evolved over the years because of improvements in the understanding of disease natural history, systemic chemotherapy and biologic treatment options, regional therapies, and technical aspects of liver operations. When classifying liver tumors as resectable both technical and oncologic aspects must be considered. This was summarized well in a consensus statement from the Americas Hepato-Pancreato-Biliary Association in 2012 (**Box 1**).[42] Technical considerations include ability to achieve negative margins, size of future

---

Box 1
Defining resectability in patients with colorectal liver metastasis

Patient selection criteria for potentially curative resection of hepatic metastases
  Ability to obtain R0 resection: no tumor present at margin
  Adequate postoperative liver volume and function
  • At least 20% of total liver volume with normal function
  • At least 30% if any chemotherapy-associated liver injury
  • At least 40% if any hepatic fibrosis or cirrhosis from other causes
  • At least two functional contiguous segments with intact portal and arterial inflow, venous outflow, and biliary drainage
  Limited extrahepatic disease that is resectable
  • No portal lymphadenopathy or multiple metastatic sites
  Limited progression if received preoperative chemotherapy
  • No development of new hepatic lesions
  Medically fit to undergo a major operation

Data from Schwarz R, Abdalla E, Aloia T, et al. AHPBA/SSO/SSAT sponsored consensus conference on the multidisciplinary treatment of colorectal cancer metastases. HPB (Oxford) 2013;15(2):89–90; and Adams R, Aloia T, Loyer E, et al. Selection for hepatic resection of colorectal liver metastases: expert consensus statement. HPB (Oxford) 2013;15(2):91–103.

liver remnant, and necessity for functional vascular inflow and vascular/biliary outflow. Oncologic aspects include patient selection and recognizing markers of aggressive biology including progressive disease on chemotherapy and the presence of extrahepatic disease including resectability and location.[43] Patients who are borderline or unresectable based on these factors are most appropriately given systemic therapy first.

Understanding prognostic factors that impact survival after surgical resection of CRLM is critical to aid decision-making, and outcomes vary from median survival greater than 7 years with 5-year survival of 64% to median survival less than 1 year with 5-year survival at 2%.[44] This wide spectrum of outcomes depends on multiple factors including margin status, nodal status of the primary tumor, presence of extrahepatic disease, less than 12-month disease-free interval, number of hepatic tumors, size of largest tumor, and CEA level.[6] Multiple large single-center cohort studies describe outcomes for patients after surgical resection of CRLM including 5-year survival estimates up to 50% and low rates of surgical mortality less than 3% (**Table 2**).

Technical Strategies for Resection

Strategies for hepatic resection are determined by the volume and anatomic distribution of disease. A less than major or hepatic parenchyma-sparing partial hepatectomy is feasible in 30% to 50% of cases.[46] The remainder requires formal lobar (right or left) hepatectomy or extended resection. Resection strategies that spare liver parenchyma are associated with lower rates of postoperative complication, specifically decreased major morbidity (34% vs 25%), rates of postoperative liver failure (2% vs 7%), and length of intensive care unit care.[48,49] Resection of a primary tumor can be done in combination with minor hepatectomy or major hepatectomy; however, risks increase with the latter in terms of mortality (1.4% vs 8.3%) and major morbidity (15.1% vs 36.1%).[50] Sparing of hepatic parenchyma also increases salvage options for patients who recur in the liver after initial resection.[49]

More advanced strategies are required when dealing with higher volume of total liver tumor or bilobar liver disease; many of these patients are left with too small liver remnant after resection if only extended hepatectomy is considered. Two-stage hepatectomy is an option available at experienced hospitals and is associated with excellent survival outcomes but high morbidity and mortality. In the first stage, the final future liver remnant (usually segments 2 and 3) is cleared of disease typically through minor nonanatomic resection or ablation techniques. The right portal vein is then ligated intraoperatively or embolized percutaneously after the operation; sometimes portal branches to segment 4 are also treated with embolization.[51] This causes hypertrophy of the future liver remnant during the next 6 to 12 weeks. Interval CT scans can document the kinetic growth rate of the liver, and a rate of greater than 2% per week is associated with low rates of liver failure after the second stage of resection.[52] In the second stage, an extended (usually right) hepatectomy is done to remove all remaining tumors. Dropout after the first stage because of tumor progression occurs in up to 35% of patients. Prognostic factors for dropout include CEA greater than 30, tumor size greater than 4 cm, greater than 12 cycles of chemotherapy, or progression during first-line treatment.[53] Completion of the second stage has a distinct survival advantage of median 37 months compared with 16 months for those who only complete the first stage.[54] The two-stage hepatectomy carries a 6.4% 90-day mortality rate and 26% major complication rate. A 5-year survival rate of 64% in those who complete the second stage reinforces the benefit of hepatic metastasectomy in those with CRLM.[55]

Table 2
Outcomes of curative intent liver resection of colorectal metastases

Series Author, Year	Patients (n)	Median DFS (mo)	DFS (%)	Median OS (mo)	OS (%)	Operative Mortality Rate (%)	Major Complication Rate (%)	Minor Resection Rate (%)
Fong et al,[6] 1999	1001	—	—	69	5-y: 37 10-y: 22	2.8	31	37
Pawlik et al,[45] 2005	557	—	—	74	5-y: 58	0.9	—	42.7
Nordlinger et al,[17] 2008; Nordlinger et al,[18] 2013 (RCT)	364	11–18	3-y: 28.1–36.2	54.3–61.3	5-y: 47.8–51.2	1.3	16–25	21
Rees et al,[44] 2008	929	—	—	42.5	5-y: 36 10-y: 23	1.5	25.9	36.2
de Jong et al,[46] 2009	1669	23	5-y: 30	36	5-y: 47.3	—	—	55
House et al,[47] 2010	1600	—	5-y: 33	64	5-y: 43	1	44	39

Abbreviations: DFS, disease-free survival; RCT, randomized controlled trial.

Minimally invasive techniques of liver resection have gained popularity in highly specialized centers showing improved outcomes compared with open operations. In general, laparoscopic liver resection is associated with reduced blood loss because of the tamponade effect of pneumoperitoneum, reduced length of stay, and reduced opioid requirements.[56] Large cohort, although retrospective, studies show similar oncologic outcomes including R0 resection rates between minimally invasive and open hepatectomy.[57–59] It has been suggested that laparoscopic liver resection techniques require advanced training and a learning curve of 60 major hepatectomies before decreasing morbidity and mortality to acceptable rates of 17.2% and 3.4%.[60]

One of the challenges in management for patients who receive chemotherapy before hepatic resection is the disappearing metastasis. With impressive response rates to modern chemotherapy, 10% to 38% of CRLM disappear after treatment with chemotherapy especially those less than 2 cm in size.[61] Disappearance on imaging studies does not correlate with certain pathologic response because up to 80% of such tumors may have residual tumor cells; therefore, the general recommendation is to still remove them if found intraoperatively.[62] Pathologic complete response occurs in 9% of tumors and is an excellent prognostic factor with 5-year survival of 75%.[63]

For patients who initially present with unresectable CRLM, rates of conversion to resectable with chemotherapy range from 17% to 40%, and most eventually undergo margin-negative resection with 5-year survival rates around 30%. This population has a high frequency of disease recurrence.[64] Recurrence after hepatectomy for CRLM overall occurs in 60% to 70% of patient.[46] In those who recur with liver only or liver-predominant disease, repeat hepatectomy may be feasible in up to 27%.[65] Major morbidity and mortality rates are similar to the primary hepatectomy at 23% and 1.2%.[66] Outcomes favor repeat hepatectomy with 5-year survival at 54% compared with 45% in those who do not undergo repeat hepatectomy (the authors admit the high selection bias in this statement).[67] Prognostic factors for better survival after repeat hepatectomy include initial R0 resection, longer interval between hepatectomy operations, no extrahepatic disease, and younger patients.[68]

Adjuncts to Resection

Radiofrequency ablation (RFA) or microwave ablation (MWA) used in place of resection for resectable liver disease has not been studied to date and is not recommended because of the higher recurrence rates and inferior disease control.[69] However, the use of ablation techniques in combination with surgical resection may allow for local therapy for CRLM for patients who are not candidates for surgical resection alone.[69,70] Ablation therapies are also helpful for patients who cannot tolerate major resection with small central liver tumors. Ablation therapies can also be used for patients with unresectable disease. The use of RFA with systemic chemotherapy in the setting of unresectable disease is associated with higher progression-free survival at 3 years (27.6%) compared with systemic chemotherapy alone (10.6%) and better 5-year OS (43.1% vs 30.3%).[71,72] Local recurrence rates after ablation are typically less than 10% and are especially low for tumors less than 3 cm in size.[73,74] Patients who undergo a combination of hepatic resection and ablation instead of two-stage hepatectomy have similar median OS around 35 months with low complication and mortality rates.[75,76] A relative contraindication to ablation is use for central tumors near major biliary structures.

Hepatic arterial infusion pump for regional liver chemotherapy therapy is a well-studied and viable adjuvant treatment to hepatic resection for CRLM.[77] The operation entails implantation of a catheter into the gastroduodenal artery connected to a subcutaneously placed pump. The most common regional chemotherapy used is 5-fluoro 2-deoxyuridine (FUDR), which may also be combined with systemic chemotherapy. FUDR intratumoral drug levels are 400 times higher than systemic therapy administration alone. A randomized controlled trial by Kemeny and colleagues[78,79] showed improved 2-year overall survival of 86% versus 74% compared with systemic chemotherapy alone with improved 10-year survival rates of 41.1% versus 27.2%. Comparisons of outcomes using modern chemotherapy regimens have also confirmed survival advantages.[80] The use of infusion pumps has been limited to a few experienced centers thus far, and technical complications may occur in 12% to 41% of patients.[81] Liver toxicity manifested as abnormal liver enzymes occurs in 42% and is managed by pump dexamethasone administration and FUDR dose reductions. Irreversible biliary toxicity is a rare but devastating complication.[82]

Multidisciplinary management of patients with CRLM is critical including involvement of a surgical oncologist or hepatobiliary surgical expert even for patients with initially unresectable disease. With high response rates to modern systemic chemotherapy, some patients convert to resectable, at which surgical input is needed. Interval imaging of liver metastases for patients receiving chemotherapy should occur every 6 to 12 weeks especially for those with a realistic hope of eventual surgical resection or other local or regional therapies. For patients who do not achieve resectable status, multiple other therapeutic options exist for CRLM and are indicated in the setting of liver only or liver-predominant disease (**Table 3**). These options should be understood by the surgeon including indications, mechanism of action, risks and

Table 3
Treatment options for unresectable liver metastasis as conversion or palliative therapies

Treatment Option	Therapeutic Use
Systemic chemotherapy	FOLFOX, FOLFIRI, CAPEOX, FOLFOXIRI ± bevacizumab or panitumumab/cetuximab (KRAS WT) • Phase III CELIM and BOXER trials[83,84]: 71%–78% response rate and 28%–40% converted to resectable
RFA	Locoregional therapy: percutaneous using ultrasound/CT guidance or laparoscopic • Phase II trial[72]: improved 5-y survival 43.1% compared with 30.3% with systemic treatment alone
Stereotactic body radiotherapy	Locoregional therapy using 34–75 Gy delivered in 3–6 fractions • Phase II trial[85]: 2-y local control 91%, 2-y OS and PFS 65% and 35%
Y-90 selective internal radiotherapy	Locoregional therapy using glass or resin beads with Y-90 delivered through the hepatic artery, doses of 100–3000 Gy that penetrates 2.5–11 mm • Phase III trials currently ongoing: EPOCH, FOXFIRE, SIRFLOX
Isolated hepatic perfusion	Open operation infuses melphlan or oxaliplatin through the hepatic artery • Phase I trial[86]: oxaliplatin used, 66% response rate
Drug-eluting beads preloaded with irinotecan (TACE - DEBIRI)	Locoregional therapy of drug-eluting beads delivered through the hepatic artery to the entire right or left lobe of the liver • Phase III RCT[87]: improved OS (22 vs 15 mo) and PFS (7 vs 4 mo) with TACE-DEBIRI over systemic FOLFIRI
Hepatic artery infusion pump	FUDR infused through the hepatic artery used in combination with systemic chemotherapy for palliative therapy or conversion to resectability • Phase II trial[88]: overall response rate of 76% with 47% converted to resectable in a median of 6 mo

Abbreviations: PFS, progression-free survival; RCT, randomized controlled trial; Y-90, yttrium-90.

toxicities, and general outcomes so the surgeon's opinion in multidisciplinary discussions is informed and balanced.

SURGICAL MANAGEMENT OF PERITONEAL METASTASES

Peritoneal carcinomatosis (PC) from CRC is a result of peritoneal cavity invasion by the primary tumor either through direct extension or seeding during surgical removal.[89] This occurs in 11% of patients overall (5.9% metachronous).[90] PC has previously been believed to represent a terminal event in the continuum of systemic disease with interventions having little effect on outcome. However, there is a distinct population of patients who may achieve durable cancer control with combination therapies.

Patients with peritoneal metastases have worse outcomes compared with other sites of metastatic disease. In a study of 10,635 patients combining accrual of 13 phase 3 clinical trials, 11% were found to have peritoneal metastases in combination with another organ, and 2% had peritoneal metastasis only.[91] OS was better in those with nonperitoneal metastasis (HR, 0.7). Those with peritoneal metastasis and two or more additional sites had the worst prognosis (HR, 1.4). There were significantly more patients with BRAF mutations (18%) in the peritoneal disease group than in nonperitoneal metastasis (12%).[91] Furthermore, a large case series of patients with isolated PC showed a median survival of 5.2 to 12.6 months without treatment.[92] Survival after treatment with chemotherapy for PC is not well documented because most large clinical trials have low numbers of patients with only peritoneal metastases. One study of 364 patients pooled from phase 3 clinical trials found a median survival of 12.7 months and progression-free survival of 5.8 months, significantly shorter than in patients without PC.[93] This study also suggested treatment with infusional FOLFOX superior to FOLFIRI (HR, 0.62) as first-line treatment. The addition of biologic agents, such as bevacizumab or cetuximab, improves survival when added to modern chemotherapy regimens, even in patients with PC.[94]

Cytoreductive Surgery and Hyperthermic Intraperitoneal Chemotherapy

Use of hyperthermic intraperitoneal chemotherapy (HIPEC) began in 1980 and has since gained steady acceptance as an adjunct to surgical cytoreduction for selected patients with PC from a variety of malignancies.[95] Cytoreductive surgery (CRS) is defined by removal of all visible tumor; addition of HIPEC in theory helps to destroy the remaining microscopic disease. The principles of cytoreduction include removal of all tumors in the abdomen including peritoneal stripping from parietal and visceral peritoneum to no gross tumor (completeness of cytoreduction [CC]-0) and greater and lesser omentectomy. These techniques were popularized by Sugarbaker[96] and have become readily adopted in most peritoneal surface malignancies. All bowel resection is performed and left in discontinuity until after HIPEC. Tumors of the small bowel mesentery are either enucleated to preserve bowel blood supply or destroyed using cautery or bipolar ablation devices. The entire abdomen is explored and all adhesions are taken down to allow maximal perfusion of all abdominal surfaces with HIPEC. Achieving a CC-0 (no gross residual tumor) or CC-1 (tumor nodules <2.5 mm) is considered optimal and is associated with improved survival compared with CC-2 (2.5 mm to 2.5 cm residual tumor size) and CC-3 (>2.5 cm residual tumor). The beneficial cutoff of 2.5 mm may be related to the maximum effective depth of chemotherapy penetration into tumor.[97] The American Society of Peritoneal Surface Malignancies consensus recommends standards for use of HIPEC (**Table 4**).[98] The drug of choice in the United States is mitomycin C, compared with many centers in Europe, which favor oxaliplatin.[98]

Table 4
HIPEC treatment options comparing the ASPSM consensus guidelines with other treatment options

	ASPSM Consensus	Alternatives Used
HIPEC method	Closed	Open
Chemotherapeutic agent	MMC	Oxaliplatin, carboplatin, doxorubicin, irinotecan, bidirectional chemotherapy
Dosage	40 mg	MMC 15–25 mg/m^2, oxaliplatin 460 mg/m^2
Timing of drug delivery	30 mg at time 0; 10 mg at 60 min	All at time 0
Volume of perfusate	3 L	2–5 L
Inflow temperature	42°C	40°C–43°C
Duration of perfusion	90 min	30–120 min

Abbreviations: ASPSM, American Society of Peritoneal Surface Malignancies; MMC, mitomycin C.

Patient Selection and Outcomes

Selection of patients appropriate for CRS and HIPEC is the cornerstone of best outcomes and less morbidity (**Box 2**). Although criteria vary among centers, the overarching theme is to select patients for CRS in whom complete cytoreduction can be achieved. Consensus guidelines from the American Society of Peritoneal Surface Malignancies were developed to somewhat standardized the range of techniques used to allow for fair comparison of patient outcomes.[98]

Critical to patient selection is the use of the peritoneal carcinomatosis index (PCI), which has shown to be an important prognostic factor.[99] The index divides the abdomen into 13 different regions and the amount of disease in each region is given a score of 0 to 3 for a maximum of 39. A PCI of 15 used as a cutoff divides 5-year survival into 48% (PCI <15) and 12% (PCI >15), with all patients in the greater than 15 group having small bowel involvement that limited complete cytoreduction. A similar score that incorporates PCI with symptoms and tumor histology called the Peritoneal Surface Disease Severity Score accurately defined population subsets with markedly different prognoses.[100] The median survival of the lowest score group was 86 months compared with 28 months in the highest score group.

Outcomes after CRS and HIPEC for patients with colorectal peritoneal metastatic disease have been shown in several studies of highly selected patients. A single clinical trial published in 2003 compared systemic chemotherapy followed by CRS and HIPEC with systemic chemotherapy with or without palliative surgery[101] and found median survival

Box 2
Patient selection criteria for CRS for colorectal peritoneal carcinomatosis

Low-volume disease that is completely resectable (R0)
• No retroperitoneal or portal lymphadenopathy

Minimally symptomatic

Abdominal-only disease
• Hepatic metastasis easily resectable with minor hepatectomy or amenable to ablation

Stable disease (no progression) with chemotherapy

Medically fit to undergo a major operation

of 22.3 months using CRS/HIPEC compared with 12.6 months with palliative treatments only. Those with more than six regions of the abdominal cavity involved or with gross disease left had poor prognosis despite aggressive surgery. Another study had similar findings of 5-year survival at 51% for patients treated with systemic chemotherapy, CRS, and HIPEC compared with 13% if treated by chemotherapy alone.[102]

Studies also suggest that outcomes after CRS and HIPEC continue to improve. As acceptance of the technique has increased, technical experience with the operation and patient management experience have expanded. Operations to achieve adequate cytoreduction and HIPEC may take 7 to 10 hours with median hospital lengths of stay at 12 to 17 days.[103] The operation also carries a high morbidity in the 30% to 40% range with stoma creation rates from 10% to 20% and readmission of 11%.[104] Most complications and death stem from intestinal leak/fistula and sepsis. Despite the risk, median survival rates over 30 to 40 months in many studies justify the use of CRS and HIPEC in selected patients (**Table 5**).

Approximately 16% of patients achieve prolonged cancer control after CRS/HIPEC, with PCI of less than 10 highly associated with best outcome.[110] Another study found the presence and number of lymph nodes at the time of primary resection and CRS/HIPEC to be most predictive of recurrence.[111] When patients recur repeat CRS/HIPEC can rarely be performed (6.2%) but when feasible may yield median OS of 39 to 57.6 months and 2-year survival of 44% to 50% (reported in small numbers of patients).[112]

Table 5
Outcomes of large case series with complete cytoreduction and HIPEC

Series Author, Year	Patients (n)	Perfusion Technique	Median OS (mo)	5-y Survival (%)	Operative Mortality Rate (%)	Major Morbidity Rate (%)
Glehen et al,[105] 2004	506 (28 institutions)	HIPEC and EPIC, multiple drugs	32.4	31	4	22.9
Verwaal et al,[106] 2008 (only RCT)	105	Open, MMC	48	45	8	19
Elias et al,[107] 2010	523 (23 institutions)	HIPEC and EPIC, multiple drugs	30.1	27	3.3	31
Ung et al,[108] 2013	211	HIPEC (MMC) or EPIC (IP 5-FU)	46.8	42	1	44.3
Kuijpers et al,[109] 2013	660	Open, MMC and oxaliplatin	33	31	3	34
Esquivel et al,[100] 2014	705	Oxaliplatin or MMC	41	58	—	—
Levine et al,[103] 2014	248	MMC	—	15	3.8	42

Abbreviations: EPIC, Early Postoperative Intraperitoneal Chemotherapy; MMC, mitomycin C; RCT, randomized controlled trial.

SURGICAL MANAGEMENT OF PULMONARY METASTASIS

Lung metastases occur overall in 10% to 20% of patients with CRC with approximately 11% as synchronous and 5.8% metachronous in terms of timing.[113] Metastasis to the lung is rarely the only site of disease (1.7%–7.2%).[114] Patients with rectal cancer are two to three times more likely to develop lung metastasis than those with colon cancer, and more distal rectal cancers have increased risk.[115] Molecular markers including *RAS* mutations, *CXCR7* expression, and *WNT* pathway activity are also associated with a pattern of predominant lung metastatic disease.[116] Overall 5-year survival is poor at 1.9% to 6.9% with 14- to 24-month median survival for those with any lung disease, and prognosis declines as the number of extrapulmonary disease sites increases.

Case series describing outcomes after pulmonary metastasectomy for metastatic CRC show low rates of mortality and complications and median time to recurrence up to nearly 3 years in some studies (**Table 6**). Another review of published series found 5-year survival ranged from 24% to 56% after surgical resection of pulmonary metastasis from CRC.[123] Similar to hepatic resection for metastatic disease, overall recurrence rates are high, up to 80% after 2 years.[124] An important study, the Pulmonary Metastasectomy in Colorectal Cancer Trial (PulMiCC, ClinicalTrials.gov: NCT01106261), began enrolling in 2010 in European centers and has a planned completion date of 2020.

Multidisciplinary evaluation of patients with lung metastasis is just as critical as for those with CRLM. Some general principles of patient selection for pulmonary metastasectomy and particularly poor prognostic features in these patients are shown (**Table 7**). Because the incidence of isolated pulmonary metastasis is low, consideration of pulmonary metastasectomy generally depends on outcomes of therapy for other sites with a median interval of 28 months between chemotherapy and resection of a primary tumor to lung resection.[125] Parenchymal sparing "wedge resection" techniques are used in 70% of patients with resection of clinically suspicious lymph nodes in 40%.[118,119] Routine lymphadenectomy is not necessary; however, lymph node sampling for suspicious nodes identified preoperatively or intraoperatively should be done because identification of thoracic lymph node disease has significant prognostic value.[126]

Table 6
Outcomes of lung metastasis resection for curative intent

Case Series Author, Year	Patients (n)	Median RFS (mo)	RFS (%)	Median OS (mo)	OS (%)	Operative Mortality Rate (%)	Major Complication Rate (%)
Kanemitsu et al,[117] 2004	313	—	—	38.4	5-y: 38.3	1.3	—
Onaitis et al,[118] 2009	378	24	3-y: 28	—	3-y: 78	1	10
Borasio et al,[119] 2011	137	35.6	3 y: 51.1	36.2	5-y: 55.4	0	13.1
Blackmon et al,[120] 2012	229	19.4	—	70.1	5-y: 55.4	0	1.7
Zampino et al,[121] 2014	199	35	—	50.4	5-y: 43	0	—
Hernandez et al,[122] 2016	522	28.3	—	54.9	5-y: 46.1	0.38	15.7

Abbreviation: RFS, recurrence-free survival.

Table 7	
Patient selection criteria for curative resection and poor prognostic features of pulmonary metastasis	
Patient Selection Criteria	**Poor Prognostic Features**
• Margin-negative resection feasible (no limit on number of tumors) • Control of primary tumor • No extrapulmonary disease (or resectable liver disease) • Able to tolerate pulmonary resection (wedge or single lobe in 80%–90% of patients)	• Increasing number of pulmonary metastases • Synchronous presentation • Short disease-free interval (<24 mo) • Elevated CEA level • Hilar or mediastinal lymph nodes • Presence of extrathoracic disease (except liver metastasis)

Patients who undergo surgical treatment of pulmonary metastasis have commonly undergone prior hepatic resection for CRLM (around 29%).[125] Studies have shown these patients to have median OS at 41 to 46 months and 5-year survival of 39%.[127,128] Outcomes after resection of liver and lung metastasis are similar to those with liver-only disease who undergo hepatic resection.[129] It may also be reasonable to consider resection of lung metastasis if other local therapy options are available for hepatic metastatic disease, such as ablation using RFA or MWA or stereotactic body radiotherapy.[130]

SUMMARY

Effective surgical treatment options exist for patients with metastatic CRC to the liver, peritoneum, and lung. Such therapies have improved over the past 20 years and are safe. These treatments are most often given in conjunction with chemotherapy to maximize survival and decrease recurrence rates. The opinions of surgical and medical oncologists are necessary pieces of the multidisciplinary team. For patients with metastasis not amenable to surgical resection initially, an important goal remains eventual metastasectomy if feasible based on response. Most patients treated with surgical resection of metastatic disease recur, and therefore future studies must continue to focus on improved biologic and systemic therapies.

REFERENCES

1. Kopetz S, Chang GJ, Overman MJ, et al. Improved survival in metastatic colorectal cancer is associated with adoption of hepatic resection and improved chemotherapy. J Clin Oncol 2009;27(22):3677–83.
2. Mohammad WM, Balaa FK. Surgical management of colorectal liver metastases. Clin Colon Rectal Surg 2009;22(4):225–32.
3. Fakih MG. Metastatic colorectal cancer: current state and future directions. J Clin Oncol 2015;33(16):1809–24.
4. Kohne CH, Cunningham D, Di Costanzo F, et al. Clinical determinants of survival in patients with 5-fluorouracil-based treatment for metastatic colorectal cancer: results of a multivariate analysis of 3825 patients. Ann Oncol 2002;13(2):308–17.
5. Miller G, Biernacki P, Kemeny NE, et al. Outcomes after resection of synchronous or metachronous hepatic and pulmonary colorectal metastases. J Am Coll Surg 2007;205(2):231–8.
6. Fong Y, Fortner J, Sun RL, et al. Clinical score for predicting recurrence after hepatic resection for metastatic colorectal cancer: analysis of 1001 consecutive cases. Ann Surg 1999;230(3):309–18 [discussion: 318–21].

7. Winter J. Metastatic malignant liver tumors: colorectal cancer. In: Blumgart LH, editor. Blumgart's surgery of the liver, pancreas and biliary tract. 5th edition. Philadelphia: Elsevier; 2012. p. 1290–1304.e1294.

8. Enquist IB, Good Z, Jubb AM, et al. Lymph node-independent liver metastasis in a model of metastatic colorectal cancer. Nat Commun 2014;5:3530.

9. Vakiani E, Janakiraman M, Shen R, et al. Comparative genomic analysis of primary versus metastatic colorectal carcinomas. J Clin Oncol 2012;30(24):2956–62.

10. Varghese S, Burness M, Xu H, et al. Site-specific gene expression profiles and novel molecular prognostic factors in patients with lower gastrointestinal adenocarcinoma diffusely metastatic to liver or peritoneum. Ann Surg Oncol 2007;14(12):3460–71.

11. Morris VK, Lucas FA, Overman MJ, et al. Clinicopathologic characteristics and gene expression analyses of non-KRAS 12/13, RAS-mutated metastatic colorectal cancer. Ann Oncol 2014;25(10):2008–14.

12. Hugen N, van de Velde CJ, de Wilt JH, et al. Metastatic pattern in colorectal cancer is strongly influenced by histological subtype. Ann Oncol 2014;25(3):651–7.

13. Yaeger R, Cowell E, Chou JF, et al. RAS mutations affect pattern of metastatic spread and increase propensity for brain metastasis in colorectal cancer. Cancer 2015;121(8):1195–203.

14. Qiu M, Hu J, Yang D, et al. Pattern of distant metastases in colorectal cancer: a SEER based study. Oncotarget 2015;6(36):38658–66.

15. Adam R, Bhangui P, Poston G, et al. Is perioperative chemotherapy useful for solitary, metachronous, colorectal liver metastases? Ann Surg 2010;252(5):774–87.

16. Nanji S, Cleary S, Ryan P, et al. Up-front hepatic resection for metastatic colorectal cancer results in favorable long-term survival. Ann Surg Oncol 2013;20(1):295–304.

17. Nordlinger B, Sorbye H, Glimelius B, et al. Perioperative chemotherapy with FOLFOX4 and surgery versus surgery alone for resectable liver metastases from colorectal cancer (EORTC Intergroup trial 40983): a randomised controlled trial. Lancet 2008;371(9617):1007–16.

18. Nordlinger B, Sorbye H, Glimelius B, et al. Perioperative FOLFOX4 chemotherapy and surgery versus surgery alone for resectable liver metastases from colorectal cancer (EORTC 40983): long-term results of a randomised, controlled, phase 3 trial. Lancet Oncol 2013;14(12):1208–15.

19. Primrose J, Falk S, Finch-Jones M, et al. Systemic chemotherapy with or without cetuximab in patients with resectable colorectal liver metastasis: the New EPOC randomised controlled trial. Lancet Oncol 2014;15(6):601–11.

20. Gruenberger B, Tamandl D, Schueller J, et al. Bevacizumab, capecitabine, and oxaliplatin as neoadjuvant therapy for patients with potentially curable metastatic colorectal cancer. J Clin Oncol 2008;26(11):1830–5.

21. Vigano L, Capussotti L, De Rosa G, et al. Liver resection for colorectal metastases after chemotherapy: impact of chemotherapy-related liver injuries, pathological tumor response, and micrometastases on long-term survival. Ann Surg 2013;258(5):731–40 [discussion: 741–2].

22. Welsh FK, Tilney HS, Tekkis PP, et al. Safe liver resection following chemotherapy for colorectal metastases is a matter of timing. Br J Cancer 2007;96(7):1037–42.

23. Kishi Y, Zorzi D, Contreras CM, et al. Extended preoperative chemotherapy does not improve pathologic response and increases postoperative liver insufficiency after hepatic resection for colorectal liver metastases. Ann Surg Oncol 2010;17(11):2870–6.

24. Robinson SM, Wilson CH, Burt AD, et al. Chemotherapy-associated liver injury in patients with colorectal liver metastases: a systematic review and meta-analysis. Ann Surg Oncol 2012;19(13):4287–99.

25. Manfredi S, Lepage C, Hatem C, et al. Epidemiology and management of liver metastases from colorectal cancer. Ann Surg 2006;244(2):254–9.
26. Adam R, de Gramont A, Figueras J, et al. Managing synchronous liver metastases from colorectal cancer: a multidisciplinary international consensus. Cancer Treat Rev 2015;41(9):729–41.
27. Sagar J. Colorectal stents for the management of malignant colonic obstructions. Cochrane Database Syst Rev 2011;(11):CD007378.
28. Wolf PS, Park JO, Bao F, et al. Preoperative chemotherapy and the risk of hepatotoxicity and morbidity after liver resection for metastatic colorectal cancer: a single institution experience. J Am Coll Surg 2013;216(1):41–9.
29. Feng Q, Wei Y, Zhu D, et al. Timing of hepatectomy for resectable synchronous colorectal liver metastases: for whom simultaneous resection is more suitable–a meta-analysis. PLoS One 2014;9(8):e104348.
30. Martin RC, Augenstein V, Reuter NP, et al. Simultaneous versus staged resection for synchronous colorectal cancer liver metastases. J Am Coll Surg 2009;208(5): 842–50 [discussion: 850–2].
31. Ferretti S, Tranchart H, Buell JF, et al. Laparoscopic simultaneous resection of colorectal primary tumor and liver metastases: results of a multicenter international study. World J Surg 2015;39(8):2052–60.
32. Poultsides GA, Servais EL, Saltz LB, et al. Outcome of primary tumor in patients with synchronous stage IV colorectal cancer receiving combination chemotherapy without surgery as initial treatment. J Clin Oncol 2009;27(20):3379–84.
33. Tarantino I, Warschkow R, Worni M, et al. Prognostic relevance of palliative primary tumor removal in 37,793 metastatic colorectal cancer patients: a population-based, propensity score-adjusted trend analysis. Ann Surg 2015; 262:112–20.
34. Faron M, Pignon JP, Malka D, et al. Is primary tumour resection associated with survival improvement in patients with colorectal cancer and unresectable synchronous metastases? A pooled analysis of individual data from four randomised trials. Eur J Cancer 2015;51:166–76.
35. Clancy C, Burke JP, Barry M, et al. A meta-analysis to determine the effect of primary tumor resection for stage IV colorectal cancer with unresectable metastases on patient survival. Ann Surg Oncol 2014;21(12):3900–8.
36. Ahmed S, Fields A, Pahwa P, et al. Surgical resection of primary tumor in asymptomatic or minimally symptomatic patients with stage IV colorectal cancer: a Canadian province experience. Clin Colorectal Cancer 2015;14(4):e41–7.
37. Ghiringhelli F, Bichard D, Limat S, et al. Bevacizumab efficacy in metastatic colorectal cancer is dependent on primary tumor resection. Ann Surg Oncol 2014;21(5):1632–40.
38. Saltz LB, Clarke S, Diaz-Rubio E, et al. Bevacizumab in combination with oxaliplatin-based chemotherapy as first-line therapy in metastatic colorectal cancer: a randomized phase III study. J Clin Oncol 2008;26(12):2013–9.
39. Power DG, Kemeny NE. Chemotherapy for the conversion of unresectable colorectal cancer liver metastases to resection. Crit Rev Oncol Hematol 2011;79(3): 251–64.
40. Shindoh J, Loyer EM, Kopetz S, et al. Optimal morphologic response to preoperative chemotherapy: an alternate outcome end point before resection of hepatic colorectal metastases. J Clin Oncol 2012;30(36):4566–72.
41. Tomlinson JS, Jarnagin WR, DeMatteo RP, et al. Actual 10-year survival after resection of colorectal liver metastases defines cure. J Clin Oncol 2007; 25(29):4575–80.

42. Adams RB, Aloia TA, Loyer E, et al. Selection for hepatic resection of colorectal liver metastases: expert consensus statement. HPB (Oxford) 2013;15(2):91–103.

43. Carpizo DR, Are C, Jarnagin W, et al. Liver resection for metastatic colorectal cancer in patients with concurrent extrahepatic disease: results in 127 patients treated at a single center. Ann Surg Oncol 2009;16(8):2138–46.

44. Rees M, Tekkis PP, Welsh FK, et al. Evaluation of long-term survival after hepatic resection for metastatic colorectal cancer: a multifactorial model of 929 patients. Ann Surg 2008;247(1):125–35.

45. Pawlik TM, Scoggins CR, Zorzi D, et al. Effect of surgical margin status on survival and site of recurrence after hepatic resection for colorectal metastases. Ann Surg 2005;241(5):715–22 [discussion: 722–4].

46. de Jong MC, Pulitano C, Ribero D, et al. Rates and patterns of recurrence following curative intent surgery for colorectal liver metastasis: an international multi-institutional analysis of 1669 patients. Ann Surg 2009;250(3):440–8.

47. House MG, Ito H, Gönen M, et al. Survival after hepatic resection for metastatic colorectal cancer: trends in outcomes for 1,600 patients during two decades at a single institution. J Am Coll Surg 2010;210(5):744–52, 752–5.

48. Memeo R, de Blasi V, Adam R, et al. Parenchymal-sparing hepatectomies (PSH) for bilobar colorectal liver metastases are associated with a lower morbidity and similar oncological results: a propensity score matching analysis. HPB (Oxford) 2016;18(9):781–90.

49. Mise Y, Aloia TA, Brudvik KW, et al. Parenchymal-sparing hepatectomy in colorectal liver metastasis improves salvageability and survival. Ann Surg 2016;263(1):146–52.

50. Reddy SK, Pawlik TM, Zorzi D, et al. Simultaneous resections of colorectal cancer and synchronous liver metastases: a multi-institutional analysis. Ann Surg Oncol 2007;14(12):3481–91.

51. Clavien PA, Petrowsky H, DeOliveira ML, et al. Strategies for safer liver surgery and partial liver transplantation. N Engl J Med 2007;356(15):1545–59.

52. Shindoh J, Truty MJ, Aloia TA, et al. Kinetic growth rate after portal vein embolization predicts posthepatectomy outcomes: toward zero liver-related mortality in patients with colorectal liver metastases and small future liver remnant. J Am Coll Surg 2013;216(2):201–9.

53. Imai K, Benitez CC, Allard MA, et al. Failure to achieve a 2-stage hepatectomy for colorectal liver metastases: how to prevent it? Ann Surg 2015;262(5):772–8 [discussion: 778–9].

54. Lam VW, Laurence JM, Johnston E, et al. A systematic review of two-stage hepatectomy in patients with initially unresectable colorectal liver metastases. HPB (Oxford) 2013;15(7):483–91.

55. Brouquet A, Abdalla EK, Kopetz S, et al. High survival rate after two-stage resection of advanced colorectal liver metastases: response-based selection and complete resection define outcome. J Clin Oncol 2011;29(8):1083–90.

56. Nguyen KT, Marsh JW, Tsung A, et al. Comparative benefits of laparoscopic vs open hepatic resection: a critical appraisal. Arch Surg 2011;146(3):348–56.

57. Martinez-Cecilia D, Cipriani F, Vishal S, et al. Laparoscopic versus open liver resection for colorectal metastases in elderly and octogenarian patients: a multi-center propensity score based analysis of short- and long-term outcomes. Ann Surg 2017;265(6):1192–200.

58. Zeng Y, Tian M. Laparoscopic versus open hepatectomy for elderly patients with liver metastases from colorectal cancer. J Buon 2016;21(5):1146–52.

59. Allard MA, Cunha AS, Gayet B, et al. Early and long-term oncological outcomes after laparoscopic resection for colorectal liver metastases: a propensity score-based analysis. Ann Surg 2015;262(5):794–802.

60. Vigano L, Laurent A, Tayar C, et al. The learning curve in laparoscopic liver resection: improved feasibility and reproducibility. Ann Surg 2009;250(5):772–82.

61. Bischof DA, Clary BM, Maithel SK, et al. Surgical management of disappearing colorectal liver metastases. Br J Surg 2013;100(11):1414–20.

62. Benoist S, Brouquet A, Penna C, et al. Complete response of colorectal liver metastases after chemotherapy: does it mean cure? J Clin Oncol 2006;24(24):3939–45.

63. Blazer DG 3rd, Kishi Y, Maru DM, et al. Pathologic response to preoperative chemotherapy: a new outcome end point after resection of hepatic colorectal metastases. J Clin Oncol 2008;26(33):5344–51.

64. Devaud N, Kanji ZS, Dhani N, et al. Liver resection after chemotherapy and tumour downsizing in patients with initially unresectable colorectal cancer liver metastases. HPB (Oxford) 2014;16(5):475–80.

65. Butte JM, Gonen M, Allen PJ, et al. Recurrence after partial hepatectomy for metastatic colorectal cancer: potentially curative role of salvage repeat resection. Ann Surg Oncol 2015;22(8):2761–71.

66. Lam VW, Pang T, Laurence JM, et al. A systematic review of repeat hepatectomy for recurrent colorectal liver metastases. J Gastrointest Surg 2013;17(7):1312–21.

67. Wicherts DA, de Haas RJ, Salloum C, et al. Repeat hepatectomy for recurrent colorectal metastases. Br J Surg 2013;100(6):808–18.

68. Battula N, Tsapralis D, Mayer D, et al. Repeat liver resection for recurrent colorectal metastases: a single-centre, 13-year experience. HPB (Oxford) 2014;16(2):157–63.

69. Abdalla EK, Vauthey JN, Ellis LM, et al. Recurrence and outcomes following hepatic resection, radiofrequency ablation, and combined resection/ablation for colorectal liver metastases. Ann Surg 2004;239(6):818–25 [discussion: 825–7].

70. Eltawil KM, Boame N, Mimeault R, et al. Patterns of recurrence following selective intraoperative radiofrequency ablation as an adjunct to hepatic resection for colorectal liver metastases. J Surg Oncol 2014;110(6):734–8.

71. Ruers T, Punt C, Van Coevorden F, et al. Radiofrequency ablation combined with systemic treatment versus systemic treatment alone in patients with non-resectable colorectal liver metastases: a randomized EORTC Intergroup phase II study (EORTC 40004). Ann Oncol 2012;23(10):2619–26.

72. Ruers T, Van Coevorden F, Punt CJ, et al. Local treatment of unresectable colorectal liver metastases: results of a randomized phase II trial. J Natl Cancer Inst 2017;109(9).

73. Tanis E, Nordlinger B, Mauer M, et al. Local recurrence rates after radiofrequency ablation or resection of colorectal liver metastases. Analysis of the European Organisation for Research and Treatment of Cancer #40004 and #40983. Eur J Cancer 2014;50(5):912–9.

74. Kingham TP, Tanoue M, Eaton A, et al. Patterns of recurrence after ablation of colorectal cancer liver metastases. Ann Surg Oncol 2012;19(3):834–41.

75. Faitot F, Faron M, Adam R, et al. Two-stage hepatectomy versus 1-stage resection combined with radiofrequency for bilobar colorectal metastases: a case-matched analysis of surgical and oncological outcomes. Ann Surg 2014;260(5):822–7 [discussion: 827–8].

76. Pawlik TM, Izzo F, Cohen DS, et al. Combined resection and radiofrequency ablation for advanced hepatic malignancies: results in 172 patients. Ann Surg Oncol 2003;10(9):1059–69.

77. Lewis HL, Bloomston M. Hepatic artery infusional chemotherapy. Surg Clin North Am 2016;96(2):341–55.

78. Kemeny N, Huang Y, Cohen AM, et al. Hepatic arterial infusion of chemotherapy after resection of hepatic metastases from colorectal cancer. N Engl J Med 1999;341(27):2039–48.

79. Kemeny NE, Gonen M. Hepatic arterial infusion after liver resection. N Engl J Med 2005;352:734–5.

80. House MG, Kemeny NE, Gonen M, et al. Comparison of adjuvant systemic chemotherapy with or without hepatic arterial infusional chemotherapy after hepatic resection for metastatic colorectal cancer. Ann Surg 2011;254(6):851–6.

81. Allen PJ, Nissan A, Picon AI, et al. Technical complications and durability of hepatic artery infusion pumps for unresectable colorectal liver metastases: an institutional experience of 544 consecutive cases. J Am Coll Surg 2005; 201(1):57–65.

82. Cercek A, D'Angelica M, Power D, et al. Floxuridine hepatic arterial infusion associated biliary toxicity is increased by concurrent administration of systemic bevacizumab. Ann Surg Oncol 2014;21(2):479–86.

83. Folprecht G, Gruenberger T, Bechstein WO, et al. Tumour response and secondary resectability of colorectal liver metastases following neoadjuvant chemotherapy with cetuximab: the CELIM randomised phase 2 trial. Lancet Oncol 2010;11(1):38–47.

84. Wong R, Cunningham D, Barbachano Y, et al. A multicentre study of capecitabine, oxaliplatin plus bevacizumab as perioperative treatment of patients with poor-risk colorectal liver-only metastases not selected for upfront resection. Ann Oncol 2011;22(9):2042–8.

85. Scorsetti M, Comito T, Tozzi A, et al. Final results of a phase II trial for stereotactic body radiation therapy for patients with inoperable liver metastases from colorectal cancer. J Cancer Res Clin Oncol 2015;141(3):543–53.

86. Zeh HJ, Brown CK, Holtzman MP, et al. A phase I study of hyperthermic isolated hepatic perfusion with oxaliplatin in the treatment of unresectable liver metastases from colorectal cancer. Ann Surg Oncol 2009;16(2):385–94.

87. Fiorentini G, Aliberti C, Tilli M, et al. Intra-arterial infusion of irinotecan-loaded drug-eluting beads (DEBIRI) versus intravenous therapy (FOLFIRI) for hepatic metastases from colorectal cancer: final results of a phase III study. Anticancer Res 2012;32(4):1387–95.

88. D'Angelica MI, Correa-Gallego C, Paty PB, et al. Phase II trial of hepatic artery infusional and systemic chemotherapy for patients with unresectable hepatic metastases from colorectal cancer: conversion to resection and long-term outcomes. Ann Surg 2015;261(2):353–60.

89. Glehen O, Osinsky D, Beaujard AC, et al. Natural history of peritoneal carcinomatosis from nongynecologic malignancies. Surg Oncol Clin N Am 2003;12(3): 729–39, xiii.

90. Kerscher AG, Chua TC, Gasser M, et al. Impact of peritoneal carcinomatosis in the disease history of colorectal cancer management: a longitudinal experience of 2406 patients over two decades. Br J Cancer 2013;108(7):1432–9.

91. Franko J, Shi Q, Meyers JP, et al. Prognosis of patients with peritoneal metastatic colorectal cancer given systemic therapy: an analysis of individual patient data from prospective randomised trials from the Analysis and Research in Cancers

of the Digestive System (ARCAD) database. Lancet Oncol 2016;17(12): 1709–19.

92. Jayne DG, Fook S, Loi C, et al. Peritoneal carcinomatosis from colorectal cancer. Br J Surg 2002;89(12):1545–50.

93. Franko J, Shi Q, Goldman CD, et al. Treatment of colorectal peritoneal carcinomatosis with systemic chemotherapy: a pooled analysis of north central cancer treatment group phase III trials N9741 and N9841. J Clin Oncol 2012;30(3): 263–7.

94. Klaver YL, Simkens LH, Lemmens VE, et al. Outcomes of colorectal cancer patients with peritoneal carcinomatosis treated with chemotherapy with and without targeted therapy. Eur J Surg Oncol 2012;38(7):617–23.

95. Spratt JS, Adcock RA, Muskovin M, et al. Clinical delivery system for intraperitoneal hyperthermic chemotherapy. Cancer Res 1980;40(2):256–60.

96. Sugarbaker PH. Peritonectomy procedures. Ann Surg 1995;221(1):29–42.

97. Glehen O, Gilly FN. Quantitative prognostic indicators of peritoneal surface malignancy: carcinomatosis, sarcomatosis, and peritoneal mesothelioma. Surg Oncol Clin N Am 2003;12(3):649–71.

98. Turaga K, Levine E, Barone R, et al. Consensus guidelines from the American Society of Peritoneal Surface Malignancies on standardizing the delivery of hyperthermic intraperitoneal chemotherapy (HIPEC) in colorectal cancer patients in the United States. Ann Surg Oncol 2014;21(5):1501–5.

99. da Silva RG, Sugarbaker PH. Analysis of prognostic factors in seventy patients having a complete cytoreduction plus perioperative intraperitoneal chemotherapy for carcinomatosis from colorectal cancer. J Am Coll Surg 2006; 203(6):878–86.

100. Esquivel J, Lowy AM, Markman M, et al. The American Society of Peritoneal Surface Malignancies (ASPSM) multiinstitution evaluation of the Peritoneal Surface Disease Severity Score (PSDSS) in 1,013 patients with colorectal cancer with peritoneal carcinomatosis. Ann Surg Oncol 2014;21(13):4195–201.

101. Verwaal VJ, van Ruth S, de Bree E, et al. Randomized trial of cytoreduction and hyperthermic intraperitoneal chemotherapy versus systemic chemotherapy and palliative surgery in patients with peritoneal carcinomatosis of colorectal cancer. J Clin Oncol 2003;21(20):3737–43.

102. Elias D, Lefevre JH, Chevalier J, et al. Complete cytoreductive surgery plus intraperitoneal chemohyperthermia with oxaliplatin for peritoneal carcinomatosis of colorectal origin. J Clin Oncol 2009;27(5):681–5.

103. Levine EA, Stewart JH 4th, Shen P, et al. Intraperitoneal chemotherapy for peritoneal surface malignancy: experience with 1,000 patients. J Am Coll Surg 2014;218(4):573–85.

104. Jafari MD, Halabi WJ, Stamos MJ, et al. Surgical outcomes of hyperthermic intraperitoneal chemotherapy: analysis of the American College of Surgeons national surgical quality improvement program. JAMA Surg 2014;149(2):170–5.

105. Glehen O, Kwiatkowski F, Sugarbaker PH, et al. Cytoreductive surgery combined with perioperative intraperitoneal chemotherapy for the management of peritoneal carcinomatosis from colorectal cancer: a multi-institutional study. J Clin Oncol 2004;22(16):3284–92.

106. Verwaal VJ, Bruin S, Boot H, et al. 8-year follow-up of randomized trial: cytoreduction and hyperthermic intraperitoneal chemotherapy versus systemic chemotherapy in patients with peritoneal carcinomatosis of colorectal cancer. Ann Surg Oncol 2008;15(9):2426–32.

107. Elias D, Gilly F, Boutitie F, et al. Peritoneal colorectal carcinomatosis treated with surgery and perioperative intraperitoneal chemotherapy: retrospective analysis of 523 patients from a multicentric French study. J Clin Oncol 2010;28(1):63–8.

108. Ung L, Chua TC, David LM. Peritoneal metastases of lower gastrointestinal tract origin: a comparative study of patient outcomes following cytoreduction and intraperitoneal chemotherapy. J Cancer Res Clin Oncol 2013;139(11):1899–908.

109. Kuijpers AM, Mirck B, Aalbers AG, et al. Cytoreduction and HIPEC in the Netherlands: nationwide long-term outcome following the Dutch protocol. Ann Surg Oncol 2013;20(13):4224–30.

110. Goere D, Malka D, Tzanis D, et al. Is there a possibility of a cure in patients with colorectal peritoneal carcinomatosis amenable to complete cytoreductive surgery and intraperitoneal chemotherapy? Ann Surg 2013;257(6):1065–71.

111. Baumgartner JM, Tobin L, Heavey SF, et al. Predictors of progression in high-grade appendiceal or colorectal peritoneal carcinomatosis after cytoreductive surgery and hyperthermic intraperitoneal chemotherapy. Ann Surg Oncol 2015;22(5):1716–21.

112. Williams BH, Alzahrani NA, Chan DL, et al. Repeat cytoreductive surgery (CRS) for recurrent colorectal peritoneal metastases: yes or no? Eur J Surg Oncol 2014;40(8):943–9.

113. Mitry E, Guiu B, Cosconea S, et al. Epidemiology, management and prognosis of colorectal cancer with lung metastases: a 30-year population-based study. Gut 2010;59(10):1383–8.

114. Tan KK, Lopes Gde L Jr, Sim R. How uncommon are isolated lung metastases in colorectal cancer? A review from database of 754 patients over 4 years. J Gastrointest Surg 2009;13(4):642–8.

115. Chiang JM, Hsieh PS, Chen JS, et al. Rectal cancer level significantly affects rates and patterns of distant metastases among rectal cancer patients post curative-intent surgery without neoadjuvant therapy. World J Surg Oncol 2014; 12:197.

116. Moorcraft SY, Ladas G, Bowcock A, et al. Management of resectable colorectal lung metastases. Clin Exp Metastasis 2016;33(3):285–96.

117. Kanemitsu Y, Kato T, Hirai T, et al. Preoperative probability model for predicting overall survival after resection of pulmonary metastases from colorectal cancer. Br J Surg 2004;91(1):112–20.

118. Onaitis MW, Petersen RP, Haney JC, et al. Prognostic factors for recurrence after pulmonary resection of colorectal cancer metastases. Ann Thorac Surg 2009; 87(6):1684–8.

119. Borasio P, Gisabella M, Bille A, et al. Role of surgical resection in colorectal lung metastases: analysis of 137 patients. Int J Colorectal Dis 2011;26(2):183–90.

120. Blackmon SH, Stephens EH, Correa AM, et al. Predictors of recurrent pulmonary metastases and survival after pulmonary metastasectomy for colorectal cancer. Ann Thorac Surg 2012;94(6):1802–9.

121. Zampino MG, Maisonneuve P, Ravenda PS, et al. Lung metastases from colorectal cancer: analysis of prognostic factors in a single institution study. Ann Thorac Surg 2014;98(4):1238–45.

122. Hernandez J, Molins L, Fibla JJ, et al. Role of major resection in pulmonary metastasectomy for colorectal cancer in the Spanish prospective multicenter study (GECMP-CCR). Ann Oncol 2016;27(5):850–5.

123. Pfannschmidt J, Dienemann H, Hoffmann H. Surgical resection of pulmonary metastases from colorectal cancer: a systematic review of published series. Ann Thorac Surg 2007;84(1):324–38.

124. Tampellini M, Ottone A, Bellini E, et al. The role of lung metastasis resection in improving outcome of colorectal cancer patients: results from a large retrospective study. Oncologist 2012;17(11):1430–8.
125. Embun R, Fiorentino F, Treasure T, et al. Pulmonary metastasectomy in colorectal cancer: a prospective study of demography and clinical characteristics of 543 patients in the Spanish colorectal metastasectomy registry (GECMP-CCR). BMJ Open 2013;3(5) [pii:e002787].
126. Gonzalez M, Poncet A, Combescure C, et al. Risk factors for survival after lung metastasectomy in colorectal cancer patients: a systematic review and meta-analysis. Ann Surg Oncol 2013;20(2):572–9.
127. Gonzalez M, Robert JH, Halkic N, et al. Survival after lung metastasectomy in colorectal cancer patients with previously resected liver metastases. World J Surg 2012;36(2):386–91.
128. Zabaleta J, Aguinagalde B, Fuentes MG, et al. Survival after lung metastasectomy for colorectal cancer: importance of previous liver metastasis as a prognostic factor. Eur J Surg Oncol 2011;37(9):786–90.
129. Andres A, Mentha G, Adam R, et al. Surgical management of patients with colorectal cancer and simultaneous liver and lung metastases. Br J Surg 2015; 102(6):691–9.
130. Comito T, Cozzi L, Clerici E, et al. Stereotactic ablative radiotherapy (SABR) in inoperable oligometastatic disease from colorectal cancer: a safe and effective approach. BMC Cancer 2014;14:619.

Lymph Node Metastasis in Colorectal Cancer

Ming Jin, MD, PhD[a], Wendy L. Frankel, MD[b],*

KEYWORDS

- Colon cancer • Metastatic lymph node • Staging • Tumor deposit
- Micrometastasis • Lymph node ratio • Rectal cancer • Neoadjuvant treatment effect

KEY POINTS

- Pathologic lymph node staging remains crucial for colon cancer prognosis. Per American Joint Committee on Cancer (AJCC) 7th and 8th editions, it is important to obtain at least 12 lymph nodes in resections intended for cure.
- Although the definition of tumor deposits has evolved over the years, interpretation challenges and interobserver variability still exist.
- Lymph nodes with isolated tumor cells are designated as N0; micrometastases are designated as N1. Additional use of special/ancillary techniques is not recommended for detection.
- Although not included in AJCC TNM staging, many studies have shown that lymph node ratio provides useful prognostic stratification in addition to the number of positive lymph nodes.
- The evaluation of lymph nodes after neoadjuvant treatment in rectal cancer can be challenging; finding of viable tumor cells is essential to classify a lymph node as positive.

INTRODUCTION

Surgical resection remains the most effective therapy for colon cancer. Pathologic findings in surgical resection specimens are the best predictor of prognosis. As in any organ system, cancer staging, the assessment of primary tumor (T), lymph node metastasis (N), and distant metastasis (M) is an important task for pathologists and treating clinicians. The College of American Pathologists (CAP) cancer protocol recommends using the American Joint Committee on Cancer (AJCC) TNM staging system and the International Union Against Cancer, but does not preclude the use of other staging systems. In this review, the authors focus on lymph node (LN)

Disclosure Statement: M. Jin and W.L. Frankel have nothing to disclose.
[a] Department of Pathology, The Ohio State University Wexner Medical Center, S305E Rhodes Hall, 450 West 10th Avenue, Columbus, OH 43210, USA; [b] Department of Pathology, The Ohio State University Wexner Medical Center, 129 Hamilton Hall, 1645 Neil Avenue, Columbus, OH 43210, USA
* Corresponding author.
E-mail address: wendy.frankel@osumc.edu

Surg Oncol Clin N Am 27 (2018) 401–412
https://doi.org/10.1016/j.soc.2017.11.011
1055-3207/18/© 2017 Elsevier Inc. All rights reserved.

surgonc.theclinics.com

metastasis in colorectal cancer using the AJCC staging criteria,[1–4] CAP cancer protocol,[5] as well as the literature. Several key or controversial topics including LN staging, tumor deposit (TD), micrometastasis, LN ratio, and neoadjuvant treatment effect in rectal cancer are discussed. Updates from the AJCC 8th edition are included.

CONTENT
American Joint Committee on Cancer Lymph Node Staging

The LN is the most common site of metastasis. Tumor spreads to LN via the lymphatic vessels usually in order of proximity to the primary site. LN (N category) staging includes information on whether the cancer has spread to regional LNs and how many LNs are involved. The regional LNs are designated based on the anatomic subsite of the large intestine.[4,5] These regional LNs are located along the course of the major vessels supplying the large intestine. LN outside the regional drainage area of the primary tumor should be characterized as distant metastasis (M category). Although colonic and rectal cancer can metastasize to almost any organ, the liver and lungs are the most common distant organ metastatic sites.

Required number of total lymph nodes
To accurately evaluate the LN metastasis, as many LNs as possible should be assessed to determine the N stage. Both the total number of regional LNs removed and the number of positive LN involved are prognostically important and thus should be reported. Studies have shown that the total number of LN removed correlates with survival, likely because of optimal mesenteric resection by the surgeon and increased accuracy in staging.[6,7] In colorectal cancer resections that are intended for cure, AJCC 7th and 8th editions state it is important to obtain and examine at least 12 LNs. The prior 6th edition suggested a range of 7 to 14 LNs that should be obtained. Even if less than the suggested number of LNs is identified, actual N stage rather than Nx should be provided.

There are many factors that can impact LN recovery, including patient age, gender, body habitus; immune response; tumor site, size, and length of colon resected; the experience of surgeon; and the diligence and experience of pathology grossing personnel.[8] In addition, the new classification of TD leads to a reduction in the total number of LNs identified because of reclassification of some LN as TD.[9] CAP cancer protocol suggests that if fewer than 12 LNs are found, reexamining the specimen for additional LN, with or without enhancement techniques, should be considered.

Some studies aimed at increasing LN yield and stage accuracy have been reported, but no major changes have been made recently in standard grossing protocols. Fat clearing can help in some cases, but is not the standard of care. Recently, Lisovsky and colleagues[10] reported that emphasis on the number of LNs examined from primary nodal basin (<5 cm away from the tumor edge) and a "second look" protocol (a second search performed in cases that were N0 after the first search) improve nodal staging. Another group concluded that the method of methylene blue intra-arterial staining (methylene blue injection into an artery in the resected colorectal specimen) significantly improved staging accuracy by finding more small-diameter LNs.[11] Additional evidence is necessary before any changes are made in the standard protocols.

American Joint Committee on Cancer N staging definition
Table 1 illustrates colon cancer AJCC N staging comparison among 6th, 7th, and 8th editions.

Compared with the 6th edition, the 7th edition further subdivides N1 into N1a, N1b, and N1c; and N2 into N2a and N2b. N1c is a newly introduced category

Table 1
Colon cancer American Joint Committee on Cancer N staging in 6th, 7th, and 8th editions

N Category	6th (2002)	7th (2010)	8th (2018)
NX	RLN cannot be assessed	RLN cannot be assessed	RLN cannot be assessed
N0	RLN = 0	RLN = 0	RLN = 0
N1	RLN = 1–3	RLN = 1–3	RLN = 1–3
N1a	—	*RLN = 1*	RLN = 1
N1b	—	*RLN = 2–3*	RLN = 2–3
N1c	—	*RLN = 0, TD in subserosa, mesentery, or nonperitonealized pericolonic or perirectal/mesorectal tissue*	RLN = 0, TD in subserosa, mesentery, or nonperitonealized pericolonic or perirectal/mesorectal tissue
N2	RLN ≥4	RLN ≥4	RLN ≥4
N2a	—	*RLN = 4–6*	RLN = 4–6
N2b	—	*RLN ≥7*	RLN ≥7

Abbreviation: RLN, regional lymph node.
Italic indicates change/clarification from prior edition.
Data from Refs.[2–4]

in the 7th edition, which is defined by TD in subserosa, mesentery, or nonperitonealized pericolonic or perirectal/mesorectal tissue without any regional nodal metastasis.

The 8th edition does not have significant changes in N staging definitions compared with the 7th edition, but rather clarifications. The expert panel attempted to clarify some issues that have remained challenging in previous editions, such as TDs and micrometastases. Small-vessel and large venous invasion involvement are recommended to be collected as registration data in addition to TDs.

The impact of N category on prognostic stage groups
Table 2 lists the 6th, 7th, and 8th edition of colon cancer AJCC prognostic stage groups. As illustrated in this table, the 7th edition includes significant changes (T and N regrouping), particularly in patients with stage II and III disease. Although these complex modifications aim to improve overall prognostic assessment, studies have shown that they do not address all survival discrepancies.[12]

Tumor Deposit

Tumor deposit definition evolution
TDs are discrete tumor nodules without histologic evidence of a residual LN identified in the pericolonic or perirectal tissue away from the leading edge of the tumor and are not infrequent in colon cancer resection specimens. Chen and colleagues[13] demonstrated that approximately 10% of colorectal cancers have TDs, and 2.5% of colon cancer and 3.3% of rectal cancer have TDs without positive LNs. The classification of these tumor nodules as TDs versus LNs has been debated over the years. TDs are thought to either represent discontinuous tumor spread, a totally replaced LN, venous invasion with extravascular extension,

Table 2
Colon cancer American Joint Committee on Cancer prognostic stage groups (6th, 7th, 8th editions)

Stage	6th (2002)			7th (2010)			8th (2018)		
	T	N	M	T	N	M	T	N	M
0	Tis	N0	M0	Tis	N0	M0	Tis	N0	M0
I	T1, T2	N0	M0	T1, T2	N0	M0	T1, T2	N0	M0
IIA	T3	N0	M0	T3	N0	M0	T3	N0	M0
IIB	T4	N0	M0	*T4a*	N0	M0	T4a	N0	M0
IIC	—	—	—	*T4b*	N0	M0	T4b	N0	M0
IIIA	T1, T2	N1	M0	T1, T2	*N1/N1c*	M0	T1, T2	N1/N1c	M0
				T1	*N2a*	M0	T1	N2a	M0
IIIB	T3, T4	N1	M0	*T3, T4a*	*N1/N1c*	M0	T3, T4a	N1/N1c	M0
				T2, T3	*N2a*	M0	T2, T3	N2a	M0
				T1, T2	*N2b*	M0	T1, T2	N2b	M0
IIIC	Any T	N2	M0	*T4a*	*N2a*	M0	T4a	N2a	M0
				T3, T4a	*N2b*	M0	T3, T4a	N2b	M0
				T4b	*N1-N2*	M0	T4b	N1-N2	M0
IVA	Any T	Any N	M1	Any T	Any N	*M1a*	Any T	Any N	M1a
IVB				Any T	Any N	*M1b*	Any T	Any N	M1b
IVC				—	—	—	Any T	Any N	*M1c*

Italic indicates change from prior edition.
Data from Refs.[2–4]

and/or less commonly, small-vessel or perineural invasion. The concept of TD was first introduced to the AJCC/TNM staging system in the 5th edition (1997). The classification was determined by TD size (tumor nodule >3 mm was considered regional LN metastasis; tumor nodule ≤3 mm was considered a discontinuous extension and classified in the T category). In the 6th edition (2002), the classification was based on the form and contour of the TD rather than the size (tumor nodule with the form and smooth contour of an LN is considered LN; tumor nodule with irregular contour was classified in the T category as either discontinuous spread or venous invasion). In the 7th (2010) edition, the size and shape or contour are not criteria, but TD is simply defined by no evidence of residual LN tissue, but within the lymphatic drainage of the primary carcinoma. The new nodal subclassification category N1c is used if there is TD but no concurrent positive LN. N1c category was created to allow data collection and outcome analysis in the hopes of better understanding the prognostic significance. Of note, N1c is not worse by definition than N1a or N1b. The number of TDs should not be added to the number of LNs for assessing adequacy of LN dissection. The number of LN and TD is reported separately. In the 8th edition, the fundamental definition of TD is not changed compared with the 7th edition, but rather clarified. If a vessel wall or neural structure is identifiable, the nodule should be classified as lymphovascular invasion or perineural invasion correspondingly. To help vessel wall identification, the use of special stains such as the elastin stain may be considered to supplement the routine H&E stains. In addition, 1 to 4 TDs or 5 or more TDs should be recorded. **Table 3** and **Fig. 1** illustrate TD definition evolution in the AJCC 5th to 8th editions. **Fig. 2** demonstrates examples of easily identified LN and TD.

Table 3
Tumor deposits evolution in American Joint Committee on Cancer 5th, 6th, 7th, and 8th editions

AJCC Edition	LN vs TD Definition	Impact on T Stage
5th (1997)	Size rule: Tumor nodule >3 mm: LN metastasis Tumor nodule ≤3 mm: T category as discontinuous extension	May upgrade T
6th (2002)	Contour rule: The form and smooth contour of an LN: LN metastasis; Irregular contour: T category as either discontinuous spread or venous invasion	May upgrade T
7th (2010)	Histologic evidence of residual LN: Yes: LN metastasis No but within the lymphatic drainage: TD; introducing N1c	Not affected
8th (2018)	Histologic evidence of residual LN: No change compared with the 7th Add clarification: for vessel identification, H&E, elastin, and any other stains can be used; 1–4 TDs or 5–8 TDs should be recorded	Not affected

Data from Refs.[1–4]

Prognostic significance of tumor deposit

Many studies have shown that the presence of TDs is associated with advanced tumor growth and reduced disease-free and overall survival.[9,14–18]

As illustrated in **Table 3**, in the 5th and 6th editions, the presence of TD may upstage T stage; however, in the 7th and 8th editions, TD is classified in the N category and its presence does not change the T staging. If one or more TDs are identified in the absence of identifiable LN metastasis, the N stage should be categorized as N1c. This rule applies irrespective of T category. Similar to N1a or N1b, the presence of N1c upstages to stage III in the prognostic stage group (see **Table 2**), which would otherwise be I or II, and adjuvant therapy is warranted. If TDs coexist with LN

5TH: >3 mm = LN   6TH: smooth contour = LN   7TH & 8TH: no histologic evidence of LN = TD

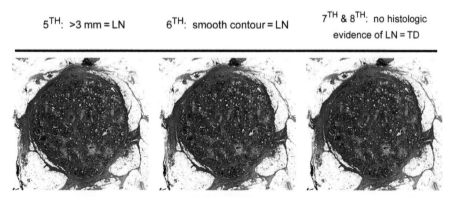

Fig. 1. AJCC TD definition evolution (5th–8th editions) (H&E stains, original magnification × 20). The tumor nodule is defined as metastatic LN by the 5th edition based on size, metastatic LN by the 6th edition based on smooth contour, and TD by the 7th and 8th editions based on the absence of histologic evidence of LN.

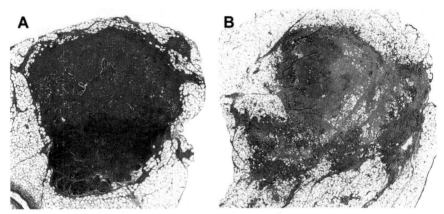

Fig. 2. Examples of easily identified metastatic LN (*A*) and TD (*B*) (H&E stains, original magnification × 20).

metastasis, their presence does not affect the N staging, which is still determined by the number of positive LNs. The number of TDs is not added to the number of positive LNs.

Ueno and colleagues[19] have shown that an increasing number of TDs was significantly relevant to adverse survival outcome. The authors' prior study found that N1c patients had significantly worse 5-year overall survival compared with N0 patients with similar T and M status and concluded that TDs predict worse patient outcome as least similarly to positive LNs.[9] Although their data were limited, it showed the cutoff points of 4 TDs and 5 TDs resulted in significant differences in survival in N1c patients, providing some support of the cutoff point chosen on the basis of N stage system of N1 (LN <4) versus N2 (positive LN ≥4).[9] Both the AJCC 7th and 8th editions recommend reporting the number of TDs, whereas the 8th edition specifically states that 1 to 4 TDs or 5 or more TDs should be recorded.

Interpretation challenges

Interobserver variability remains in interpreting TDs even among pathologists with an interest in gastrointestinal pathology.[20] It is apparent that the determination of TD sometimes remains subjective, and no single criterion or group of criteria are

Table 4
Tumor deposit interpretation challenges and possible solutions

Challenges	Possible Solutions
TD vs discontinuous tumor spread	No consensus on minimum distance between TD and tumor Deeper sectioning
TD vs totally replaced LN	Determine whether residual LN architecture present Helpful features[15]: • Round shape • Peripheral lymphocyte rim/lymphoid follicles • Possible subcapsular sinus • Residual LN in surrounding fibroadipose tissue • Thick capsule
TD vs venous invasion	Deeper sectioning and/or elastin stain

universally used or agreed upon, but awareness of the potential challenges and possible solutions may help interobserver variability. Standardization will permit the collection of useful data for future prognostic significance analyses. **Table 4** includes several challenges and corresponding possible solutions, which are further described in later discussion. In summary, TD should only be diagnosed when no definitive discontinuous tumor spread, LN, perineural, or venous invasion is identified.

Tumor deposit versus discontinuous tumor spread Sometimes it is difficult to determine if a tumor nodule near the leading edge of the tumor should be called a TD or considered discontinuous tumor spread. Studies have attempted to define the minimum distance between a TD and the leading edge of the tumor and determine prognostic significance,[12] but no set distance has been agreed upon. Deeper sectioning may be helpful to demonstrate continuity with the leading edge of the tumor rather than a TD[21,22] **(Fig. 3)**.

Tumor deposit versus totally replaced lymph node A multi-institutional interobserver variability study conducted by the authors' group demonstrated that the helpful features to identify residual LNs that are often used in aiding the distinction include round shape, peripheral lymphocyte rim, peripheral lymphoid follicles, possible subcapsular sinus, and residual LN in surrounding fibroadipose tissue and thick capsule[20] **(Fig. 4)**. Although smooth contour is not a criterion for LN in the AJCC 7th edition, pathologists continue to use this feature from the 6th edition. Round shape was ranked the most important characteristic used by pathologists with an interest in gastrointestinal pathology when faced with a challenging metastatic nodule.

Tumor deposit versus venous invasion In the AJCC 7th and 8th editions, it is recommended that venous invasion should be reported separately from small-vessel vascular invasion. Small-vessel invasion is defined by tumor involvement of thin-walled vessels and has been shown to be an independent indicator of LN metastasis or other adverse outcomes. Venous invasion is defined by tumor involving endothelial lined spaces with an identifiable smooth muscle layer or elastic lamina. Although the significance of intramural venous invasion is unclear, extramural venous invasion has been demonstrated to be an independent adverse prognostic factor. Deeper sectioning and special stains for elastin have been reported as helpful ancillary

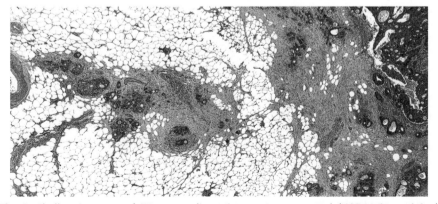

Fig. 3. Challenging case of TD versus discontinuous tumor spread (H&E stains, original magnification × 20). A tumor nodule (*left*) is identified near the leading edge of the tumor (*right*). Deeper levels did not show continuous tumor spread.

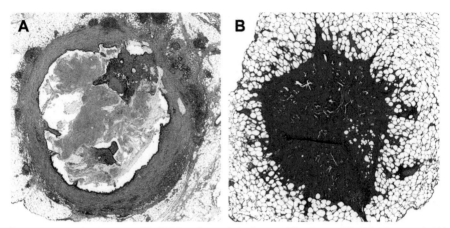

Fig. 4. Metastatic LN versus TD (H&E stains, original magnification × 20). (*A*) Metastatic LN is favored due to round shape, thick capsule, and peripheral lymphoid follicles; (*B*) TD is favored due to lack of identifiable LN tissue/architecture.

methods to identify venous invasion.[23,24] Features suspicious for venous invasion include "orphan arteriole" sign (tumor nodules adjacent to arterioles) and "protruding tongue sign" (elongated tumor nodules extending into pericolonic fat from the muscularis propria).

Isolated Tumor Cells and Micrometastases

The prognostic significance of isolated tumor cells (ITCs) or micrometastases in colon cancer remains controversial. ITCs are defined as single cancer cells or small clusters of tumor cells measuring ≤0.2 mm and classified as N0 (i+). Micrometastases are defined as tumor clusters measuring greater than 0.2 mm but ≤2.0 mm in greatest dimension, and classified as N1 (mic). A recent systematic review and meta-analysis showed that micrometastases are a significantly poor prognostic factor.[25] Per AJCC 8th edition, these micrometastases may be designated as N1 (mic), but they may be better considered standard positive LNs. In fact, most pathologists have always considered these to be positive LNs. On the other hand, the prognostic value of ITCs is less clear. Studies using additional special/ancillary techniques (pancytokeratin immunohistochemical stain) to increase ITC identification and sentinel LN mapping have been reported.[26,27] The data are insufficient, and the real biological significance of these ITCs remains unclear. At this time, the use of special/ancillary techniques is not recommended for the identification of micrometastases or ITCs in LN.

Lymph Node Ratio

Although LN status remains one of the most powerful prognostic indicators in colon cancer, the prognostic significance of metastatic lymph node ratio (LNR), defined as the ratio of positive LN over total LN examined, remains controversial.[28–31] Although the underlying mechanisms are not entirely clear, studies have shown that the number of normal LNs retrieved from the resection specimens conveys important prognostic information in both stage II and stage III colon cancer.[6,7] A systematic review of 16 studies focusing on patients with stage III colon and rectal cancer treated without neoadjuvant therapy demonstrated that LNR provided superior prognostic stratification compared with the number of positive LNs.[29] A recent prospective study demonstrated that metastatic LNR in stage III rectal cancer was a valuable prognostic factor even with less than 12 LNs retrieved.[32] Ozawa and colleagues[33] suggested that LNR was also a potent prognostic indicator for stratification in patients with stage IV colon cancer who had undergone curative resection. Although the data need to be substantiated by other large studies, Isik and colleagues[34] defined LNR of 0.25 as the prognostic cutoff value for patients with stage III colon cancer. LNR remains a controversial area, and reporting of LNR is not currently part of the AJCC staging system.

Neoadjuvant Treatment Effect in Rectal Cancer

Neoadjuvant chemoradiation therapy is considered standard of care for rectal adenocarcinomas, and it is associated with significant tumor response and downstaging. The resection specimens from these patients should be examined thoroughly to assess treatment response, residual disease, and nodal status. Challenging issues discussed subsequently include the total number of LNs required, the interpretation of acellular mucin, and measuring response after therapy.

Required number of total lymph nodes

LNs may be more difficult to identify in resection specimens from patients who have received neoadjuvant therapy. Per AJCC, there is no required number of total LNs

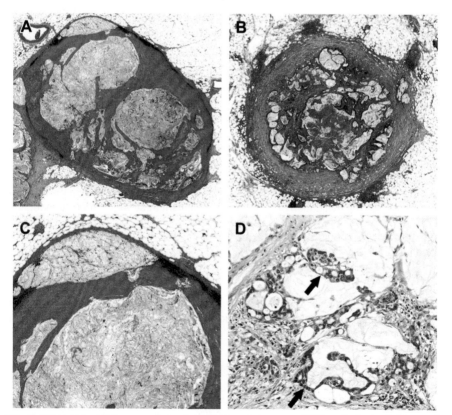

Fig. 5. Metastatic LN in neoadjuvant treated rectal cancer (H&E stains). Acellular mucin without viable tumor cells is not considered positive LN (*A* × 20; *C* × 100). The determination of positive LN requires the presence of viable tumor cells (*B* × 20; *D* × 100; *arrows*, the viable tumor cells).

in rectal cancer resections that are intended for palliation or have received neoadjuvant therapy; fewer LNs may be obtainable or acceptable. In routine practice, pathologists obtain as many LNs as they can and commonly reexamine specimens when less than 12 LNs are identified. A recent article suggests a minimum of 12 LN is necessary and improves staging.[35]

Acellular mucin
Acellular mucin pools found in LNs from colorectal specimens after neoadjuvant therapy are considered negative and are not counted as positive LNs. Only LNs with viable tumor cells are considered positive for metastasis (**Fig. 5**). The approach to evaluation of acellular mucin in LNs is similar to the assessment of the primary tumor for as assigning pT stage where viable cells are a necessary finding in mucin pools to consider as involved by tumor.

Regression assessment after neoadjuvant therapy
The evaluation of the response to neoadjuvant therapy is focused on the primary tumor, not the LNs nor other metastatic sites. However, a recent study has shown that LN regression grade should be considered a prognostic indicator of response to neoadjuvant therapy in patients with rectal cancer.[36] Large-scale and prospective studies are needed to confirm this finding.

SUMMARY

There remain several challenging and controversial topics in staging LN in colon and rectal cancer. AJCC N staging has changed over the years and will continue to be modified as new data are compiled. Although as many LNs as possible should be obtained, the minimum total LN number recommended remains 12. The AJCC 8th edition does not change the TD definition from the 7th edition, and interpretation challenges and interobserver variability continue to exist. Deeper sectioning and special/ancillary techniques may be of use. LNs with ITCs are designated as N0 (i+). LN micrometastases (traditionally designated as N1 [mic]) may be better considered standard positive LNs. Additional use of special/ancillary techniques is not recommended for ITCs or micrometastases detection. LN ratio is not included in AJCC TNM staging system, but there is some evidence for useful prognostic stratification in addition to the number of positive LNs. The evaluation of LNs after neoadjuvant treatment in rectal cancer can be challenging. In these cases, LN can be difficult to identify, but a careful dissection to include all LNs should be undertaken. The finding of viable cells in mucin pools is essential to classify an LN as positive.

ACKNOWLEDGMENTS

M. Jin and W.L. Frankel gratefully acknowledge Shawn Scully and Wendy Karavolos of the Department of Pathology at The Ohio State University Wexner Medical Center for providing editorial assistance.

REFERENCES

1. Fleming ID, Cooper JS, Hensen DE, et al. AJCC cancer staging manual. 5th edition. Philadelphia: Lippincott-Raven Publishers; 1997. p. 83–8.
2. Greene FL, Page DL, Fleming ID, et al. AJCC cancer staging manual. 6th edition. New York: Springer-Verlag; 2002. p. 113–24.
3. Edge SB, Byrd DR, Compton CC, et al. AJCC cancer staging manual. 7th edition. New York: Springer-Verlag; 2010. p. 143–64.

4. Jessup JM, Goldberg RM, Asare EA, et al. AJCC cancer staging manual. 8th edition. New York: Springer-Verlag; 2017. p. 251–74.
5. Kakar S, Shi C, Berho ME, et al. College of American Pathologists Cancer Protocol for the Examination of Specimens from patients with primary carcinoma of the colon and rectum. (Version: Colon Rectum 4.0.0.0, Protocol Posting Date: June 2017). Available at: http://www.cap.org/ShowProperty?nodePath=/UCMCon/ContributionFolders/WebContent/pdf/cp-colon-17protocol-4000.pdf.
6. Johnson PM, Porter GA, Ricciardi R, et al. Increasing negative lymph node count is independently associated with improved long-term survival in stage IIIB and IIIC colon cancer. J Clin Oncol 2006;24(22):3570–5.
7. Swanson RS, Compton CC, Stewart AK, et al. The prognosis of T3N0 colon cancer is dependent on the number of lymph nodes examined. Ann Surg Oncol 2003;10(1):65–71.
8. Frankel WL, Jin M. Serosal surfaces, mucin pools, and deposits, oh my: challenges in staging colorectal carcinoma. Mod Pathol 2015;28(Suppl 1):S95–108.
9. Jin M, Roth R, Rock JB, et al. The impact of tumor deposits on colonic adenocarcinoma AJCC TNM staging and outcome. Am J Surg Pathol 2015;39(1):109–15.
10. Lisovsky M, Schutz SN, Drage MG, et al. Number of lymph nodes in primary nodal basin and a "second look" protocol as quality indicators for optimal nodal staging of colon cancer. Arch Pathol Lab Med 2017;141(1):125–30.
11. Reima H, Saar H, Innos K, et al. Methylene blue intra-arterial staining of resected colorectal cancer specimens improves accuracy of nodal staging: a randomized controlled trial. Eur J Surg Oncol 2016;42(11):1642–6.
12. Hari DM, Leung AM, Lee JH, et al. AJCC Cancer Staging Manual 7th edition criteria for colon cancer: do the complex modifications improve prognostic assessment? J Am Coll Surg 2013;217(2):181–90.
13. Chen VW, Hsieh MC, Charlton ME, et al. Analysis of stage and clinical/prognostic factors for colon and rectal cancer from SEER registries: AJCC and collaborative stage data collection system. Cancer 2014;120(Suppl 23):3793–806.
14. Nagtegaal ID, Quirke P. Colorectal tumour deposits in the mesorectum and pericolon; a critical review. Histopathology 2007;51(2):141–9.
15. Puppa G, Ueno H, Kayahara M, et al. Tumor deposits are encountered in advanced colorectal cancer and other adenocarcinomas: an expanded classification with implications for colorectal cancer staging system including a unifying concept of in-transit metastases. Mod Pathol 2009;22(3):410–5.
16. Tong LL, Gao P, Wang ZN, et al. Is the seventh edition of the UICC/AJCC TNM staging system reasonable for patients with tumor deposits in colorectal cancer? Ann Surg 2012;255(2):208–13.
17. Ueno H, Hashiguchi Y, Shimazaki H, et al. Peritumoral deposits as an adverse prognostic indicator of colorectal cancer. Am J Surg 2014;207(1):70–7.
18. Ueno H, Mochizuki H, Hashiguchi Y, et al. Extramural cancer deposits without nodal structure in colorectal cancer: optimal categorization for prognostic staging. Am J Clin Pathol 2007;127(2):287–94.
19. Ueno H, Mochizuki H, Shirouzu K, et al. Actual status of distribution and prognostic impact of extramural discontinuous cancer spread in colorectal cancer. J Clin Oncol 2011;29(18):2550–6.
20. Rock JB, Washington MK, Adsay NV, et al. Debating deposits: an interobserver variability study of lymph nodes and pericolonic tumor deposits in colonic adenocarcinoma. Arch Pathol Lab Med 2014;138(5):636–42.
21. Puppa G. Enhanced pathologic analysis for pericolonic tumor deposits: is it worth it? Am J Clin Pathol 2010;134(6):1019–21.

22. Wunsch K, Muller J, Jahnig H, et al. Shape is not associated with the origin of pericolonic tumor deposits. Am J Clin Pathol 2010;133(3):388–94.
23. Kirsch R, Messenger DE, Riddell RH, et al. Venous invasion in colorectal cancer: impact of an elastin stain on detection and interobserver agreement among gastrointestinal and nongastrointestinal pathologists. Am J Surg Pathol 2013; 37(2):200–10.
24. Messenger DE, Driman DK, Kirsch R. Developments in the assessment of venous invasion in colorectal cancer: implications for future practice and patient outcome. Hum Pathol 2012;43(7):965–73.
25. Sloothaak DA, Sahami S, van der Zaag-Loonen HJ, et al. The prognostic value of micrometastases and isolated tumour cells in histologically negative lymph nodes of patients with colorectal cancer: a systematic review and meta-analysis. Eur J Surg Oncol 2014;40(3):263–9.
26. Protic M, Stojadinovic A, Nissan A, et al. Prognostic effect of ultra-staging node-negative colon cancer without adjuvant chemotherapy: a prospective national cancer institute-sponsored clinical trial. J Am Coll Surg 2015;221(3):643–51 [quiz: 783–5].
27. Estrada O, Pulido L, Admella C, et al. Sentinel lymph node biopsy as a prognostic factor in non-metastatic colon cancer: a prospective study. Clin Transl Oncol 2017;19(4):432–9.
28. Berger AC, Sigurdson ER, LeVoyer T, et al. Colon cancer survival is associated with decreasing ratio of metastatic to examined lymph nodes. J Clin Oncol 2005;23(34):8706–12.
29. Ceelen W, Van Nieuwenhove Y, Pattyn P. Prognostic value of the lymph node ratio in stage III colorectal cancer: a systematic review. Ann Surg Oncol 2010;17(11): 2847–55.
30. Lee SD, Kim TH, Kim DY, et al. Lymph node ratio is an independent prognostic factor in patients with rectal cancer treated with preoperative chemoradiotherapy and curative resection. Eur J Surg Oncol 2012;38(6):478–83.
31. Manilich EA, Kiran RP, Radivoyevitch T, et al. A novel data-driven prognostic model for staging of colorectal cancer. J Am Coll Surg 2011;213(5):579–88, 588.e1-2.
32. Madbouly KM, Abbas KS, Hussein AM. Metastatic lymph node ratio in stage III rectal carcinoma is a valuable prognostic factor even with less than 12 lymph nodes retrieved: a prospective study. Am J Surg 2014;207(6):824–31.
33. Ozawa T, Ishihara S, Nishikawa T, et al. Prognostic significance of the lymph node ratio in stage IV colorectal cancer patients who have undergone curative resection. Ann Surg Oncol 2015;22(5):1513–9.
34. Isik A, Peker K, Firat D, et al. Importance of metastatic lymph node ratio in non-metastatic, lymph node-invaded colon cancer: a clinical trial. Med Sci Monit 2014;20:1369–75.
35. Wexner SD, Berho ME. The rationale for and reality of the new national accreditation program for rectal cancer. Dis Colon Rectum 2017;60(6):595–602.
36. Choi JP, Kim SJ, Park IJ, et al. Is the pathological regression level of metastatic lymph nodes associated with oncologic outcomes following preoperative chemoradiotherapy in rectal cancer? Oncotarget 2017;8(6):10375–84.

Moving?

Make sure your subscription moves with you!

To notify us of your new address, find your **Clinics Account Number** (located on your mailing label above your name), and contact customer service at:

Email: journalscustomerservice-usa@elsevier.com

800-654-2452 (subscribers in the U.S. & Canada)
314-447-8871 (subscribers outside of the U.S. & Canada)

Fax number: 314-447-8029

Elsevier Health Sciences Division
Subscription Customer Service
3251 Riverport Lane
Maryland Heights, MO 63043

Printed and bound by CPI Group (UK) Ltd, Croydon, CR0 4YY

03/10/2024

01040400-0017